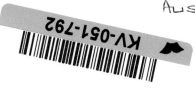

ALISON MASSEY.

Oncology for Nurses and Health Care Professionals

Second Edition

Volume 2

Care and Support

Oncology for Nurses and Health Care Professionals

Second Edition

Volume 2

Care and Support

Series Editor

ROBERT TIFFANY OBE RGN, RCNT, FRCN

Director of In-patient Services/Chief Nursing Officer,
The Royal Marsden Hospital, London and Surrey,
and President, International Society of Nurses in Cancer Care

Volume Editor

PAT WEBB RGN, RNT, DipN(London), DipSocRes

Senior Nurse – Education,
The Royal Marsden Hospital, London and Surrey
and Marie Curie Memorial Foundation, London

Harper & Row Publishers, London
In co-publication with
Beaconsfield Publishers, Beaconsfield

Philadelphia San Francisco
New York   London
St. Louis   Singapore
Sydney   Tokyo

First edition printed 1978
Reprinted 1989

Harper & Row Ltd
Middlesex House
34–42 Cleveland Street
London
W1P 5FB

British Library Cataloguing in Publication Data

Oncology for nurses and health care professionals – 2nd ed.
Vol. 2: Care and support
1. Man. Cancer – for nursing
I. Tiffany, Robert   II. Webb, Pat
616.99·4·00 24613

ISBN 0-06-318418-4

Typeset in Baskerville 11/13pt
by Burns and Smith, Derby.
Printed in Great Britain
at the Alden Press, Oxford.

CONTENTS

Preface

Cancer is one of the major health problems of our times. A cancer patient is not merely an individual with a diseased body; he is also a person with a thinking mind and a stirring soul. He has attitudes and aptitudes, interests and instincts, hopes and dreams, which are all affected by his condition. There is a need for a close partnership of all who are engaged in different aspects of caring for the cancer patient if we are to achieve a health care system that will meet their demands.

The purpose of this three volume work is to provide a concise and comprehensive introduction to oncology for nurses and other health care professionals. The presentation of the various subjects was entrusted to a team of authors chosen for their expertise in their own profession and oncology. Although each chapter reflects the unique point of view of its author or authors, they share the same commitment to total patient care based upon a multidisciplinary approach. A certain amount of overlap and repetition may at times be apparent to the reader. The content of each volume has been arranged so that each chapter may stand in its entirety, enabling the book to be used for reference purposes. A list of references and suggestions for further reading are given at the end of most chapters to assist the reader in further study of the theme taken by the author.

The volumes as a whole should be of particular value to trained health care professionals who want to continue and develop their work in oncology, and to those taking courses of study in oncology such as are those developed by the National Boards for Nursing, Midwifery and Health Visiting of the United Kingdom, various universities and other institutes of higher education.

While the scientific knowledge-base to treat and care for cancer patients is of paramount importance, patients and their families also need to be supported through their experience of cancer. The chronic nature of cancer means that no-one else but the patient can feel the fear, isolation, anxiety and indeed the physical symptoms of cancer. No-one can remove the social disruption to his life and that of his family or other relationships, at a time when cohesion and unity is needed. However, health professionals have a vital role to care for and support patients and their families throughout their experience of cancer. Such support requires considerable resource from carers. Volume 2 provides the reader with a comprehensive overview of issues related to care and support from those who are practising it in their everyday work.

Robert Tiffany
Director of In-patient Services/
Chief Nursing Officer
The Royal Marsden Hospital
London and Surrey

Pat Webb
Senior Nurse — Education
The Royal Marsden Hospital
London and Surrey
and Marie Curie Foundation London

Acknowledgements

As Series Editor, I am indebted to a large number of people for the completion of this three volume work.

It is my pleasure to thank the contributors for their willing co-operation and my colleagues and friends at The Royal Marsden Hospital for their continued help and support.

I offer my Volume Editors, Phylip Pritchard, Pat Webb and Derryn Borley, my highest praise for their enthusiasm, encouragement, vigour and attention to detail, for without them these books would not have been possible.

Lynne Montgomery and Renate Low, as Secretarial Assistants to the project, deserve special mention for their hard work and patience, particularly in the apparently endless retyping of early drafts.

Special thanks also go to the Librarians at the Royal College of Nursing and the Institute of Cancer Research for their painstaking efforts to track down the most elusive references.

Finally, my gratitude to Lindsey Pegus, Head of the Medical Art Department at The Royal Marsden Hospital, and her colleagues in Medical Photography for their help with the artwork and photographs included in these volumes.

Robert Tiffany
Director of In-patient Services/Chief Nursing Officer,
The Royal Marsden Hospital, London and Surrey,
and President, International Society of Nurses in Cancer Care

Chapter 1

The Sociological Impact of Cancer

ROBIN PUGSLEY BM, BS, BMedSci, FSMC, FBOA,
BOpth Optics
Physician, London

and

JENNY PARDOE MA, CQSW
Director
Care and Counsel, London

Introduction

Sociology is the scientific study of the social behaviour of human beings. It
is concerned with social interaction.

(Leonard, 1966)

Social interaction should be divided into three main categories: that of
one individual with another; of the individual with such institutions as
the family; and, third, interaction of the individual with society in
general. Indeed it might be held that sociology has a major part to play
in the demystification of our social world by showing how social and
cultural history form the basis for what is happening around us today.
In other words, attitudes and behaviour patterns that people exhibit in
a particular society at a particular time are very much the result of a
combination of gradually evolving patterns of co-operation with others
in general, and of personal experience of a family setting in particular.
Any society needs a clearly defined structure that the majority of its
members accept and use as guidelines of behaviour. These rules can
be roughly divided into two main types, namely the laws of the land,
which enable differentiation between what is considered illegal and
what is not, and a set of accepted customs which, although they are
equally powerful in regulating behaviour, are more likely to be based
to a greater extent on life experience.

This chapter deals with the social impact of cancer on individual
patients, their families and the society in which they live.

Illness, Disease and the Sick Role

The concept of illness has a number of facets:

1. It is usually unexpected, a state entered into involuntarily by the person concerned.
2. It is commonly understood to be undesirable by both those affected and those around them, leading to an expectation that the sick person should do all he or she can to get better as soon as possible and enlist all appropriate forms of outside help.
3. The confirmation of illness causes an increase of general anxiety.
4. Illness is usually manifest by a group of physical symptoms and signs in the person afflicted, combined with alterations in accepted social behaviour in both the sick and healthy members of society.

It could be said that all of the above constitute the reaction to a process of disease, which can be defined as the physical disturbance of the organs in the body. This is often the result of exposure to an outside influence whether that be a bacterial infection as in pneumonia, or an environmental hazard such as in asbestosis. Perhaps it should be said at this point that there is the added dimension of mental illness. Its causation has been debated at length – whether it should be regarded as a reaction to stress in life or the result of a disease process. The answer is still not clear.

When an individual becomes diseased, the person will exhibit the patterns of an illness and usually adopt the sick role. The 'role' is used to describe the part an individual plays when certain factors are present. For example, the captain of a ship fulfils a number of day-to-day roles which are concerned with getting his vessel from A to B safely. In addition to these he has another role in that he may perform a marriage ceremony. It is a transitory one as the occasion demands.

Thus it is the same with the sick role. The concept was first introduced by Parsons (1951) and is seen to be a role that is adopted either when a diagnosis is made or sometimes before if the individual has perceived a significant change in himself/herself. The illness is then confirmed and the individual acquires the legitimate status of being ill and, therefore, qualifies for the sick role.

To acquire this role usually involves a surrendering of independent functioning, which has benefits as well as drawbacks. On becoming diseased an individual will be looked after either by family and friends or by professional health care staff, sometimes in an institution if the person's condition is considered appropriate. They will be cared for at a time when they are vulnerable and may not be able to look after themselves. They will no longer be expected to cope with all of life's responsibilities whether these be minor ones, such as what to eat and when to eat it, or more major ones such as whether they are expected to continue to go to work. All of this can help relieve anxiety at a time when they are feeling unwell.

The person who is ill gives up a certain amount of independence because he or she understands, consciously or unconsciously, that it is an effective social mechanism to gain appropriate help and, equally important, the individual anticipates that he or she will soon be able to take back full responsibility and control after the illness has resolved. In other words, only part of the independence is surrendered and then on the implicit understanding that it is a temporary arrangement.

In summary, then, there are three main concepts to consider: that of *illness* which can be thought of as the expression, in both physical and non-physical terms, of an underlying disease process; the *sick role* which establishes the individual's right to alter his or her behaviour and be looked after; *society's response*, which comprises an affirmation of the sick role and recognition of a duty to provide extra-familial support.

The Individual's Response

The word 'cancer' is used as an umbrella term for a whole range of disease processes all having certain common histological features but presenting in many different ways. Cancers range from the rodent ulcer on an elderly person's cheek, which can be cured completely, to very fast growing tumours that are resistant to all forms of treatment and prove rapidly fatal. Despite the increasing body of knowledge about the causes and treatment of cancer, there remains a unique air of fear when the diagnosis is made. This is a reaction based on centuries of human experience, resulting in the acquisition of knowledge of how the disease progresses and the unpleasant effects it can have. One way of trying to cope with any phenomenon that is perceived as powerful and life threatening is to attempt to understand it using allegory, myth and legend. One example might be the propitiation of a volcano by sacrifices, the development by the threatened community of a behaviour pattern designed to limit the extent of damage from its activity.

THE MYTHS OF CANCER

The Alien Within

It is believed by many that cancer is not a disease at all but an alien entity that lives independently inside an individual's body. It is thought to lie dormant until the person experiences a shock of some sort which may be a fall, an accident, a blow to the body or simply bad news. Once the cancer is awakened it starts to grow inside the body until it kills the patient. An operation, a diagnostic procedure or even a fall on the ice wakes it up and, from that time, it begins to grow inside the body until it destroys the person.

Case 1

Mr A. was recalled for a bronchoscopy after attending for a chest X-ray. He described how he saw his X-ray film, which he interpreted as 'a big black thing pressing down onto the lungs and then after they had put the telescope down I spat up a bit of blood and later on they said I'd got cancer and that it had spread and that's why I was short of breath'. He had not understood, of course, that his chest film was a photographic negative and that 'the big black thing' was in fact the radiolucent inflated lungs and that the 'lungs' were his radio-opaque heart. He was convinced that the bronchoscope had prodded the cancer into life, hence the blood, and now it was growing in his lungs causing the shortness of breath.

Case 2

Miss B. was 74 years old and lived on her own in warden-supervised accommodation. She was diagnosed as suffering from carcinomatosis from a primary cancer of the stomach and found her enforced inactivity through ill-health very distressing. Although well past retirement age, prior to her illness she had been in charge of a small family office; she had been the linchpin of the entire operation and felt keenly the compound loss of health and role. These problems paled into insignificance, however, besides her worries about what 'the cancer was doing inside'. Miss B. was convinced that the cancer was a living thing inside her stomach. The pain she felt was because the cancer was entwined around her intestines gaining an ever tighter grip in its efforts to kill her. Therefore she did not want to eat. First, she did not feel hungry because her stomach was being strangled and, second, she could not eat because she understood that any food she swallowed would be used by the cancer, which would get stronger. Her job, as she saw it, was to hold out and starve the cancer to death before it could kill her.

Case 3

Mr C. had buried his father some 12 weeks before the first bereavement visit. He was very distressed at the onset of the interview and, although not unusual in itself for Mr C., there was a particular reason for it. He said at the time of his father's funeral there had been much family debate about whether his father's body should be buried or cremated. The rest of the family were in favour of cremation but he had insisted his father had wanted to be buried. The family knew he had been the favourite and therefore acceded. Now, 12 weeks later, he felt he had made a dreadful mistake; he could not visit the grave at all because he was fearful that the cancer had continued to grow and somehow entered the ground. He felt that he now understood why cremation had become popular in modern times; it was to ensure that cancer was completely destroyed.

Case 4

Mrs D. had very advanced cancer of the stomach. She was being well looked after by her three grown-up daughters and the physical symptoms were well managed. She was a devout Roman Catholic and her priest was a great support to her and her family. One day on a routine visit, the daughters were found weeping on the sofa saying that they could not carry on with their mother's care. In the conversation that followed they said that they had been told by a neighbour that when someone had cancer they split open at the moment of death. The previous evening the film *Alien* had been shown on television, and the scene in which an alien creature burst out of the body of one of the crew had graphically confirmed what they had been told.

These four case histories may seem bizarre and atypical but when patients and their families feel safe enough to disclose their inner fears, then it is towards these sorts of concepts that their minds turn. A very significant number of people believe that cancer is an independent alien being that causes pain when it grabs part of the body and, if it happens to seize a blood vessel, then it causes a haemorrhage.

The Wages of Sin

Cancer is also frequently assumed to be a punishment for past sins. Trying to find the reason for the unexplained and notions of self-blame occupy a large part of any psychologists's involvement in ideas of sickness and disease. We shall not develop that particular theme as it is addressed elsewhere. Suffice it to say that concepts of guilt and its expiation through suffering are commonplace.

Contagion

It is commonly believed that cancer is in some way catching and, as Sontag (1977) comments, 'a surprisingly large number of people with cancer find themselves being shunned by relatives and friends and are objects of practices of decontamination by members of their household, as if cancer, like tuberculosis, were an infectious disease'.

Case 5

When asked how she thought she had become ill, Mrs E. said that three months previously she had gone on a council holiday for the elderly. She had thoroughly enjoyed it but on returning had felt ill and had been to see her general practitioner about her cough. He had sent her for tests which confirmed what she already suspected – that she had cancer of the lung. The reason for her suspicion was that she had been told that the previous occupant of her room had had cancer. Mrs E. was convinced that she had caught cancer from sleeping on the same pillows.

Occasionally, there are misunderstandings that feed into these erroneous beliefs.

Case 6

Mr F., aged 57 years, had been in hospital for three weeks and was about to be discharged. He had been admitted for tests following an acute onset of breathlessness and bronchoscopy had revealed a large carcinoma of the lung. While in hospital an incidentally resistant streptococcal infection had necessitated his isolation for a few days but now discharge plans could be made. The usual arrangements for meals-on-wheels and home-help were put into action but a few days later a worried home-help organizer telephoned back to the hospital insisting that she must have a doctor's letter stating that Mr F. was not infectious. A neighbour visiting Mr F. while in hospital had seen him being barrier nursed and had talked about this to a friend who was the home help assigned to Mr F. Along the line the fact had been translated into the fantasy that Mr F.'s cancer was the sort 'you could catch' and that he would always have to be kept 'in quarantine'.

The Sex of Cancer

Cancer is often attributed with either male or female characteristics in that male cancers are understood to be the sort that do not spread and can be cut out, with a reasonable chance of survival, but female cancers spread and, therefore, have a much worse prognosis.

The Family's Reaction

The term 'family' is used to cover a wide range of social groupings. It is popularly understood to mean people living together who are either married or related to each other. A number of different sorts of family types have been described (Bott, 1957). All family groups have a physical and a non-physical structure. With reference to the former, there are two main considerations – geography and the number of generations.

UNDER ONE ROOF

'Book Ends' (Figure 1.1)

In this household there are members of only one generation, whether they be two siblings or a married couple without children.

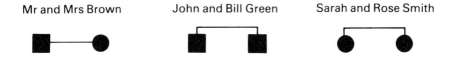

Figure 1.1 'Book ends' – households with two members of one generation only.

The Nuclear Family (Figure 1.2)

This is the family type that springs most readily to mind in the late twentieth century comprising, as it does, a husband and wife and their children. In other words, there are two generations living together.

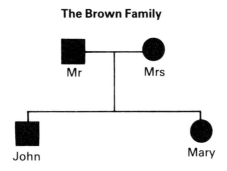

Figure 1.2 The nuclear family.

The Extended Family (Figure 1.3)

In this family, there are more than two generations with an inevitable increase in the number of people living in the home.

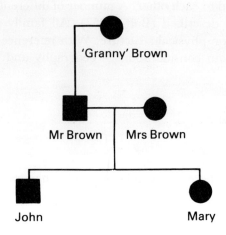

Figure 1.3   The extended family living under one roof.

UNDER MORE THAN ONE ROOF

The Extended Family (Figure 1.4)

The generational pattern is the same as before, the only difference being that the various family members live in different homes.

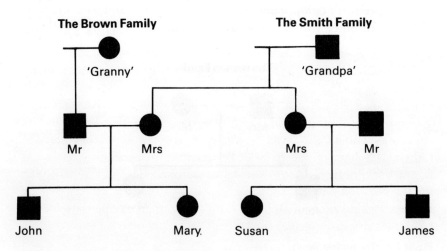

Figure 1.4   The extended family living under more than one roof.

The Tribal Family (Figure 1.5)

This sort of grouping is, in effect, a type of extended family. In this case there is often a strong family head, either a matriarch or a patriarch, surrounded by a number of family groupings. They all live geographically near to one another and there is free traffic of adults and children between their various homes.

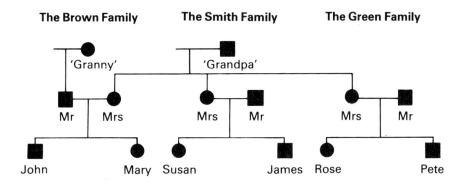

Figure 1.5   The tribal family.

Finally, there are households which comprise friends and/or lovers who, although having no blood tie, are commonly accepted to be a family group.

The non-physical family structure is built up of a combination of social and emotional roles: examples of the former being mother, father, husband, and wife; and of the latter, leader, housekeeper, clown and arbiter. Each individual may assume more than one role at a time and these may change with time and circumstances.

All families have a history of their own. This may go back many generations and be the subject of frequent discussion round the meal table, with a strong oral tradition passed down from generation to generation, imbuing family members with a comfortable sense of continuity and of the family's ability to survive all outside threats. Others will have a much more fragmented understanding of their family background — there may be gaps in knowlege or just no one to tell the story. In either case, myths can and do develop, either from the frequent telling of a much loved family tale or to compensate for the lack of history essential for the sense of belonging needed to bind them together.

This knowledge of family history becomes a strong force when the family is faced with a crisis such as one of its significant members becoming ill. Individuals will fall back on tried and tested remedies and proven ways of coping with stress and problems. 'Let's telephone Auntie Mabel, she's looked after two brothers with cancer, she will know what to do.' If, however, the family has no Auntie Mabel then its members are thrown back on their own resources and may face the whole issue as a new experience for everyone involved.

THE CANCER FAMILY

Cancer is often seen to run in families and indeed there is some evidence that for particular types of cancer there may be either a direct inheritance or inheritance of a gene that predisposes an individual to risk from an environmental factor. However, frequently it is no more than the chance finding that it will occur in families with a large number of members, cancer being a relatively common disease. Although the different members of the family may have suffered from different types of cancer, the understanding will be that they are in some way linked and hence the phenomenon of a 'cancer family'. Patients will say that they expected to have cancer because 'it's in the family' or alternatively that they were shocked by the diagnosis because 'there was no cancer in my family'. Clearly, this label may well be known outside the family and have far-reaching consequences.

In summary, the way in which a family responds to the crisis of cancer appearing in its midst depends on a large number of factors. These range from the number of people living under the same roof, through the strengths and weaknesses of their individual relationships to their past experience in their own lives and in those of preceding generations. It follows that those families with a tried and tested coping mechanism based on good relationships between their members will manage the effects of cancer far better than a fragmented family with a long history of being unable to cope. The way in which different families manage will impinge on the community in which they live. The reaction caused will depend to some extent on intrafamilial patterns but also on the reaction of society to cancer.

Community Reactions

A community has been defined as a geographical area in which a particular group of people live, often having been brought up there

(Willmott, 1963). They are familiar with the physical terrain but have also developed a complex network of interpersonal relationships which reinforce their feeling of belonging. These relationships will be both intra- and extrafamilial. It is essential that such a community develops mechanisms to maintain its integrity if it is to continue to protect and support its members.

These mechanisms have slowly evolved to combat anything that is a potential threat to that community. In other words, they are the response to any process that appears to challenge that which is perceived as necessary for its stability, or considered 'normal' by the majority of its members. Erving Goffman (1968) describes the process as one of stigmatization and explains that if an individual who might otherwise be regarded as quite acceptable in society develops a trait that is seen as a threat, then he or she can be shunned by the other members of the group. The individual carries a stigma – 'an undesired differentness'.

Individually and collectively, in groups and in neighbourhoods, there is a concept of what is normal and there is a natural inclination for individuals to congregate with those who share a similar perception. When a challenge is posed to what the core group holds to be its concept of normality, the group members will defend their position by outlawing the challenge as abnormal. If it is an individual who is seen as posing such a threat, that person will be stigmatized as not belonging and, therefore, undesirable.

Clearly such a rejection of anything or anyone perceived to be a threat was developed as a very powerful protective mechanism for the group, and nowhere would this have been more effective than in combating disease. In primitive communities, to reject any member who was ill has the effect of limiting the spread of infection and thus helps to preserve the corporate health of the community. It is important to bear in mind that this system probably evolved, particularly in the beginning, in a largely unconscious way, as the result of trial and error. Early civilizations would have learned that it was dangerous to associate with a member of the community whose behaviour had changed in a particular way or who had developed recognizable physical signs and symptoms of disease.

As our knowledge increased about the meaning of these changes and the concept of cure by specific treatments evolved, this reflex protective mechanism was modified. No longer were sick people totally rejected, although limitations were placed on them. In return for being provided with care and shelter, the recipients were expected to honour their part of the bargain by behaving in a specific way. Thus lepers were cared for in colonies but were expected to keep themselves apart, warning others of their approach by ringing a bell to prevent any accidental contamination. As civilization developed, the primitive response to shun disease and evict the sick from the community became modified by an emerging concept of corporate responsibility. It might be argued that the hospitals came into being as a further response by the community – the institutionalization of disease. In many societies the sick were cared for by religious communities as a practical demonstration of their faith. Many of the early monasteries had infirmaries and much of primitive medication evolved from the study of herbal remedies, an accepted discipline of monastic life.

The history of illness in our society could be said to follow a distinct pattern of appearance and disappearance of various diseases, usually as much a response to public health measures as specified cures. There has been a series of epidemics, by nature infective, such as leprosy, the Black Death, cholera, typhoid, smallpox, syphilis, pulmonary tuberculosis and Asian flu, and currently there is the possibility of AIDS being added to that list.

As far as cancer is concerned, the ability to make the diagnosis had to await the development of the technical facilities, such as the microscope, so that many forms of tumour previously thought to be due to other causes could be redesignated. This may well be one reason that the response in sociological terms to this distinct disease entity has been so complex. Another is the result of the psychological effect of the diagnosis (see Chapter 2). The third important aspect is the prevailing impression that, unlike infections, the medical profession has been unable to effect a cure. All these factors combine to make cancer a unique and very powerful threat.

The response has been equally powerful and concentrated on the two main aspects: that a cure must be found and that because the prognosis is so poor, the care of those dying from cancer must be of a much higher standard. This resulted in the creation of such organizations as the Imperial Cancer Research Fund, a new branch of medicine called oncology, and the development of establishments like the Marie Curie Foundation and Cancer Relief Macmillan Fund. To these were added hospices, based on the original mediaeval model of provision of care for pilgrims, many of whom were making their journey in the hope of relief from physical suffering.

Conclusion

Society's response to cancer is, at its most primitive, a subconcious desire to avoid the sufferer – the remaining vestige of the primitive but still powerful protective herd instinct. This has gradually been modified by the real and mythological experience of individual patients and their families. It is this interplay between the old and the new parts of consciousness that, even though often remaining at the subconscious level, may be at the centre of the difficulties that arise for all concerned.

Case 7

Mr H. had drunk in the same public house for some 25 years. He was well known as a local character, had his own seat and tankard and was generally well liked. Initially everyone in the pub was very upset to hear that he was in hospital and had been diagnosed as suffering from cancer. They had a whip round and sent him fruit and flowers and made sure that transport was provided for his wife to and from the ward when she went to visit him. Mr H. underwent major surgery and this was followed by intensive chemotherapy. Eventually he recovered sufficiently to be discharged home. When he went to the pub he found things had changed. People looked embarrassed, pretended they had not seen him and when he approached them, seemed very anxious to get away. After a week or two, the publican called at his home and asked if Mr H. would mind coming in for a drink at lunchtime only. After a very awkward conversation it became clear that the customers were finding it very difficult to be near him. Apparently they found his appearance very distressing and some felt that they could not take the risk of drinking out of a glass he might have used previously. Some of them had even gone so far as to say that they came to the pub to enjoy themselves and could not do that if Mr H. was there. His presence made them feel self-conscious about being seen to be laughing and enjoying life while he, quite clearly, was having a very difficult time.

References

Bott, E. (1957) *Family and Social Networks*, Tavistock Publications, London.
Goffman, E. (1968) *Stigma*, Pelican Books, London.
Leonard, P. (1966) *Sociology in Social Work*, Routledge & Kegan Paul, London.
Parsons, T. (1951) *The Social System*, The Free Press, Glencoe.
Sontag, S. (1977) *Illness as Metaphor*, Allen Lane, New York.
Willmott, P. (1963) *The Evolution of a Community*, Routledge & Kegan Paul, London.

Chapter 2

The Psychological Impact of Cancer

STIRLING MOOREY BSc, MB, BS, MRCPsych
Lecturer in Psychological Medicine
The Royal Marsden Hospital, London and Surrey and Institute of Psychiatry,
London

Introduction

It has long been known that cancer and its treatment can be a source of great mental anguish, yet it is only recently that attempts have been made to investigate and alleviate the psychological distress associated with cancer. Denial of the extent of patients' psychological suffering and assumptions that depression must be inevitable and 'rational' in life-threatening illness may have contributed to the lack of interest in this area. Over the last 10 years, however, research has shown that although the majority of people cope well with the stresses of cancer, a substantial number have difficulties that are amenable to some form of psychological help. Derogatis *et al.* (1983) found that 44 per cent of 215 unselected admissions to three centres in the USA had clinically significant psychiatric disorders. Most of these were adjustment reactions but 18 per cent had pure major depression and 7 per cent a pure anxiety state. Farber *et al.* (1984) studied 141 patients attending a Canadian oncology outpatient clinic and reported 34 per cent with 'a high and clinically significant level of psychological distress'.

Although psychological disturbance seems to be highest at key points in the course of the illness, such as diagnosis and recurrence, it can persist for some time. One to two years after mastectomy 22–25 per cent of women are still suffering from depression (Morris *et al.*, 1977; Maguire *et al.*, 1978). These studies have highlighted the problems which patients experience, but relatively little is known about the way people again and again bear the burdens that cancer imposes on them without breaking down. To understand the psychological impact of cancer one must begin by reviewing what is known about the process of adjustment and coping which all patients go through, and use this as a way of examining the psychological reactions found at different stages of the disease.

A consideration of the psychological impact of cancer must restrict itself to the way the person reacts emotionally to the stress of cancer. Psychological disorders in some patients are caused by physical factors, for example drug toxicity, metabolic disturbance, cerebral metastases. While trying to understand a patient's distress from a psychological viewpoint, the health care professional must always have a high index of suspicion for organic mental disorder. If any doubt exists about the cause of psychological disturbance, a psychiatric assessment should be sought.

Cancer does not occur in a vacuum, and the psychological impact on the family is as important as the effects on the patient. A section of this chapter, therefore, is devoted to what is known about the effects of cancer on the family. Finally, consideration is given to the ways in which health care professionals can participate in the psychological management of the patient. Among the issues to be addressed are:

1. appraisal and coping;
2. psychological reactions to the early stages of cancer;
3. psychological effects of cancer treatments;
4. psychological effects of advanced cancer;
5. psychological impact on the family;
6. psychological management of the patient with cancer.

Appraisal and Coping

In order to understand the psychological impact of cancer, it is useful to have a model of the way people react to stressful events. Lazarus and Folkman (1984) have proposed a three-stage model for coping with stress:

1. *Primary appraisal* – is there a threat?
2. *Secondary appraisal* – what can be done about it?
3. *Coping* – implementing strategies for coping.

This process of appraisal and coping is a continuing series of reactions to the different stresses which cancer imposes and will vary with the course of the illness. At the time of diagnosis the person needs to decide how life threatening the illness is; the initial reaction, as Greer (1985) remarked, is to view the diagnosis of cancer as a 'catastrophic threat tantmount to a death sentence'. With further information about the type of cancer and the treatment available many people change their appraisal to a more optimistic one. During treatment a new series of stresses are faced. Surgery such as mastectomy poses a threat to a woman's self-image and the degree of threat will depend on the importance of physical appearance, and of the breast in particular, to the woman's self-esteem. Other types of threat are encountered in terminal illness, where the patient no longer has to find ways of tolerating the uncertainty of cancer prognosis but has to come to terms with death itself. Increasing evidence is available that cure also creates its own pressures. In all these situations the psychological impact of the disease is mediated by the person's interpretations and evaluations of what is happening, together with the capacity, real and perceived, for coping.

THE MEANING OF CANCER

The threat to life is the most difficult aspect of cancer for most patients to face. The way in which this is dealt with will be influenced by how threatening cancer is seen to be (primary appraisal) and the belief that patients have in their own, their family's and their doctor's ability to cope with this threat (secondary appraisal). Greer, Morris and Pettingale (1979) identify four categories of 'mental adjustment to cancer' along these lines:

1. *Fighting spirit.* The patient fully accepts the diagnosis of cancer, adopts an optimistic attitude, seeks information about cancer and is determined to fight the disease. Example: 'I won't let cancer beat me'.
2. *Denial.* The patient either rejects the diagnosis of cancer or denies/minimizes its seriousness. Example: 'The doctors just took my breast off as a precaution'.
3. *Fatalism.* The patient accepts the diagnosis, does not seek further information and adopts a fatalistic attitude. Example: 'I know what it is, I know it's cancer, but I've got to carry on as normal, there's nothing I can do'.
4. *Helplessness/hopelessness.* The patient is engulfed by knowledge of the diagnosis; his/her daily life is disrupted by a preoccupation with cancer and dying. Example: 'There's nothing they can do, I'm finished' (Greer and Watson, 1987).

In a study of the effects of these different attitudes to cancer 69 women with early breast cancer were assessed three months after mastectomy. A structured interview was used to allocate each patient to one of the four categories. At 5- and 10-year follow-ups those patients who had an attitude of denial or fighting spirit orginally were significantly more likely still to be alive. In these two categories 55 per cent of patients were alive with no recurrence after 10 years, compared with only 22 per cent of patients who showed fatalism or a helpless/hopeless response (Pettingale *et al.*, 1985). Di Clemente and Temoshok (1985) found that in patients with malignant melanoma women showing fatalism and men with high helplessness/hopelessness scores had more rapid disease progression over 18–29 months. In both these studies the psychological variables were found to be independent of biological prognostic factors. One prospective study (Cassileth *et al.*, 1985) has failed to confirm these results but is not strictly comparable because the patients were assessed using different instruments from these studies and the group had advanced rather than early stage disease.

It is too early to make any judgements about the effect of these attitudes on the prognosis of cancer but they may have important influences on patients' ability to cope with the psychological impact of the disease. A questionnaire measure of mental adjustment has recently been developed (Mental Adjustment to Cancer (MAC) Scale) which includes a fifth category of 'anxious preoccupation'. Using the MAC scale, together with the Hospital Anxiety and Depression Scale (Zigmond and Snaith, 1983), the anxious preoccupation response has been found to be significantly associated with anxiety scores and the fatalistic and helpless responses correlated with depression scores (Watson *et al.*, 1988).

WAYS OF COPING

It seems that patients who see cancer as a challenge, and feel they may have some influence over the disease, have a better adjustment. There is much less clear idea about which methods of coping work best – probably because these are even more dependent on the personality of the patient and the demands of the disease at any given time. Friedman (1980) reviewed the literature and proposed ten major coping strategies which she used as the basis for suggestions on how nurses and other health care professionals might help cancer patients' own coping strategies:

1. seeking information;
2. turning to others for support;
3. following orders, having faith in professionals;
4. denying, escaping;

5. finding meaning for the disease and making the most of life;
6. preparing for death;
7. returning to employment;
8. relying on past coping strategies;
9. tension-reducing strategies such as smoking, drinking, overeating, focusing on physical symptoms;
10. blaming oneself, someone or something else.

Whether a strategy is effective or not depends on the circumstances in which it is used. At times adopting a confronting attitude to the disease and using strategies like information-seeking and planning positive activities may be most helpful. In other situations the disease may seem very much out of the person's control, in which case more palliating strategies aimed at tension reduction and controlling emotional reactions may be more appropriate.

The position of denial as a response to cancer is an interesting and important one. Traditionally denial has been seen as an undesirable defence mechanism. Greer's work shows that it may be functionally useful to some patients and it seems likely that most people use some form of denial during the course of the illness. Denial of cancer and denial of the consequences of the disease should be distinguished. The former is becoming rarer, but the latter is still commonly seen in cancer patients. It is not clear if denial is the correct term for this. Most patients who have been told that their illness is terminal are able to discuss their prognosis rationally, but for most of the time live as if they did not have a terminal illness. This is often a process of conscious avoidance of thinking about cancer, which has the advantage of allowing the person to get on with daily life. With some patients it may be difficult to distinguish denial from fighting spirit. One patient with advanced breast cancer said, 'I know they've told me there's nothing more they can do, but I won't accept that I'm going to die'. This form of denial should not be rigorously challenged unless there is clear evidence that the patient is suffering as a result, for example refusing treatment or becoming psychologically disturbed.

Psychological Reactions to the Early Stages of Cancer

The beginning of a person's psychological adjustment to cancer usually occurs well before the diagnosis. Aitken-Swan and Paterson (1955) found that most patients with breast cancer, but only a minority of patients with other cancer, suspected their diagnosis. Despite discovering breast lumps many women delay before consulting their doctors. Up to one-quarter of women may delay more than three or four months (Green, 1976; Margarey *et al.*, 1977). In the study by Green (1976) the principal reasons given for delay were fear of diagnosis and fear of disfigurement from mastectomy. This is a clear example of how denial and avoidance can be maladaptive. Health education has reduced the number who delay, but a proportion of patients still delay for too long before coming for treatment.

Once cancer has been diagnosed, the processes of appraisal and coping come into play as discussed already. At this early stage many patients go through a normal stress reaction, which is similar in form to that seen in victims of other traumas (Horowitz, 1979). During adjustment the patient experiences many conflicting emotions of numbness, disbelief, anger and protest, fear, hope and despair (Sutherland and Orbach, 1953; Peck, 1972). It can be a time of emotional turmoil and disorganization. Most people see their world shattered, and issues about death which have been avoided are suddenly staring them in the face. Part of the stress reaction involves a desperate attempt to give sense and meaning to a world which has fallen apart. Some writers have suggested that these emotional reactions follow a particular sequence but evidence for fixed stages through which everyone must pass is not strong (Silver and Wortman, 1980).

It is not surprising that this is a time of emotional turmoil since within a few days a patient can move from suspicion of cancer to diagnosis and the beginning of treatment. The emotional reactions are responses to the stress which is most salient at any given time. In breast cancer, for instance, the stress response preoperatively is predominantly one of anxiety, with insomnia and difficulty in concentrating on routine matters – a response to the uncertainty of the situation. Post-mastectomy patients often suffer a period of depression and grieving for the loss of the breast (Holland and Mastrovito, 1980). The severity and duration of this acute distress vary from one person to another, but are usually short-lived. Penman (1979) found that most women who had undergone mastectomy returned to normal home life within one to three months of the operation.

Facing a diagnosis of cancer is a time of reappraisal of priorities and life itself but the occasion of recurrence of the disease may be a time of even greater psychological disturbance. Silberfarb *et al.* (1980) found depression and anxiety to be more frequent in patients at the time of recurrence than in the terminal stage of the illness. The shattering effect of disease recurrence is illustrated by the case of a woman with breast cancer who initially had a positive attitude to the disease and set herself a limit of a year in which to get well saying to herself, 'I'll do that when I'm back to my old self'. Local recurrence of the cancer came just before her year was up and resulted in a catastrophic reaction. Professionals are aware of, and sympathetic to, the shock associated with diagnosis of cancer but not always as vigilant to the psychological effects if the disease recurs.

WHEN STRESS REACTIONS NEED MORE SPECIALIZED HELP

While this acute phase of adaptation to cancer is an entirely normal phenomenon there may be occasions when the individual needs more specialized help to pass through it. If the distress is so severe that the patient's life is disrupted or the ability to understand and make reasoned judgements about treatment is adversely affected, intervention is necessary. Referral to a psychiatrist or counsellor may be indicated. Usually a short period of counselling, occasionally in conjunction with medication such as anxiolytic drugs, is sufficient to help the person through the crisis.

Psychological Effects of Cancer Treatments

It is often difficult to distinguish between the effects of diagnosis and of treatment on a person's emotional state. Treatment is usually instituted soon after diagnosis and the person has to deal with the two together. The implications of treatment, however, are very different from the implications of diagnosis. While some patients can face the possibility of death stoically, they find the side-effects of treatment intolerable. For many people with cancer the physical symptoms experienced at the time of treatment are relatively minor compared to the side-effects of therapy. Surgery is usually seen as a necessary evil and the thought that cancer has been removed is often a relief, but radiotherapy and chemotherapy do not always have such obviously visible results.

SURGERY

Mastectomy is the surgical treatment which has been studied most extensively and is therefore used most as an example. A woman undergoing mastectomy has to face the removal of a body part which is associated with femininity in both its sexual and maternal aspects. For some, the loss produces a grief reaction which can become an overt depressive illness. Women may feel less attractive and find it difficult to look at the mastectomy scar. With the improvement in practical advice and counselling for breast cancer patients, women with breast cancer feel better informed and less alone but many problems still occur. Anxiety, depression and sexual problems are found in a substantial minority of patients following mastectomy (Morris *et al.*, 1977; Maguire *et al.*, 1978). When dealing with individual patients it is useful to remember that emotional reactions are not stereotyped. The breast is not a symbol of sexuality for all women. Fallowfield *et al.* (1986) recently found the same incidence of psychological symptoms in a group treated with lumpectomy plus radiotherapy as in a group of women treated with mastectomy. In the lumpectomy group the benefit of less mutilating surgery was offset by the fear that the less radical form of surgery did not remove all the cancerous cells.

Other surgical procedures have not been so thoroughly investigated. Studies of colostomy patients have shown an incidence of psychological problems of between 25 and 50 per cent (Devlin *et al.*, 1971; Wirsching *et al.*, 1975; Eardley *et al.*, 1976). Depression, reduced social activities and sexual difficulties were particularly common. High rates of depression and work problems are found in patients who have undergone laryngectomy (Barton, 1965; Drummond, 1967).

RADIOTHERAPY

Nausea and fatigue are common side-effects of radiotherapy (Peck, 1972; Hughes, 1982). It may be difficult sometimes to distinguish these symptoms from the lethargy experienced in depressive reactions. In other patients the fatigue caused by radiotherapy may be misinterpreted as being due to the cancer or a sign of personal inadequacy. Schmale *et al.* (1982) found that agitation, withdrawal, non-engagement with the doctor and unrealistic expectations about treatment predicted psychosocial adjustment to radiotherapy.

CHEMOTHERAPY

Maguire *et al.* (1980) found that adjuvant chemotherapy following mastectomy resulted in a significant increase in the incidence of depression, anxiety and sexual problems when compared with mastectomy alone. This was particularly so in patients who experienced drug toxicity. Hughes (1987) has suggested that this form of adjuvant chemotherapy may be less well tolerated than chemotherapy given as the sole treatment because the latter produces a noticeable improvement in physical symptoms, whereas the former is usually given when the patient's symptoms have been relieved by surgery. Many patients experience anxiety just before their attendance for each course of chemotherapy. Rarely does it become so severe that they cannot attend for treatment. In some cases the thought of attending for chemotherapy can bring on the side-effects of the treatment. This anticipatory or conditioned nausea occurs in 10–15 per cent of patients. Sometimes an anxiolytic such as lorazepam, given prior to attendance, can reduce the symptoms. Psychological interventions, including relaxation and systematic desensitization, have been shown to be effective (Burish and Lyles, 1979; Morrow and Morrell, 1982). Despite these adverse effects of chemotherapy, it should be remembered that the treatment may also have a positive psychological effect. Hughes (1985) found that lung cancer patients who were receiving palliative therapy had less depression and fewer communication problems than those receiving no treatment at all. The act of prescribing chemotherapy can function as a message that there is still hope, or that the patient has not been abandoned.

Psychological Effects of Advanced Cancer

Active and advancing disease presents different problems for the patient than does early disease. Many of the feared consequences have now come about and it is physical symptoms of pain, weakness and anorexia which cause the most distress. Again the important factor to consider is the meaning of the cancer and its symptoms for the particular patient. For some patients it is the fear of a painful lingering death which frightens them, but for others it is the limitations they face as a result of their symptoms which is frustrating and humiliating. In a study of 62 oncology inpatients Bukberg *et al.* (1984) found that depression was associated with increasing levels of physical disability. The limitations which physical disability placed on them lead some patients to give up even those activities they are still able to do, thus contributing to a spiral of depression. Working with these patients to help them make the most of their activities, within the confines of the disease, may help to give them a sense of control over their lives and contribute to improving their quality of life.

There is not space here to consider the psychological aspects of terminal illness in detail; the experience of dying has been investigated and described by several authors (Glaser and Strauss, 1966, 1968; Kubler-Ross, 1969; Hinton, 1972). For a more recent introduction to the problems encountered by patients, families and professionals who have to deal with death, referral should be made to Stedeford (1984).

Psychological Impact on the Family

Little is known about the frequency of psychological disturbance among family members. Coursey *et al.* (1975) reported that the level of anxiety is often higher in the immediate family member than in patients themselves. Partners go through the same reactions to cancer as the patients, but their need to provide support often prevents them from being able to express their feelings very openly. During treatment the patient may no longer be able to carry out his or her normal role and the stresses on the partner consequently may be great. A patient with lung metastases from breast cancer had always been the dominant partner. Her increasing breathlessness and disability threw her husband into a panic. He compensated by becoming the perfect nurse, constantly being at her bedside, seeing to her every need. Periodically his own dependency needs would emerge, and he collapsed. This resulted in his wife resuming her dominant role briefly until the cycle repeated itself. This unsatisfactory state of affairs continued until her death. Some partners refuse to change their habits — sometimes as a way of coping with the stress of cancer. The young husband of a woman with a thymoma refused to visit the hospital and when his wife came home, made no allowances for her illness, expecting her to look after the house and the children as before. This extreme avoidance seemed to be the only way he could cope with her illness.

One area of marital disturbance that has been researched is that of sexual relationships. When patients with benign breast disease were compared with patients who had undergone mastectomy 18–33 per cent of the cancer patients reported serious sexual problems compared with only 8–10 per cent of controls (Morris *et al.,* 1977; Maguire *et al.,* 1978). Other surgical procedures are associated with impaired sexual functioning, including colostomy for rectal cancer (Devlin *et al.*, 1971), limb amputation for sarcoma (Sugarbaker *et al.*, 1982) and orchidectomy for teratoma (Reiker *et al.*, 1985). The common factor here is the body image problems which any major surgery of this kind creates. Patients view themselves as sexually less attractive or, more subtly, may see themselves less potent or less feminine. The problems the patient experiences are compounded if there are also communication problems. An example of this is seen with the husband who does not initiate love-making after his wife's mastectomy because he is not sure that she is well enough. If he does not give his reasons for this, the wife may misinterpret his behaviour as a sign that he no longer finds her attractive. When he does show an interest in sex she rebuffs him, hurting his feelings and reducing the likelihood that he will initiate further love-making. As with other psychological problems in cancer, providing information about these sorts of reactions to mastectomy and encouraging an early return to to sex, can go a long way to preventing sexual difficulties.

When facing death, communication about the diseases and the future becomes even more painful. In a study of couples facing death Stedeford (1981) found 83 per cent of patients and 68 per cent of spouses were satisfied with the quality of communication between them about the illness. In only 63 per cent of marriages were both content. Satisfaction did not correlate with quality of marriage and some couples who were particularly close just could not bring themselves to talk about what was happening to them.

It is remarkable how well many relatives cope with the burdens cancer places on them. In some cases marriages may actually improve as a result of one partner having cancer (Hinton, 1981; Hughes, 1987) and, despite the enormous strains, the divorce rates for long-term survivors do not seem to be higher than for the normal population (Forbair *et al.*, 1986).

Psychological Management of the Patient with Cancer

FACILITATING THE PROCESS OF ADJUSTMENT

Many of the patients encountered by health service professionals are in crisis. They are trying to come to terms with the implications of cancer for themselves and their family. This is a natural process of adjustment in which the patient is actively engaged, but there are ways in which he or she can be helped through this process. The first step involves understanding some of the patient's emotional reactions. Anxiety is the commonest emotion at the time of diagnosis and it is important to be aware of some of its effects. The turmoil that patients often experience is associated with poor concentration and difficulty in encoding information so that some of the important facts about the disease and its treatment may not be readily grasped. In the consultation with the doctor, the patient's state of mind will also make it more difficult to remember facts and to ask important questions. Skilful information-giving is one way of reducing the stress of the situation. Health care professionals need to describe procedures clearly and repeatedly in order to get the point across. It is helpful to ask the patient what he or she understands from the explanation that has been given. This feedback allows any misconceptions to be corrected, and also gives the carer clues to the patient's fears.

Nichols (1984) includes a useful section on 'informational care' in his guide for psychological care in physical illness. He uses the mnemonic 'II FAC' for information giving: I – initial information check (what does the patient know?), I – information exchange, FAC – final accuracy check (what does the patient understand from what you have said?). There is considerable evidence that stress can be reduced if the person is prepared for the problems he or she is going to encounter. For instance, Ridgeway and Mathews (1982) demon-strated that hysterectomy patients who had received educational counselling or coaching in coping strategies, experienced less preoperative anxiety and needed less postoperative analgesia than patients who had been left to cope on their own. The person with cancer has to live with daily uncertainty about the future; appropriate information about treatments and their side-effects can help to make the patient's world a little more predictable.

Information does not have to be confined to the physical aspects of the disease. Patients who are referred for psychiatric help frequently express guilt about feeling anxious or depressed, or berate themselves for not accepting their illness stoically. Yet most of them are simply experiencing a more severe form of what everyone with cancer goes through at some stage. Telling patients that these feelings are normal can bring them enormous relief. Taking a little time to share information with them about others who have felt and behaved similarly, can reduce guilt feelings. Providing it is handled sensitively, another patient who has gone through a similar operation can on occasion be as useful as a professional counsellor in this situation. Booklets on the effects of treatment are becoming easily available and provide a quick way of getting across some of the basic information (see Chaper 6).

The professional dealing with someone who is trying to come to terms with cancer needs to have good interpersonal skills. These are easier to recognize than describe, but there does seem to be consensus that abilities in listening and showing empathy are important components. Oncology is a busy and 'urgent' speciality. It is easy to get caught up in the urgency of treatment and not listen to what the patient has to say. Nurses often see patients at just the time when they need to tell someone of their fear and desperation. Taking time to listen is not a luxury. There is evidence that half an hour of non-directive counselling preoperatively can have a lasting effect on psychological adjustment (Burton and Parker, 1988). Ten minutes may be sufficient for someone to talk about his or her most important worries and this investment of time could well prevent a crisis at a later date. The answers you get depend on the sort of questions you ask. Here are some questions which are unlikely to lead to a discussion of emotions:

'How are we today Mrs. Smith, alright? Good.'

'You're doing really well. You're looking much better this morning. How are you feeling?'

The first question left no room for an answer. The second gave a clear message that the questioner knew what answer the patient was expected to give. The following interventions might leave more space for a discussion of emotions:

'I noticed you were crying yesterday. Everyone goes through bad patches just after their operation, would you like to talk?'

'How are you feeling?'

Questions that are open ended and based on feelings are more likely to lead to a talk about emotions. It is very important to give the patient time to answer, even if this seems to take a long time. If the initial answer is superficial like 'I'm fine', waiting a little longer or asking a more specific question such as 'How are you feeling in yourself?' or 'How are your spirits?' may allow the person to speak freely. Patients should never be forced to talk about emotions. If they do not pick up on such opportunities to speak about feelings their privacy should be respected.

It is not only the way in which questions are worded that can block communication. Subtle non-verbal messages can also be very important. One patient described how her fear of radiotherapy was worsened by seeing the radiographers rushing out of the treatment room. She mistook their hurry as a sign that radiotherapy was so dangerous they could not wait in the room even for a few seconds. The busier staff look, the less likely patients are to bring their worries to them. Another non-verbal block is the positioning of the interviewer. If the patient is in bed, anyone standing over him or her is automatically in a position of power. To create a more equal and more trusting relationship it is necessary to kneel or sit down to be at the same level as the patient.

Some of these communication issues are considered in detail in Chapter 5. What is more important here is to consider how communication can help or hinder the patient's psychological adaptation. The great fear about communicating is that there is so little time available. If the patient starts talking about emotions there will not be the time or expertise to cope. In most cases the patient is already working hard to come to terms with the situation. Having someone to express their feelings to for just a few minutes, can help patients to see that their coping efforts are on the right track. Patients who become very distressed may need longer or they may need referral to a psychological service, where this is available.

Helping adaptation includes:

1. *Providing information*:
    (a) information on disease and treatment;
    (b) information on emotional reactions.

2. *Communication skills*:
    (a) use of open questions;
    (b) avoidance of false reassurance;
    (c) reflecting back what the patient says.

RECOGNIZING PSYCHOLOGICAL MORBIDITY

There are no hard and fast rules for distinguishing normal fear and sadness from anxiety and depression or deciding when an opinion from a specialist is needed. Emotional distress seems to form a continuum from normal reactions to frank, psychiatric disorder. Sometimes a patient's reaction to the stress of cancer diagnosis is so severe that it warrants psychiatric treatment. At other times normal adjustment reactions continue long beyond the immediate stress and turn into depression or anxiety. Penman (1979) reported that women at high risk of distress four months post-mastectomy could be identified by the less effective coping strategies they employed just after the operation. Other factors which have been shown to be associated with poor psychosocial adjustment are anxiety, depression, previous psychiatric treatment and lack of employment (Schonfield, 1972; Morris *et al.*, 1977; Bloom, 1982). Mood disturbances are the commonest psychological disorders encountered in patients with cancer.

DEPRESSION

Depression is characterized by a pervasive feeling of sadness, which is often resistant to circumstances. In severe depression there may be a daily variation in mood, with the morning being the time of lowest mood. In addition to the mood disturbance there are motivational, cognitive and physiological symptoms of depression. There is a loss of interest in surroundings and an inability to get pleasure from previously enjoyable activities, often associated with a feeling that these activities are no longer important in the face of a future of pain and death. Hopelessness about the cancer may infiltrate other areas of the patient's life, for example the depressed teratoma patient who feels there is no point in going back to work. Hopelessness may be so extreme that the patient feels suicidal. Suicide is not common in cancer patients, but the professional should be aware of this risk in all depressed patients. In depression the world looks bleak and one's own weaknesses and flaws stand out. The depressed cancer patient may blame himself or herself for the illness, or dwell on past indiscretions which now seem terrible crimes. Severe depression is not difficult to recognize but forms of depression in which the mood disturbance is less obvious may easily be missed in busy clinics or wards.

Physiological changes in depression present a problem since there is an overlap with the symptoms of the disease. Sleep disturbance, in the form of early morning wakening or difficulty in getting off to sleep, can also be associated with pain. Loss of appetite and weight loss are also symptoms of cancer as well as often occurring during treatment with radiotherapy or chemotherapy. Lethargy and tiredness are again symptoms of both depression and cancer. Table 2.1 summarizes some of the features which should alert the health care professional to the possibility of depression in a cancer patient.

The scope of this chapter does not allow for a detailed investigation of the origins of depression but it must be remembered that physical as well as psychological causes may often be important. Treatment with cytotoxic drugs can cause depression. Organic brain disease due to cerebral metastases, hypercalcaemia or other metabolic disturbances may be associated with depression in cancer patients. This is another reason why it is important to detect depression and not just assume that it is inevitable that all cancer patients will feel depressed.

Table 2.1   *Identifying depression*

(1)	Patient is withdrawn and does not engage in ward or home routine.
(2)	Patient is unduly tearful, miserable, slowed down.
(3)	Patient reports lack of interest, a wish not to see visitors, inability to feel strong emotions or get pleasure out of things.
(4)	Patient shows excessive guilt or self-criticism.
(5)	Past psychiatric history.

ANXIETY

Anxiety is a natural response to threat, and as such is felt by most cancer patients at some time in the course of their illness. In some people it may become so persistent and disabling that it requires treatment. The patient is usually fearful, apprehensive and tense. Frequently the cancer completely absorbs the patient's thoughts, to the extent that he or she is preoccupied continually by thoughts of painful treatments, recurrence or worsening of the disease and a fear of being unable to cope.

As with depression, physical symptoms of anxiety may be confused with those of the disease. Signs of autonomic overactivity such as palpitations, tremor, sweating and dry mouth may all be seen. It is not difficult usually to detect a clinically significant anxiety state since the patient will present with considerable physical and psychological complaints.

FAILURE TO RECOGNIZE PSYCHOLOGICAL DISTURBANCE

It has already been seen how certain behaviours by carers can make it more difficult for patients to discuss their fears. This becomes particularly important when considering the need to identify psychopathology in patients with cancer. Maguire (1985) describes a process which he calls 'distancing', where staff use mechanisms to

keep the emotional life of their patients at arm's length. The closed
questions examined earlier are a form of distancing, in which the
patient is given the message 'You're alright really'. Selective attention
is a mechanism in which the emotional side of the patient is just
ignored. The carer only hears the physical complaints of the patient,
but does not ask for any information on psychological symptoms.
Sometimes the professional jumps in too quickly with statements like
'You'll get well, don't worry' or gives reassurance about physical
symptoms without acknowledging that the patient's real distress is
psychological. Some of the reasons for this distancing have been
outlined already. Maguire (1985) mentions fear of being overloaded,
fear of being unable to answer difficult questions, fear of being unable
to cope with strong emotions and fear of getting too close, as important
contributors to the lack of awareness of emotional disturbance in
cancer patients. The remedy for this is not simple. Better training in
communication and counselling skills may reduce the tendency to
avoid asking questions about emotions. Skills training using simulated
patient interviews can help nurses working in cancer patients' own
homes to identify the need for psychiatric assessment.

TREATMENT OF PSYCHOLOGICAL DISORDERS

When a major psychological problem has been identified it is
appropriate to refer to a specialist, whether this is a nurse counsellor,
psychologist or psychiatrist. It is important to remember that the role
of the health care professional does not end here. The patient will often
still be having treatment and it is essential for the teams dealing with
the patient's physical and psychological well-being to liaise closely.
Some of the methods of treatment available for distressed cancer
patients are reviewed briefly below.

Counselling

'Counselling' is a difficult term to define. It usually refers to a mixture
of practical advice about the illness and emotional support. This most
often follows 'non-directive' lines, allowing patients to talk through
their problems in a sympathetic atmosphere. Although there is a high
degree of consumer satisfaction there is no evidence to support the idea
that counselling of all patients prevents mood disorder. Maguire *et al.*
(1980) found that a nurse counsellor was able to detect and refer
patients with depression and anxiety at any early stage. On the whole,

patients with clinically significant psychiatric disorder should receive more specialized help.

Psychological Intervention

A number of studies investigating the effects of psychological treatments for cancer patients have been reviewed by Watson (1983) and Greer (1985). Treatments have followed psychodynamic, behavioural and cognitive therapy approaches. Behavioural treatments have focused on specific problems such as pain (Spiegel and Bloom, 1983), conditioned nausea (Burish and Lyles, 1979) or insomnia (Stam and Bultz, 1986) with some initially promising results. Tarrier *et al.* (1983) describes a cognitive behavioural treatment for patients with breast cancer which includes stress management and identification and modification of reversible negative changes that had occurred since mastectomy, for example withdrawal (Tarrier *et al.*, 1983; Tarrier and Maguire, 1984). A study at The Royal Marsden Hospital, funded by the Cancer Research Campaign, is investigating the effectiveness of six sessions of a cognitive behavioural therapy called 'adjuvant psychological therapy' (APT). The behavioural techniques used include relaxation training and activity scheduling. The cognitive component of the therapy teaches patients to monitor and challenge their negative thoughts about cancer and thereby helps to foster a fighting spirit. Wherever possible, patients are seen with their spouse, partner or friend to help communication.

Drug Treatment

Depression in cancer patients has shown to be responsive to antidepressant medication (Costa *et al.*, 1985). There is some evidence that in patients with major depression, drugs and psychological treatment may be accumulative in their therapeutic effects. The newer tetracyclic antidepressant mianserin has been used in clinical trials with depressed cancer patients. This drug has the advantage of fewer side-effects than more established antidepressants such as amitriptyline.

Anxiety may often be helped by benzodiazepines but these drugs lose their effectiveness over time and can produce tolerance. They are best used as a short-term measure. The importance of psychological treatments for anxiety should not be underestimated. With phobic anxiety or conditioned nausea, relaxation training and systematic desensitization have been found to be effective.

Summary

The psychological impact of cancer on patients and their families has been considered for various stages of the disease: diagnosis, treatment and advanced disease. A model which emphasizes the meaning of cancer for the individual has been suggested, and this may help health care professionals to understand some of the idiosyncrasies of patients' emotional reactions. Most people go through a process of adjustment to the stresses of cancer and emerge with a degree of adaptation. For a substantial minority, psychological symptoms will persist or recur at other stress points in the course of the disease. If their problems are recognized early these patients can benefit from psychiatric help. Some ways in which nurses and other professionals can identify psychological disturbance and facilitate adjustment are covered, with special consideration for the role of communication skills as an essential component of psychological care for the patient with cancer.

Acknowledgements

This chapter was made possible by the generous support of the Cancer Research Campaign. I wish to thank my colleagues at The Royal Marsden Hospital for their help in its preparation.

References

Aitken-Swan, J. and Paterson, R. (1955) The cancer patient: delay in seeking advice, *British Medical Journal,* Vol. 1, pp. 623–7.

Barton, R. T. (1965) Life after laryngectomy, *Laryngoscope,* Vol. 75, pp. 1408–15.

Bloom, J. R. (1982) Social support, accommodation to stress and adjustment to breast cancer, *Social Science and Medicine,* Vol. 16, pp. 1329–38.

Bukberg, J. *et al.* (1984) Depression in hospitalised cancer patients, *Psychosomatic Medicine,* Vol. 46, pp. 199–212.

Burish, T. G. and Lyles, J. N. (1979) Effectiveness of relaxation training in reducing the aversiveness of chemotherapy in the treatment of cancer, *Journal of Behavioural Therapy and Experimental Psychiatry,* Vol. 10, pp. 357–61.

Burton, H. V. and Parker, R. W. (1988) A randomised controlled trial of pre-operative psychological preparation for mastectomy: a preliminary report, in M. Watson, S. Greer and C. Thomas (eds.) *Psychosocial Oncology,* Pergamon, Oxford, pp. 133–58.

Cassileth, B. R. *et al.* (1985) Psychological correlates of survival in advanced malignant disease? *New England Journal of Medicine,* Vol. 312, pp. 1551–55.

Costa, D. *et al.* (1985) Efficacy and safety of mianserin in the treatment of depression of women with cancer, *Acta Psychiatrica Scandinavia,* Vol. 72 (suppl. 320) pp. 85–92.

Coursey, K. *et al.* (1975) Comparative anxiety levels of cancer patients and family members, *Proceedings of the American Association for Cancer Research,* Vol. 16, p. 246.

Derogatis, L. R. *et al.* (1983) The prevalence of psychiatric disorder among cancer patients, *Journal of the American Medical Association*, Vol. 249, pp. 751–7.

Devlin, H. B. *et al.* (1971) Aftermath of surgery for ano-rectal cancer, *British Medical Journal,* Vol. iii, pp. 413–18.

Di Clemente, R. J. and Temoshok, L. (1985) Psychological adjustment to having cutaneous malignant melanoma as a predictor of follow up clinical status, *Psychosomatic Medicine,* Vol. 47, p. 81.

Drummond, S. (1967) Vocal rehabilitation after laryngectomy, *British Journal of Disorders of Communication,* Vol. 2, pp. 39–44.

Eardley, A. *et al.* (1976) Colostomy: the consequences of surgery, *Clinical Oncology,* Vol. 2, pp. 277–83.

Fallowfield, L. J. *et al.* (1986) Effects of breast conservation on psychological morbidity associated with diagnosis and treatment of early breast cancer, *British Medical Journal,* Vol. 293, pp. 1331–4.

Farber, J. M. *et al.* (1984) Psychosocial distress in oncology outpatients, *Journal of Psychosocial Oncology,* Vol. 2, pp. 109–18.

Forbair, P. *et al.* (1986) Psychological problems among survivors of Hodgkin's disease, *Journal of Clinical Oncology,* Vol. 4, pp. 805–14.

Friedman, B. A. D. (1980) Coping with cancer: a guide for health care professionals, *Cancer Nursing,* Vol. 3, no.2 pp. 105–10.

Glaser, B. G. and Strauss, A. L. (1966) *Awareness of Dying,* Aldine, Chicago.

Glaser, B. G. and Strauss, A. L. (1968) *Time for dying,* Aldine, Chicago.

Green, L. W. (1976) Site- and symptom-related factors in secondary prevention of cancer, in J. W. Cullen, B. H. Fox and R. N. Isom (eds.) *Cancer, the Behavioural Dimensions,* Raven Press, New York, pp. 45–61.

Greer, S. (1985) Cancer: psychiatric aspects, in Granville Grossman (ed.) *Recent Advances in Clinical Psychiatry,* Churchill Livingstone, Edinburgh.

Greer, S., Morris, T. and Pettingale, K. W. (1979) Psychological response to breast cancer: effect on outcome, *Lancet,* Vol. ii, pp. 785–7.

Greer, S. and Watson, M. (1987) Mental adjustment to cancer: its measurement and prognostic importance, *Cancer Surveys,* Vol. 6, no. 3, pp. 439–53.

Hinton, J. (1972) *Dying,* Penguin, Harmondsworth.

Hinton, J. (1981) Sharing or withholding awareness of dying between husband and wife, *Journal of Psychosomatic Research,* Vol. 25, pp. 337–43.

Holland, J. C. and Mastrovito, R. (1980) Psychologic adaptation to breast cancer, *Cancer,* Vol. 46, pp. 1045–52.

Horowitz, M. J. (1979) Psychological response to serious life events, in V. Hamilton and D. M. Warburton (eds.) *Human Stress and Cognition: an Information Processing Approach,* John Wiley & Sons, Chichester.

Hughes, J. E. (1982) Emotional reactions to the diagnosis and treatment of early breast cancer, *Journal of Psychosomatic Research,* Vol. 26, pp. 277–83.

Hughes, J. E. (1985) Depressive illness and lung cancer, II, Follow-up of inoperable patients, *European Journal of Surgical Oncology,* Vol. 11, pp. 21–4.

Hughes, J. E. (1987) Psychological and social consequences of cancer, *Cancer Surveys,* Vol. 6, no. 3, pp. 455–75.

Kubler-Ross, E. (1969) *On Death and Dying,* Macmillan, London.

Lazarus, R. S. and Folkman, S. (1984) *Stress, Appraisal and Coping,* Springer, New York.

Magarey, C. J. *et al.* (1977) Psychosocial factors influencing delay and breast self-examination in women with symptoms of breast cancer, *Social Science and Medicine,* Vol. 11, pp. 229-32.

Maguire, G. P. (1985) Barriers to psychology in care of the dying, *British Medical Journal,* Vol. 291, pp. 1711-13.

Maguire, G. P. *et al.* (1978) Psychiatric problems in the first year after mastectomy, *British Medical Journal,* Vol. i, pp. 963-5.

Maguire, G. P. *et al.* (1980) Psychiatric morbidity and physical toxicity associated with mastectomy, *British Medical Journal,* Vol. ii, pp. 1454-56.

Morris, T. *et al.* (1977) Psychological and social adjustment to mastectomy: a 2 year follow up study, *Cancer,* Vol. 40, pp. 2381-7.

Morrow, G. R. and Morrell, C. (1982) Behavioural treatment for the anticipatory nausea and vomiting induced by cancer chemotherapy, *New England Journal of Medicine,* Vol. 307, pp. 1476-80.

Nichols, K. A. (1984) *Psychological Care in Physical Illness,* Croom Helm, London.

Peck, A. (1972) Emotional reactions to having cancer, *American Journal of Roentgenology Radium Therapy and Nuclear Medicine,* Vol. 114, pp. 591-9.

Penman, D. (1979) Coping strategies in adaptation to mastectomy. Unpublished doctoral dissertation, Yeshiva University, New York.

Pettingale, K. W. *et al.* (1985) Mental attitudes to cancer: an additional prognostic factor, *Lancet,* Vol. i, p. 750.

Reiker, P. P. *et al.* (1985) Curative testis cancer therapy: psychosocial sequelae, *Journal of Clinical Oncology,* Vol. 3, pp. 1117-26.

Ridgeway, V. and Mathews, A. (1982) Psychological preparation for surgery: a comparison of methods, *British Journal of Clinical Psychology,* Vol. 21, pp. 271-80.

Schmale, A. H. *et al.* (1982) Pretreatment behaviour profiles associated with subsequent psychosocial adjustment in radiation therapy patients: a prospective study, *International Journal of Psychiatry in Medicine,* Vol. 12, pp. 187-95.

Schonfield, J. (1972) Psychological factors related to delayed return to an earlier lifestyle in successfully treated cancer patients, *Journal of Psychosomatic Research,* Vol. 16, pp. 41-6.

Silberfarb, P. M. *et al.* (1980) Psychosocial aspects of neoplastic disease: I. Functional status of breast cancer patients during different treatment regimens, *American Journal of Psychiatry,* Vol. 137, pp. 450-5.

Silver, R. L. and Wortman, C. B. (1980) Coping with undesirable life events, in J. Garber and M. E. P. Seligman (eds.) *Human Helplessness: Theory and Applications,* Academic Press, New York.

Spiegel, D. and Bloom, J. R. (1983) Group therapy and hypnosis reduce metastatic breast carcinoma pain, *Psychosomatic Medicine,* Vol. 45, pp. 333-9.

Stam, H. J. and Bultz, B. D. (1986) The treatment of severe insomnia in a cancer patient, *Journal of Behavioural Therapy and Experimental Psychiatry,* Vol. 17, pp. 33-7.

Stedeford, A. (1981) Couples facing death II: unsatisfactory communication, *British Medical Journal,* Vol. 283, pp. 1098-101.

Stedeford, A. (1984) *Facing Death,* Heinemann, London.

Sugarbaker, P. H. *et al.* (1982) Quality of life assessment of patients in extremity sarcoma clinical trials, *Surgery,* Vol. 91, pp. 17-23.

Sutherland, A. M. and Orbach, E. C. (1953) Psychological impact of cancer and cancer surgery, II. Depressive reactions associated with surgery for cancer, *Cancer,* Vol. 6, pp. 958-62.

Tarrier, N. and Maguire, G. P. (1984) Treatment of psychological distress following mastectomy: an initial report, *Behaviour Research and Therapy,* Vol. 22, pp. 81-4.

Tarrier, N. *et al.* (1983) Locus of control and cognitive behaviour therapy with mastectomy patients: a pilot study, *British Journal of Medical Psychology,* Vol. 56, pp. 265-70.

Watson, M. (1983) Psychosocial intervention with cancer patients: a selected review, *Psychological Medicine,* Vol. 13, pp. 839-46.

Watson, M. *et al.* (1988) Development of a questionnaire measure of adjustment to cancer: the MAC scale, *Psychological Medicine,* Vol. 18, no. 1, pp. 203-9.

Wirsching, M. *et al.* (1975) Results of psychosocial adjustment to long-term colostomy, *Psychotherapy and Psychosomatics,* Vol. 26, pp. 245-56.

Zigmond, A. S. and Snaith, R. P. (1983) The hospital anxiety and depression scale, *Acta Psychiatrica Scandinavia,* Vol. 67, pp. 361-70.

Chapter 3

Ethical Issues in Cancer Care

PETER W. SPECK MA, BSc

*Chaplain and Honorary Senior Lecturer
(General Practice Department), Royal Free Hospital, London*

The influence of the media and self-help groups in recent years has meant that the general public is far better informed about medical matters than in former years. This greater awareness has encouraged people to take a more active part in their own health care, whether by self-examination or presenting themselves for regular screening. Alongside this increased sense of responsibility have developed an awareness of the different value judgements which are made at various stages in an illness and, for some, a desire to have a greater say in decisions which relate to treatment and after-care. The British Medical Association *Handbook of Medical Ethics* (1984) draws attention to this when it states:

> Another change of attitude with ethical implications concerns claims by non-medically qualified people, that doctors should not have sole authority over diagnosis, referral, treatment, the granting of access to resources, and rehabilitation. This development has deep significance for patients, for all the health professions, and for the health services. (British Medical Association, 1984, para. 5.3)

The exploration of values in health care is, therefore, something which can involve all who are concerned with the care of sick people.

For the most part ethics is concerned with people and with issues of responsibility, duty and rights. These in turn involve consideration of confidentiality, autonomy and paternalism. This chapter is not exhaustive of all aspects but focuses on some of the basic issues which may be encountered in the care of people with cancer.

Autonomy and Respect

Many of the ethical issues in medicine focus around an understanding of the word *autonomy* and the way in which those offering health care will or will not allow those who are ill to exercise their autonomy. To be an autonomous person is to have the ability to be able to choose for oneself or to be able to create and fulfil one's own plans and ambitions. Being a person is bound up with the ability 'to stand on one's own feet' or 'to know what one wants'. Autonomy may be applauded until it involves another person's autonomy and begins to create difficulties. However, to respect a person entails taking into account the fact that that person is self-determining, self-governing and has feelings, desires and reason. This may be expressed in terms of *rights* and *duties*.

A patient's *rights* are the usual human rights of individuals:
1. the freedom to choose;
2. the rights to knowledge and dignity;
3. the right to self-determination.

A patient also has *duties*:
1. to be truthful and to disclose all relevant information fully and frankly in order that a diagnosis can be made. There is also a duty to co-operate with the physician in matters which can be demonstrated to be in the best interests of the patient;
2. the exchange between doctor and patient depends on this duty for, unless the truth is told, truth cannot be told in return. This has implications for the way in which we care for the person who happens to be ill and who may still wish to retain a measure of autonomy.

A focus for the consideration of autonomy and respect is the interaction which takes place between the sick person and a doctor, nurse, physiotherapist or pastor, especially where decisions are being made. There are several elements to this interaction.

CONFIDENTIALITY

It is implicit that whatever is shared in a consultation or visit is confidential and this is an important element in building up a relationship of trust. Within the health service any information obtained in the course of work within a hospital is confidential – even the fact that a patient has been admitted. However, most professionals work in multidisciplinary teams and so the issue arises about how much information can be shared and with whom. Each professional group has its own code of conduct which acts as a guide for practice. In the United Kingdom, for example, the United Kingdom Central Council for Nursing, Midwifery and Health Visiting (UKCC, 1984, 1987) produces a *Code of Professional Conduct* for those groups, which gives specific details on the issue of confidentiality. There are several levels of information which will be stored in many places, some more easily accessed than others, on the assumption that the patient has agreed to this sharing and that it remains confidential to the team. Consider the example of Alan. The information about him may be divided into four categories:

1. *Identification data*. Alan is a 34-year-old married man, living in an inner-city council flat. He has recently become a long-distance lorry driver. Alan has been admitted for investigation of jaundice.
2. *Medical*. Medical tests show a probable liver tumour. Examination of Alan's blood shows that he is HIV positive and carries the AIDS virus. He is known to the sexually transmitted diseases clinic.
3. *Social*. He has two children, both well, although one is due to come before the courts for shop-lifting. He has only told this to the social worker. His wife works part-time as a school dinner lady.
4. *Psychological*. He is anxious about an operation and about his child's future court appearance. He also feels anxious about keeping his job. Recently, he has suffered from impotence and this has caused stress in his marital relationship. He is embarrassed about this and does not want anyone to know. Because of extramarital relationships he has recently visited the sexually transmitted diseases clinic and feels very guilty about this. He has asked for an AIDS test because of anxiety aroused by recent publicity, but has yet to tell his wife.

Various questions arise about who should know what about Alan. Does everybody need to know everything? How much should be communicated to the occupational health department at Alan's place of work? Alan has not developed AIDS but who should know that Alan is HIV positive? There are also issues of confidentiality relating to the storage of information about Alan, and who should have access, which would need to be considered. If the diagnosis of a tumour is confirmed, how much information should Alan be given or want to know? Many of these issues will be resolved if there is good communication.

COMMUNICATION

A feature of the meeting between the sick person and those who are caring for him or her which can help to preserve autonomy and respect, is the way in which people take care over courtesy, communication and listening. This may be in very simple matters such as remembering names, introducing yourself clearly, and saying goodbye, which are all part of showing respect and acknowledging that the patient is a person. This can be especially important for those patients who suffer a malignant disease which leads to disfigurement and sometimes destroys the person's sense of identity and acceptability (Speck, 1978), or for cancer patients who are in protected environments because of a risk of infection (as in leukaemia or those undergoing treatment with high-dose chemotherapy) and are therefore isolated from others. Similarly, explaining treatment and symptoms to patients in ways they can understand without talking down to them respects their intelligence and allows them a better chance of participating in the decision-making. This is not easy but is important to the development of trust and honesty in the relationship. Perhaps the most obvious aspect of trust and honesty is in relation to telling the truth. Many sick people are trying to come to terms with uncertainty and may already know a great deal about their illness.

A person who is ill and feeling very unsure about the future will search in many ways for information that will either confirm his or her worst fears or reduce anxiety. Some of the messages received may be ambiguous or confused and thus create more anxiety. However, other communications may match the thoughts and feelings of the patient and help to make sense of what is being experienced. Some of the ways in which we receive information include:

1. direct statements from doctor, nurse or other person;
2. overheard comments made by staff, family or others;
3. changes in treatment, position of bed in ward, etc.;
4. changes in behaviour observed in other people;
5. self-diagnosis — reading medical dictionaries;
6. alterations of symptoms, especially if they do not fit in with what the patient has already been told or led to expect;
7. an alteration in the attitude of others toward the patient's future plans or job prospects.

When the initial shock of being ill has worn off, the sick person will sometimes say that deep down he or she knew that 'things were not good'. Although they may have denied their diagnosis to themselves and to others the above sources of information have often conveyed the seriousness of their condition. This may be borne out by such comments as: 'It was their eyes that told me. They smiled with their mouths, but their eyes were sad' or 'After the biopsy results came back the doctors didn't stay long with me, or would avoid me. I felt written off'. Sometimes it is the patient's own anxieties about death and dying which may block any real sharing and lead to evasion and avoidance of any close contact.

It is clear, therefore, that whatever is decided about sharing what is known about their prognosis, patients will already have received a lot of communication from those around them and will have made various deductions of their own. Anyone who has undergone a range of tests, investigations, operation and subsequent treatment will have reached some conclusion even if it is not discussed openly with anyone else. There cannot be set rules about what people are, or are not, told. Getting close enough to the person is the only way to resolve this question because the sort of information being given (or withheld) is best shared in a trusting, caring relationship. There also needs to be consultation with others who are providing care.

The answer to the question 'To tell or not to tell?' depends more on our preparedness to get close to those who are ill, finding out what *they* want to know, appreciating the effects of uncertainty, and then having the courage to share the reality with them. The uncertainty of the patient may be shared by the professional since the doctor may not be absolutely sure how best to interpret a set of results and therefore what to tell the patient or family. The doctor or nurse will make various value judgements before deciding how to approach the patient. Patients and their families may want answers to specific questions but the professional may only be able to answer in terms of trends and probabilities. For example, if Alan asks the doctor, 'Will I die of the tumour?', the doctor may not want to be evasive yet feel unable to give a simple 'Yes' or 'No' answer. Telling the truth is a particular aspect of the problem of uncertainty in medical care.

It is important not to tell lies to patients, but this does not imply a need to tell the *whole* truth all at once. In many situations the *whole* truth is not told for what might be described as 'very good reasons' such as 'we don't know *all* the truth,' 'the other person does not want to hear it,' 'I don't think it is appropriate'. Clearly, in deciding what to tell Alan in answer to his question, 'Will I die of cancer?' several factors need to be considered. What is the actual question that Alan is asking? Is he only expecting a 'No' or is he preparing himself for a 'Yes' or a 'Maybe'? Listening to the patient can help the professional carer to be clearer about what the question is. Timing is important since the implications of information do not always sink in at once and the facts may need to be restated several times. Telling the truth as it is should include allowing the patient some choice in the management of the condition.

Returning to Alan, it is not only the details of the tumour but the fact that he is HIV positive that may need to be shared with him. He may then decide who should be told what about his condition and by whom. It can help to reflect on various aspects of the situation before entering into discussion with a sick person or family. Is the knowledge of the possible outcome of treatment and the prognosis available to answer the questions the patient may ask? What attitudes are held concerning the sharing of information with patients; in other words are there times when one would *not* tell the truth, tell a lie, not tell the *whole* truth or confront the person with the truth? It is tempting to assume that patients and families want to know the truth, and that this will help them to cope. However, this assumes a great deal about how people might cope with the information and, for some, the information may be a great burden which cuts them off from the one person who would normally be their prime support.

PATERNALISM

Because of the different situations which have to be faced over 'truth-telling', it can be tempting to deal with it by restricting the person's autonomy and by being paternalistic. Paternalism is the protection of individuals from self-inflicted harm and decisions are taken, choices made, freedom inhibited, all for the good of the patient (as we see it). The words used can sometimes betray a paternalistic approach: 'We're going to give you a test this morning'; 'If you're good we'll let you out at the weekend'. The main problem with paternalism is that it makes decisions for others which they have a right to take for themselves: 'Just leave that to me' or 'You don't need to know all the details'. Some would argue that there is a place for paternalism. Brewin (1985) presents the argument for a degree of paternalism in medical consultations to avoid overloading patients with information that can become a burden. He argues for a balance between informed consent and protection based on better communication with more explanation for those who need it and less for those who do not.

> What we don't need is unhelpful rhetoric; a wholesale attack of trust; excessive emphasis on 'fully informed consent' and 'autonomy'; a serious

distortion of priorities with a consequent fall in standards of care...
because we are all prisoners of time, the more time we spend trying to
explain things, the less there is for other aspects of patient care.

Within the context of a team it should be possible to ensure that
someone is available to give time to the patient and thus ensure that
the above balance is correctly maintained.

CAN THE PATIENT BE PART OF THE TEAM?

An important corollary of autonomy is a consideration of the patient's
contribution to the decision-making process. This is slightly different
from 'truth-telling' in that the patient may not be given every item of
medical information but his/her views and opinions may be sought
and then represented at a team meeting. The amount of information
given to, or understood by, a patient may vary considerably and be an
important factor to consider when obtaining consent for any
procedure.

Being the patient's advocate and representing the wishes and
feelings of the sick person may be a very important role for non-
medical staff, such as a hospital chaplain, to undertake. Some patients
find it very difficult to speak out at times and may feel under a certain
amount of pressure to consent to an operation or a particular
procedure or test. It can, therefore, be appropriate for someone to
meet the ward or medical staff and discuss these issues on behalf of the
patient. It may emerge that the patient has not fully understood the
need or reason for the test or operation. In cancer care, the reasons for
a change from active to palliative treatment may not be fully
appreciated by the patient. They may refuse chemotherapy, for
example, because of unexpressed fears of side-effects. At the same time
the patient may feel great pressure to accept whatever the medical staff
offer and not to question decisions made. The pressure that the patient
is feeling may not have been recognized.

Similarly, some families can feel under pressure to give consent to a
post-mortem examination after a relative has died. Unless the coroner
is involved they can refuse permission but may not feel strong enough
to say so. Medical staff have no wish to act unethically in such matters
but may not always be aware of the pressures felt by relatives when
requests are made. Feelings may lead to a sense of *obligation* to
consent which may subsequently be regretted. There may, therefore,
be a need for someone to fulfil a vital, though at times uncontrollable,

role in ensuring that the patient's and family's rights are adequately protected.

Quality of Life

Quality of life is another fundamental concept which is reflected in so many aspects of health care though it is not so easy to define. There seems to be no universally accepted definition, though most agree that quality of life relates to the individual person, that it is best perceived by that person, it changes with time, and it must be related to all aspects of life. In Alan's case, any assessment of his quality of life would entail an understanding of his diagnosis and prognosis in respect of the liver tumour. However, one should not ignore the other factors affecting his quality of life at present: his anxiety about his child and the court appearance, his impotence and HIV positive status as well as the implications of these factors for his marriage. Apart from his physical condition and fears of a possible malignant disease, there are many other things which affect Alan's assessment of his quality of life. One way of assessing the quality is to look at the individual's hopes and aspirations in relation to that individual's actual present state. The phrase 'quality of life' is often linked with 'quantity of life' and the hope in medicine is that while seeking to improve the patient's quality of life it may also prolong survival. This may perhaps be twinned with the principle that doctors should not only 'do no harm' but should also endeavour to 'do good' by increasing the benefit to others.

Issues relating to quality and/or quantity feature strongly in connection with continuation or withdrawal of treatment and the question of whether life should be preserved at all costs. Where there is a trade-off between quality and quantity it cannot be assumed that patients will always choose quality. Thus in a study of patients with cancer of the larynx the quantity of their life was their first choice. Where there is a local cancer not extending beyond the larynx, but advanced enough to cause complete immobility of the vocal cords resulting in hoarseness of voice, a laryngectomy leads to a three year survival rate of 60 per cent, but with permanent loss of speech. Alternatively, radiation therapy offers a reduced survival (30–40 per cent in three years) but retains normal or near normal speech. Given this information 81 per cent said they would opt for surgery (with a greater survival rate) even though it would result in irreversible loss of voice (McNeil *et al.*, 1981). There may also be conflict between the needs and wishes of the patient and those of the family, especially in relation to continuing or discontinuing treatments such as chemotherapy or radiotherapy. It is also important not to confuse a low quality of life with meaninglessness or being of little worth since there may still be potential for meaning and growth, even in the face of gross disability.

Euthanasia

'Euthanasia' means death without suffering, or a good death. The term is usually qualified in various ways.

1. *Voluntary euthanasia* refers to the situation where the patient makes a conscious decision to die and requests assistance to do so. Another person is therefore asked to assist with the suicide.
2. *Involuntary euthanasia* refers to the situation where another person makes the decision that the life of the patient should be brought to an end. This use of the term would imply that ending the suffering does not have the consent of the sufferer.
3. *Active euthanasia* refers to some active step being taken to bring about the death of the sufferer, such as the administration of a drug.
4. *Passive euthanasia* refers to the situation where no active step is taken to end the person's life, but treatment may be withheld knowing that this will result in the patient's life being shortened.

There has been extensive discussion of the various aspects of euthanasia as can be seen from the texts referred to at the end of this chapter. Clearly any medical practitioner has a general duty to sustain life and to avoid giving patients anything which might be harmful. However, this should not have the effect of prolonging their suffering as is sometimes seen when mechanical aids to life are used inappropriately. It can be argued that while there is a right to live there is also a right to die, or to be allowed to die, preferably with dignity. Often when discussing our views on euthanasia it is helpful to review society's ideology and value system and consider how far it is imposed on others.

One example of this is in relation to the 'doctrine of double effect' which, in this context, is seen to mean that an action can be seen as 'good' if it is intended to give a desired effect, while recognizing that there may be harmful consequences. Thus the administration of a drug to control pain, even when it might shorten life, is seen as acceptable. The problem with the 'double effect' argument is that it assumes that certain things are always wrong in themselves. It also assumes that it is easy to distinguish between what is intended and what is merely foreseen and that such a distinction is always morally relevant. Without these assumptions there is no need for double-effect arguments. For example, when the Antarctic explorer Captain Oates walked into the snow it does not seem to matter morally whether we say he intended to die in order not to be a burden to his companions and thus foresaw his death, or whether he intended to commit suicide to save his companions. Either way it was gallant. However, those who believe that suicide is always wrong will prefer the first statement.

The doctrine of double effect is usually used in connection with discussion of acts and omissions and whether or not there is a moral difference between the two. Thus it could be thought to be morally acceptable to withhold treatment which could prolong life, but morally unacceptable to kill a patient by an act which accelerates the process of death.

Consent

Consent is a concept related to any relationship between patients and those providing health care. It may be defined as granting to someone the permission to do something he or she would not have the right to do without such permission. It is usual to find various adjectives attached to the word 'consent' in clinical practice – implied, voluntary, informed, etc.

There are many reasons why consent should be obtained and is morally desirable. It maintains respect for individual autonomy and self-determination by the sick person by allowing them to say 'Yes' or 'No'. In respect of Alan, whose history was given earlier in this chapter, his consent would be needed before his HIV-positive status was communicated to his wife. If he refused permission, then the information could not be shared. This can cause conflict for staff and it is interesting to note that while Alan's consent is required in respect of HIV status, his consent would probably not be obtained before sharing his diagnosis and prognosis of cancer of the liver with his wife. Seeking consent ensures that the patient is aware of the risks undertaken, although this is dependent on the honesty of the person who gives the information and on the sick person's ability to comprehend what is being told. Because sick people are vulnerable there needs to be a way of protecting them from duress and of ensuring that the physician, or whoever, looks at his or her own motives for suggesting the operation or procedure. Having to explain and justify the treatment can also help doctors or nurses in their own development as well as contributing to the wider debate of ethical issues among the general public. Some ethical committees, who monitor medical research, request that doctors who seek approval for ethical trials attach a statement in lay terms of the information that the doctor will give to the patient. This has a twofold effect in that the committee can see what patients will be told and it ensures that doctors also have to give careful thought as to how they will present the research protocol to the patients.

The different adjectives indicate the various ways in which 'consent' is used in health care.

Implied consent suggests that consent can sometimes be taken for granted and that specific permission does not need to be obtained. Confidentiality, certain treatments and examination or being seen by medical students in a teaching hospital are examples of implied consent. However, there must be limits to what can be assumed and implied consent should always be linked with courtesy.

Informed consent has been the subject of much discussion because of the difficulty of ensuring that the patient is adequately informed. Can a lay person ever be fully informed? How much information should a doctor reveal about possible rare side-effects? The question of competence also arises since certain groups may not be able to comprehend the information given, for example children, unconscious patients and very distressed people. Information about a potentially terminal illness will trigger off a grief reaction in anticipation of future events. The shock and disbelief associated with this can affect the patient's ability to comprehend information. This factor should be considered when seeking consent. Since patients do not always fully understand and, therefore, may have doubts, they may wish to discuss the information with other people such as the ward staff, hospital chaplain or general practitioner, etc.

Voluntary consent implies that the patient consents of his or her own free will and is not coerced or pressured. However, some decisions may seem to offer a very restricted choice since a person with an inoperable tumour may not worry about distinctions between treatment, therapeutic research and non-therapeutic research but agree to anything on offer.

For consent to be valid, therefore, there need to be both disclosure and understanding of the information shared. The consent obtained then needs to be given voluntarily and the patient should be competent to give that consent. However, attention also needs to be given to how much information is given, whether it is really understood, and whether the consent can ever be fully voluntary. Sometimes a patient will refuse to give consent for a treatment that the physician knows would be beneficial, thus creating a conflict between respect for the autonomy of the patient and desire of the physician (governed by the principle of benevolence) to help the patient.

Clinical trials also raise ethical problems because while it is necessary to make progress in understanding the nature, causation, prevention and treatment of disease, to do so may cause harm. This creates a dilemma between caring for the individual (the principle of non-maleficence or benevolence) and caring for the good of the majority (the utilitarian principle). This dilemma is seen most clearly when the health of the individual will not be promoted by the proposed treatment, although others might benefit in the future. The use of a control group or a placebo would be an example of this. A 'placebo' is a harmless pill or injection which allows assessment of the effect of 'giving something' to the patient to be compared with active treatment. In many cases the 'placebo effect' can be beneficial whereas the real drug may be of no benefit, or even harmful. The ethical problems involved are not always, therefore, straightforward and may be especially complex when one considers the vulnerability of the patient who has cancer, together with the very natural desire to try anything in the hope of finding a cure.

Conclusion

Those involved in caring for the sick may, from time to time, find that they are invited to join patients, families or other staff in examining the various ethical issues that arise in health care. This is a multidisciplinary undertaking and relates very closely to the quality of the care that is given and not just to technical excellence, important though that is. While we may not always be involved in the more dramatic ethical issues in medicine, the very nature of the caring relationship has an ethical aspect which should not be ignored, since 'only intense personalised involvement can create the moral environment in which care is not only excellent but also a true response to human need' (Levine, 1977).

References and Further Reading

Brewin, T. (1985) Truth, trust and paternalism, *Lancet*, no. 8453, pp. 490–2.

British Medical Association (1984) *The Handbook of Medical Ethics*, BMA, London, para. 5.3.

Glover, J. (1977) *Causing Death and Saving Lives*, Penguin, Harmondsworth.

Levine, M. (1977) Ethics: nursing ethics and the ethical nurse, *American Journal of Nursing*, Vol. 77, no. 5, pp. 845–9.

Lockwood, M. (ed.) (1985) *Moral Dilemmas in Modern Medicine*, Oxford University Press.

McNeil, B.J., Weichselbaum, R. and Pauker, S.G. (1981) Speech and survival. Tradeoffs between quality and quantity of life in laryngeal cancer, *New England Journal of Medicine*, Vol. 305, pp. 982–7.

Speck, P. (1978) *Loss and Grief in Medicine*, Baillière Tindall, London, p. 68.

Tschudin, V. (1986) *Ethics in Nursing*, Heinemann, London.

United Kingdom Central Council (UKCC) (1984) *Code of Professional Conduct for the Nurse, Midwife and Health Visitor*, UKCC, London.

United Kingdom Central Council (UKCC) (1987) *Confidentiality — an Elaboration of Clause 9 of the Second Edition of the UKCC's Code of Professional Conduct*, UKCC, London.

Weir, R.F. (ed.) (1986) *Ethical Issues in Death and Dying* (2nd edn.), Columbia, New York.

Chapter 4

The Principles of Cancer Education

BARBARA M. JOHNSON DipCommNurs, RGN,
QN, HVCert, TTCert
Education Adviser, South West Thames
Regional Cancer Organization

Yet cancer education is no more than a convenient label that will fit anything from a lurid and frightening poster campaign to discreet advice given by family doctors and their patients.

(Wakefield, 1962)

Background

In its stated terms, the National Health Service Act 1946 (HMSO, 1946) requires the Minister of Health to be responsible for providing a 'comprehensive health service designed to secure improvement in the physical and mental health of the people of England and Wales and the prevention, diagnosis and treatment of illness'. It is argued that even today there remains considerable doubt about the role of preventative medicine, health promotion and health education, particularly within the National Health Service (NHS) (McEwen, 1985). In 1976, the government made its second and more serious attempt to encourage health authorities to address the issue of prevention and health within the context of the delivery of care (DHSS, 1976). Until this time the National Health Service had allocated almost its entire budget to rectifying the harm induced by either personal behaviour or social and environmental factors. It is now being recognized that 'in the absence of unforeseen and economical new methods of treatment, curative medicine may be increasingly subject to the law of diminishing returns' (DHSS, 1976). This was, and still is, particularly true of the most common cancers.

Following a period of consultation in 1982 the government issued clear directives to health authorities about their role in prevention and health promotion. While warning authorities that preventative medicine and health promotion 'may not always be welcomed by those called upon to change their personal behaviour or their commercial activities' (DHSS, 1982), they were advised not to be deterred. They were charged with the responsibility of:

1. insisting that the NHS develops a commitment to policies on health promotion and preventative medicine;
2. ensuring that resources are directed to these purposes;
3. establishing priorities for programmes which meet the health interests of the local population.

By this definition prevention of illness and health promotion are perceived as an integral part of comprehensive health care. However, until recently there has been little emphasis on planned policies and co-ordination of services to secure the removal of recognized causes of disease and disability, the provision of a healthy environment, the encouragement of individuals to adopt healthy lifestyles and the control of those forces known to militate against health.

This chapter examines education about cancer in the United Kingdom within the context of prevention, health promotion and health education, as well as locating the role of the health professional within those parameters discussed.

Prevention, Health Promotion and Health Education

Historically, preventative care has focused on exhorting individuals to adopt patterns of behaviour recommended by health professionals as being the most effective way of reducing health risks, controlling the development of serious disease or, at the very least, producing the best quality of life possible for those suffering with disease (Calnan, 1982). Initially health messages were aimed at presenting factual medical information in such a way that this would initiate a shift towards 'correct' attitudes and behaviour which would, in turn, yield a reduction in morbidity and mortality – persuasive communication.

Meanwhile, educationalists have contended that education about health should be aimed at enabling people to make health choices within the constraints of their cultural, political and socioeconomic environment. Many variables are now known to influence the degree of change in an individual's attitude and behaviour when confronted by persuasive communication. Moreover, stressing the need to alter attitudes and beliefs often does not lead to a change in behaviour. Indeed, it may induce personal stress, intrapersonal conflict, arouse personal defence mechanisms, isolate the individual from his or her social group and even arouse fear over matters of relative unimportance as compared with other health needs (Green, 1970). This is of particular relevance when considering certain aspects of cancer control, for example breast self-examination, where health education has been accused of inducing anxiety in women (Frank and Mai, 1985)

The speculation and debate about defining the most effective way of gaining improvements in people's health (Seymour, 1984; Baric, 1985) have led to the development of a number of models by a variety of people including health professionals, educationalists, sociologists, psychologists, environmentalists and economists – to name but a few. The models suggest that improvements in health do not rest entirely on individual behaviour. There was, therefore, a need for people to extend their concept of health, so often linked with disease, to include social, political and economic spheres as well as education (Baric, 1985). Health promotion and education thus became the responsibility of politicians, social and political administrators, economists and industrialists as well as health professionals and educationalists.

This extended definition of health and health maintenance is described as health promotion though the relationship between health education and health promotion continues to be the subject of debate. Of the many descriptions of this relationship the following assertion is probably one of the most useful:

> The terms health promotion and health education are not interchangeable. Health promotion covers all aspects of those activities that seek to improve the health status of individuals and communities. It therefore includes both health education and all attempts to produce environmental and legislative change conducive to good health. Put another way, health promotion is concerned with making healthier choices easier choices.
>
> (Dennis *et al.*, 1982)

By this definition, health promotion describes the process of enabling people to increase control over and improve their health. Health education, however, is concerned with raising individual competence and knowledge about health and illness, and is seen by some to be an inherent part of that process (Baric, 1985).

It has been argued consistently that where it is possible, the only way to change personal behaviour with speed and efficiency is to reduce the number of available choices. For example, outlawing the import and sale of tobacco would reduce the prevalence of cigarette smoking; adding fluoride to water supplies would prevent dental caries; qualifying for child allowance by agreeing to have a cervical smear test would reduce the incidence of cervical cancer. These are but a few proposals to which politicians have been asked to address themselves or may be asked to address themselves in the future. However, such measures do infringe individual liberty and they pose serious political questions for a government. Today there still remains public dissent about seat belt legislation and yet, one could argue, it has done more for accident prevention than years of public education.

Examined from this perspective, health promotion does raise ethical issues and there is growing concern among health professionals about the moral implications of health promotion which could, after all, be described as an 'admirable enterprise' (Gillon, 1987). While the two central goals of health education are described as rational decision-making and individual autonomy, health promotion is about convincing other people that they need, or ought to have, what the salesperson or promoter wants them to have. Put another way, health promotion might be seen to be no different from commercial 'hard-sell' practices and if this is so, then health promoters need to confront some fundamental questions which the consumer has every right to ask:

- What am I being offered or sold?
- Is it necessary/do I want it?
- Does it work/do what is claimed?
- Does it do harm/could I be worse off?
- What's in it for the salesman?

(Williams, 1984)

If one considers some of these questions within the context of selling messages about cancer to the public, one might conclude that this method of inducing behaviour change raises serious questions for the promoter. What is on offer is sold to us as a means to a desired end.

WHAT AM I BEING OFFERED OR SOLD?

The previous statement may be true when coercing women into having cervical smear and breast tests or encouraging individuals to look for significant departures in well-being and seek prompt medical advice. The end might be an early diagnosis of cancer: is that a desirable thing to have?

IS IT NECESSARY? DO I WANT IT?

The second question is perhaps less difficult to answer. There is overwhelming evidence that in general people fear cancer and, of all diseases, it is for many the one they would least want to develop (Paterson and Aitken-Swan, 1954; Briggs and Wakefield, 1967; Hobbs, 1967; Williams, Cruikshank and Walker, 1972). The commodity, or state, of 'no cancer' is, therefore, attractive and desirable if that is what is being offered realistically.

DOES IT WORK? DOES IT DO WHAT IS CLAIMED?

With regard to the third question, one might ask what is the evidence for the claims being made and what guarantees are being offered? It is impossible to guarantee that the desired action will prevent the onset of cancer or at the very least cure it. One has to sell the fact, therefore, that certain behaviours may reduce the risk of disease but in the context of 'hard-sell' promotion there is no room for games of 'risk' or 'chance'.

DOES IT DO HARM? COULD I BE WORSE OFF?

One could argue that the personal cost of giving up smoking, examining breasts and skin, eating fibre and moderating alcohol intake is, to some people, greater than the benefit claimed in 'hard-sell' campaigning. It is suggested, for example, that anxiety may be raised in some women exposed to breast self-examination teaching, leaving them in a state of 'breast lump anxiety' (Frank and Mai, 1985). Furthermore it has so far not been proven that finding a breast lump early increases one's chance of cure, and yet it is suggested that many women will have to live with the fear of death for a longer time as a result of such promotion (Williams, 1984). It could be argued that with 'hard-sell' promotion there is an inherent risk of inducing people to a feeling of guilt if they do not succumb to the pressure to purchase. Like any commercial advertising subsequent behavioural change is, at best, likely to be temporary (Bjartveit, 1977). It is believed, therefore, that long-term commitment to 'sensible behaviour' is necessary if the health status of individuals is to be improved. Some would argue that this is the role of education rather than 'hard-sell' promotion but perhaps there is room for both. Either way, whatever the health educator decides, the ethical implications of promotion in relation to cancer education must be heeded.

Cancer Education

In its revised constitution the Cancer Education Co-ordinating Group (CECG) of the UK and Republic of Ireland (1985)* lists as its first objective, 'to promote the co-ordination of public and professional education as to the causes, effects, prevention and recognition of the cancers, and the treatment, care and rehabilitation of people with these diseases'. Implicit in the objective is a definition of cancer education which is congruent with the classification of health education described as being primary, secondary and tertiary prevention (Caplan, 1964). Promoting healthy lifestyles such as non-smoking, skin care and protection and high-fibre diets, is believed to prevent the onset of cancer (Doll and Peto, 1981) and constitutes primary prevention. Secondary prevention refers to a situation when an individual actually has a disease. By educating that person about the condition and what he or she can do about it, it may be possible to prevent the disease becoming chronic or irreversible and restore the person to his or her former health status. An example of secondary prevention may be to encourage the uptake of cancer screening tests and seeking prompt medical advice for any persistent departure from normal 'well-being'. Restoring good health may also involve the individual in complying with new therapy programmes as well as acquiring self-care skills, for example compliance with drug therapy.

For many people ill-health has not been, nor could it be, prevented. Such people have to live with chronic and often incurable disease. Tertiary prevention describes active rehabilitation, which includes the prevention of unnecessary socioeconomic hardship, and encouraging self-management and independence. The aim of cancer education, therefore, could be to improve the quality of health, thus contributing to the quality of life and not merely helping someone to avoid illness. However, the relationship between the provision of correct information and behavioural outcome is not as elementary as might be believed. There is much evidence (Box *et al.*, 1984; Flaherty *et al.*,

* Cancer Education Co-ordinating Group: Hon. Secretary, M. Wood, Ulster Cancer Foundation, 40/42 Eglantine Avenue, Belfast.

1987) to show that at all levels of preventative teaching there remains a consistent level of non-compliance with recommended health actions. In the past this has left health educators feeling baffled and bewildered and clearly, if they are to become more effective, it is necessary to examine the reasons why people do, as well as do not, respond to professional exhortation.

Cancer Education – The Lay Perspective

Historically cancer education campaigns have focused on increasing the general public's knowledge about the prevention, treatment and curability of cancer, thus encouraging people to adopt a more realistic and positive attitude towards cancer and its control. Public opinion surveys (Paterson and Aitken-Swan, 1954; Briggs and Wakefield, 1967; Hobbs, 1967; Williams, Cruikshank and Walker, 1972) have described the public as having an unrealistic attitude towards cancer, being 'over-pessimistic' about its prevention and treatment, and generally being too negative in its beliefs about the disease. It is assumed that this pessimistic attitude stems directly from the public's ignorance of the true scientific facts about cancer. Studies (Briggs and Wakefield, 1967; Knopf, 1976) have shown that individuals overestimate the number of cancer deaths, underestimate the number 'cured' and believe that early detection and treatment have little effect on prognosis. As discussed earlier, opinion studies have shown, without exception, that cancer is the most feared and alarming of diseases.

Apart from examining to what extent public knowledge correlates with the scientific facts about cancer, the studies have also evaluated earlier public education campaigns (Aitken-Swan and Paterson, 1959; Knopf, 1976). An interesting finding is that while there has been a marginal shift in beliefs about the value of early detection of cancer, considerable fear and anxiety persist about the disease. Meanwhile, there is little evidence to suggest that the change in opinion has generated a sizeable change in patterns of health and illness behaviour, particularly among the socially disadvantaged groups. Non-compliance has led some educators to believe that the general public does not behave appropriately because it is over-pessimistic about cancer control and that such pessimism stems from a level of ignorance which health education can rectify by presenting the scientific facts about cancer. That an individual will conform to recommended behaviour once presented with the facts has been argued at a number of different levels.

Once it was realized that increased knowledge does not necessarily redirect behaviour, interest grew in the dimensions of compliant behaviour. To some it became clear that such behaviour is dependent on a range of variables of which knowledge is only one. Variables include an individual's readiness to take action or health motivation, the perceived value of reduced threat of illness, perceived vulnerability to illness, as well as other modifying and enabling factors, such as demographic, structural and attitudinal factors (Becker *et al.*, 1977). This perspective is popularly referred to as the 'health belief model' (HBM) and more recently it has been developed to include 'locus of control' as a further important factor in predicting behaviour. It is suggested that the more a person feels powerless to control his or her own destiny the less likely that person will be to comply with health recommendations (Becker, 1979). Such an argument has serious implications for the cancer educator as many people have fatalistic beliefs about cancer and its control, 'Well – it's in all of us isn't it? It just needs triggering off – there's not much we can do to avoid it. We have it from the day we are born – what will be will be' (Calnan and Johnson, 1985).

Furthermore, social support, whether through the family or lay network, is yet another factor identified as possibly influencing behaviour. This has been observed particularly in relation to smoking cessation and breast screening (Calnan, Moss and Chamberlain, 1985).

It is suggested, however (Antonovsky and Anson, 1976), that the health belief model will only appeal to the rational, goal-directed individual as its emphasis is clearly on rational action based on the individual weighing up the costs and benefits of the recommended health action. The fundamental assumption in this model is that all individuals have the same values, interests and expectations as the professional, as well as having implicit faith in medical knowledge and expertise, thus accepting the authority of the professional. The lay person is depicted as passive and uncritical and, given the right level of information, motivation and opportunity, will comply with the recommended health actions. An alternative approach to under-standing health and illness behaviour has been described as the 'pluralist approach' (Pratt, 1976) where the individual is active and critical, manages his or her own health requirements and is discriminating in the use of medical knowledge, advice and expertise. It also suggests that the professional and layperson have differing and even conflicting perspectives and interests. The professional is seen as one source of advice within a network of consultants. There is a shift away from an emphasis on explaining behaviour in terms of medical rationality towards attempting to understand the individual's action within the parameters of his or her own logic, knowledge and beliefs. It is believed by some that this approach would be a more useful method for understanding health and illness behaviour in relation to cancer (Calnan and Johnson, 1983a).

Health knowledge has been identified as being important in the understanding of health behaviour. What is the individual's concept of health? Assumptions are often made that the public shares a common definition of health which is congruent with the medical or official health definition. But studies have shown that definitions of health range from 'feelings of well-being' to 'absence of disease' and an 'ability to function normally' (Blaxter and Paterson, 1982; Calnan and Johnson, 1985). The threshold of perception of illness is high among disadvantaged groups because the expectation that they will be susceptible to certain illnesses is an inherent part of their daily lives. This may go some way towards explaining why compliance is generally poorer in the lower socioeconomic groups. Clearly, definitions of health are dependent on what people consider to be normal health and their concept of this normality appears to be influenced by social status and position.

Health threat or vulnerability to illness is considered to be another element in health behaviour. How do people assess threats to their health? While fearing cancer, the general concern people express about cancer does not mean they believe they will develop it. 'Well, I fear getting cancer but I don't believe I will get it' (Calnan and Johnson, 1985).

The distinction between a general fear of cancer and feelings about personal vulnerability stems from people's ideas about the causes of cancer. In one study the most common theory of causality was a hereditary theory, which may be the product of the way people construct and develop their theories of causality (Calnan and Johnson, 1985). People tend to base their theories on personal experience rather than on official information. Attempts by professionals to dispel myths and misconceptions about cancer are often rejected by individuals. 'Of course, smoking is one cause. I know it is not supposed to be hereditary but I know of two people who had breast cancer and their fathers, when they were alive had it, so I believe that it is hereditary although medically speaking they say it is not. But I just have a strong belief' (Calnan and Johnson, 1983a).

The use of personal experience as a basis for making sense of health and illness is important because it is in conflict with the underlying philosophy in cancer education as already discussed, which tends to use an epidemiological model of causation.

A third element considered to be important in health behaviour is how individuals perceive their responsibility for health maintenance. Accepting personal responsibility for health lies in the belief that something can be done to prevent (or at the very least reduce the risk of) the onset of disease. Some people believe that some illnesses are caused by factors beyond their control, for example the environment, heredity factors and unknown causes. Such beliefs are particularly true in relation to the cancers. While many people may refer to causes of cancer including knocks, bumps, smoking and breast feeding, the most common explanation often given is that they do not know (Calnan and Johnson, 1983a).

To understand better why people do or do not seek medical help for signs and symptoms of cancer we are required to refer to those studies which examine lay concepts of illness and the dynamics of illness behaviour. Response to illness is described by Herzlich (1973) as falling into one of three categories:

1. inactivity or denial where illness is perceived as a destroyer;
2. fighting and controlling it where illness is explained in terms of an occupation;
3. liberation where illness relinquishes the individual from daily responsibility.

In the first group, the likelihood of people seeking medical care is remote because there is a refusal to acknowledge the problem (denial) and because little value is placed on the outcome of medical intervention. 'Well, I mean they can't really cure it (breast cancer) can they... in spite of what they tell you' (Calnan and Johnson, 1983a). However, in the second and third groups medical care is an essential component of the behaviour process and therefore people are more likely to seek it.

There are also social processes inherent in illness and help-seeking behaviour. First, the individual identifies that something is wrong and then attempts to classify it using a diagnostic label. Each individual has a unique relationship with his or her body and thus each has his or her own personal models of normal and abnormal states (Helman, 1981). Providing the public with information about the early warning signs of cancer has been an attempt by cancer educators to resolve some of the difficulty individuals may have in identifying and assessing the significance of a change in their state of well-being. However, this in itself can lead to difficulty as illustrated by the considerable variation and uncertainty about what a breast lump should look and feel like (Calnan, 1984). Some would resolve such a problem by seeking prompt medical advice – 'if in doubt, go to the doctor', whereas others might adopt a 'wait and see' policy. Deciding what action to take is further complicated by the individual's anxiety about 'wasting the doctor's time' or being seen to overutilize the service, thus being labelled a 'bad' patient.

Having recognized the existence of a problem, the individual then has to decide what to do about it – ignore the problem, wait and see what develops, self-treat or seek outside help. Uncertainty, in relation to cancer, can have an inhibiting effect especially if the individual does not believe anything can be done about it anyway. It has been suggested that people with symptoms of illness will tolerate and accommodate them because the social, psychological and economic costs of accepting the illness, the dependent sick role, and seeking medical care, far outweigh the benefits (Robinson, 1971). This may be particularly true in the case of cancer where people are confronted with the possibility of aggressive treatment, the outcome of which is often uncertain.

The Professional and Cancer Education

Little is understood about the long-term effects of propaganda campaigns or planned interventions aimed at the lay public by professional groups. Even less is known about behaviour changes which occur naturally in society. While there has, for example, been a significant change in smoking habits within certain sections of the population, the mechanism of change underlying the trend remains largely mysterious (Hunt and Macleod, 1987).

Nevertheless, in recent years there has been a growing awareness among the public of the need for more information and education about health issues. It is understood that individuals want to participate more actively in their health care (Macleod Clark and Webb, 1985) and there is now a discernible movement towards encouraging self-help as well as educating individuals to take more responsibility for their health.

Assessing the effectiveness of health professionals in health education is difficult (Calnan and Johnson, 1983b) but there is a reasonable assumption that doctors, nurses and others are well appointed to influence attitudes and engineer behavioural change.

There is increasing evidence that health education on a one-to-one basis is effective (Leigh, Walker and Janaganathan, 1977; Boore, 1978; Norell, 1979) and all health professionals who work with the public are giving information and advice as part of their everyday work. By definition this makes health professionals health educators, but because most are more comfortable with the principles of looking after the sick, they fail often to identify and exploit their educational role (Faulkner and Ward, 1983).

For some health professionals, such as health visitors, dietitians and dental hygienists, the preventative role is clearly defined and the opportunites for health education are obvious and extensive. For those concerned primarily with the management of illness and disease, the opportunity and, therefore, the role, are less obvious. Indeed sometimes health professionals may not see the role as important because they consider that if illness has occurred, health education may be 'too late'.

It is suggested that health professionals need to take deliberate steps to identify and organize health education as a conscious and inherent component in the delivery of care. However, if this challenge is to be met it is argued that radical and fundamental changes need to be made to the 'learner' curricula so that students of the health professions can identify and develop their health education skills. It is further argued that a shift in the relationship between health professional and layperson is necessary if health education is to be effective (Macleod Clark and Webb, 1985). This means a more balanced and contractual liaison where the health professional reduces the social distance by being less dominant and encourages the layperson to take a more active and critical role in the social encounter. One needs to be mindful that this role relationship will be difficult, if not impossible, for some professionals and individuals to achieve.

Health education is about communication. It is essential, therefore, that health professionals are equipped with a firm knowledge base, the confidence and determination to pass that knowledge on to others, and the skills required to put these principles into practice.

Health professionals need to think clearly beforehand about what objectives they are aiming for in a health education session. These may include raising awareness about breast screening, increasing knowledge and understanding about the effect of screening, if necessary changing negative attitudes towards screening and understanding how and where to go for a screening test. Clearly the objectives of health education must be pursued within the context of assessing the individual's needs, level of knowledge and depth of understanding.

People, and patients in particular, do have communication needs. These may include social interaction, information, advice, reassurance, discussion of treatment and prognosis, discussion of feelings and counselling (Macleod Clark and Bridge, 1981). It is therefore necessary for the professional to assess individual needs and be aware of the many factors which could influence the communication process. To be effective, health information and advice about cancer must be realistic and within the parameters of the individual's own day-to-day life.

Health education, including cancer education, at the one-to-one level can be defined as a three-stage process (Ewles and Shipster, 1981):

1. giving information or advice to an individual which relates to his or her health or illness;
2. ensuring that the individual understands and remembers the information and advice given;
3. ensuring that the individual is able to act on the information and advice given.

Studies have shown that good communication and appropriate health education can play a significant role in preventing disease, ensuring that treatment programmes are followed, improving rates of recovery, improving the use of services and controlling symptoms such as pain, stress and anxiety (Hayward, 1975; Baric and MacArthur, 1976; Leigh, Walker and Janaganathan, 1977). However, as discussed earlier in the chapter, it is necessary for the health professional to guard against making mistaken assumptions about individuals' level of comprehension and understanding of the messages, as well as their personal values and attitudes towards the messages being given, for example 'Well it's just facts – no one's proved it' (Calnan and Johnson, 1985).

Assessment is part of the communication process. At the very least assessment of individual needs and teaching requires skills of listening and attending, observing and picking up cues and questioning, as well as the skills of informing and explaining as discussed in Chapter 5.

Within the parameters of the earlier discussion, there is, perhaps, little value in trying to encourage an individual to take advantage of screening and aggressive treatment procedures if the person believes that there is no cure for cancer and that the prescribed treatment is unacceptable. It is possible, however, that by combining the skills of assessment and counselling, the health professional is able to explore and understand better the individual's feelings and beliefs about cancer screening, treatment and curability. In doing so, it may be possible to dispel any misconceptions the individual may have as well as facilitating the time and space for the person to make an informed choice between the available options. Individual attitude changes and rates of learning vary enormously.

To do this effectively, health professionals need to confront their own feelings and beliefs about cancer. Personal attitudes can be transmitted verbally and/or non-verbally during the communication process, though evidence to support the belief that negative attitudes convey 'wrong' images of cancer is difficult to find. As members of society, professionals share fundamental social beliefs. Some authors claim that public opinion about cancer merely reflects professional attitudes (Jenkins, 1979). It has been found that nurses have a more negative reaction to the word 'cancer' than to death itself (Ayers *et al.*, 1973). Professionals' feelings and beliefs about cancer are important with reference to cancer education and it is suggested that non-compliance is due in part to the nature of communication between the layperson and the professional (Hubbard, 1978). As stated previously, there is much evidence that people would like more information about their condition and treatment (Ley, 1977, 1979; Macleod Clark and Hockey, 1979), and when dissatisfied with the amount of information and instruction given they default from their doctors' instructions (Korsch, Gozzi and Francis, 1968). Authors have concluded that nurses, for example, are inadequately informed and express very negative attitudes about cancer. However, knowledge and opinion about cancer do, it seems, improve with clinical experience, though these findings may well reflect the content of cancer education for qualified professionals. While nurses may be regarded as authoritative sources of medical information and opinion by both their patients and social contacts, they often do not make a well-informed and balanced assessment of cancer. It is, therefore, questionable whether or not nurses and other health care professionals are able to motivate the public to undertake preventative care, seek early medical advice regarding suspicious symptoms and approach the whole subject of cancer with less fear. People with mistaken fears and concepts of cancer control are unlikely to be encouraged by professionals who have their own doubts, whatever the basis for these.

Differences in knowledge and opinion can also be observed between hospital and community-based nurses. Community-based nurses are more frequently exposed to the cancer patient who is terminally ill and are therefore exposed to the more negative images of cancer.

Evidence suggests that doctors, both hospital and in general practice, also have fairly negative beliefs about cancer, particularly with regard to cervical smear tests and the curability of cancer (Easson, 1967). General practitioners, however, were found to be very positive about preventative medicine particularly in relation to smoking and lung cancer prevention. There is little evidence that doctors, with the exception of a few, are actively engaged in preventative teaching. Moreover, there is evidence that they are reluctant to discuss topics or actions relevant to cancer (Bluck, 1975) and adopt policies of 'not telling' their patients their diagnosis (McIntosh, 1977). Non-disclosure of information could result from doctors sharing their patients' negative images of cancer and any disclosure of information that might imply cancer is seen by the doctors as bad news (Calnan, 1982).

Conclusion

One of the major objectives of cancer education is to change health beliefs about cancer and its control. It is estimated that one-third of the current death rate due to cancer could be prevented if people did not smoke, and that many more lives could be spared if compliance with screening programmes and earlier diagnosis could be improved.

To do this effectively the health promoter and/or health educator needs to have a better understanding of the nature of the public's beliefs about cancer and their relationship with their health and illness behaviour. To achieve this understanding it has been argued that the current approaches to compliant behaviour need to be complemented with what has been called 'the pluralist approach', which emphasizes the need to explain the layperson's concept of health and illness within his or her own frame of reference rather than imposing models of behaviour which stem from a medical perspective.

References

Aitken-Swan, J. and Paterson, R. (1959) Assessment of the results of five years of cancer education, *British Medical Journal,* Vol 1, p. 708.

Antonovsky, A. and Anson, O. (1976) Factors related to preventative health behaviour. In J.W. Cullen, B.H. Fox and R.W. Isom, (eds.) *Cancer: the Behavioural Dimensions,* Raven Press, New York.

Ayers, R. *et al.* (1973) Research in cancer nursing. In *Proceedings of the National Conference on Cancer Nursing,* American Cancer Society.

Baric, L. (1985) The meaning of words: health promotion, *Journal of the Institute of Health Education,* Vol. 23, no. 1.

Baric, L. and MacArthur, C. (1976) Health norms in pregnancy, *British Journal of Preventive and Social Medicine,* Vol. 3, no. 1, pp.30–8.

Becker, M.H. (1979) Understanding patient compliance: the contributions of attitudes and other psychosocial factors. In S.J. Cohen, (ed.), *New Directions in Patient Compliance,* Lexington Books, Lexington, USA.

Becker, M.H., Haefner, D.P., Kasl, S.V., Kirscht, J.P. *et al.* (1977) Selected psychosocial models and correlates of individual health related behaviours, *Medical Care,* Vol. 15, no. 5 (suppl.), pp. 27–46.

Bjartveit, K. (1977) The Norwegian Tobacco Act, *Health Education Journal,* Vol. 36, no. 1, pp. 3–10.

Blaxter, M. and Paterson, E. (1982) *Mothers and Daughters. A Three-generational Study of Health, Attitudes and Behaviour,* Heinemann Educational, London.

Bluck, M.E. (1975) *Public and Professional Opinion on Preventative Medicine,* Tenovus Cancer Information Centre, Cardiff.

Boore, J. (1978) *A Prescription for Recovery,* Royal College of Nursing, London.

Box, V. *et al.* (1984) Haemoccult compliance rates and reasons for non-compliance, *Public Health (London),* Vol. 98, no. 1, pp. 16–25.

Briggs, J.E. and Wakefield, J. (1967) *Public Opinion on Cancer, a Survey of Knowledge and Attitudes among Women in Lancaster,* Department of Social Research, Christie Hospital and Holt Radium Institute, Manchester.

Calnan, M. (1982) Lay beliefs and feelings about cancer. In M. Alderson, (ed.) *The Prevention of Cancer,* Edward Arnold, London.

Calnan, M. (1984) Women and medicalisation – an empirical examination of the extent of women's dependence on medical technology in the early detection of breast cancer, *Social Science of Medicine,* Vol. 18, no. 7, pp. 561–9.

Calnan, M. and Johnson, B. (1983a) Understanding non-compliance with cancer education campaigns. *UICC Technical Report Series,* Vol. 76, pp. 49–64.

Calnan, M. and Johnson, B. (1983b) Influencing health behaviour: how significant is the general practitioner? *Health Education Journal,* Vol. 42, no. 1, pp. 39–44.

Calnan, M. and Johnson, B. (1985) Health, health risks and inequalities: an exploratory study of women's perceptions, *Sociology of Health and Illness,* Vol. 7, no. 1, pp. 55–75.

Calnan, M., Moss, S. and Chamberlain, J. (1985) Explaining attendance at a breast screening clinic, *Patient Education and Counselling,* Vol. 7, no. 1, pp. 87–96.

Caplan, G. (1964) *Principles of Preventive Psychiatry,* Tavistock, London.

Dennis, J. *et al.* (1982) Health promotion in the reorganised NHS, *The Health Services,* 26 November 1982.

DHSS (1976) *Prevention and Health: Everybody's Business,* HMSO, London.

DHSS (1982) *Care in Action,* HMSO, London.

Doll, R. and Peto, R. (1981) *The Causes of Cancer,* Oxford University Press.

Easson, E.C. (1967) Cancer and the problem of pessimism, *CA. A Cancer Journal for Clinicians,* Vol. 17, pp. 7–14.

Ewles, L. and Shipster, P. (1981) *One to One: a Handbook for the Health Educator*, East Sussex Area Health Authority.

Faulkner, A. and Ward, L. (1983) Nurses as health educators in relation to smoking, *Nursing Times*, Vol. 79, no. 15, pp. 47-8.

Flaherty, C. *et al.* (1987) Approaches to clients in two breast self-examination programmes, *Health Education Journal*, Vol. 46, no. 1, pp. 23-4.

Frank, J.W. and Mai, V. (1985) Breast self-examination in young women: more harm than good? *Lancet*, Vol. ii, pp. 654-7.

Gillon, R. (1987) Health education and health promotion, *Journal of Medical Ethics*, Vol. 13, no. 1, pp. 3-4.

Green, L.W. (1970) Should health education abandon attitude-change strategies?: perspectives from recent research, *Health Education Monographs*, no. 30, Society for Public Health Education Inc., New York, pp. 25-48.

Hayward, J. (1975) *Information. A Prescription Against Pain*, Royal College of Nursing, London.

Helman, C. (1981) Disease versus illness in general practice, *Journal of the Royal College of General Practitioners*, Vol. 31, no. 230, pp. 548-52.

Her Majesty's Stationery Office (1946) National Health Service Act (1946) in *Parliamentary Government Acts*, HMSO Publications, London, chap. 49.

Herzlich, C. (1973) *Health and Illness*, Academic Press, London.

Hobbs, P. (1967) *Public Opinion on Cancer – a Survey of Knowledge and Attitudes among Women on Merseyside*, Merseyside Cancer Education Committee, Liverpool.

Hubbard, S.M. (1978) Breast cancer: nurse's role is vital in early detection. *Nursing Mirror*, 7 December 1978.

Hunt, S.M. and Macleod, M. (1987) Health and behavioural change: some lay perspectives, *Community Medicine*, Vol. 9, no. 1, pp. 68-76.

Jenkins, C.D. (1979) An approach to the diagnosis and treatment of problems of health related behaviour, *International Journal of Health Education*, Vol. 22, no. 2 (suppl.).

Knopf, A. (1976) Changes in women's opinions about cancer, *Social Science and Medicine*, Vol. 10, nos. 3-4, pp. 191-5.

Korsch, B.M., Gozzi, E.K. and Francis, V. (1968) Gaps in doctor–patient communication 1. Doctor–patient interaction and patient satisfaction, *Pediatrics*, Vol. 42, pp. 855-71.

Leigh, J.M., Walker, J. and Janaganathan, P. (1977) Effect of pre-operative anaesthetic visit on anxiety, *British Medical Journal*, Vol. 2, no. 6093, pp. 987-9.

Ley, P. (1977) Psychological studies of doctor–patient communication. In S. Rachmsan, (ed.) *Contributions to Medical Psychology*, Permagon Press, Oxford.

Ley, P. (1979) The psychology of compliance. In D. Osborne, M.M. Gruneberg and J.R. Eiser, (eds.) *Research in Psychology and Medicine*, Academy Press, London.

Macleod Clark, J. and Bridge, W. (1981) Nursing and communication. In W. Bridge and J. Macleod Clark, (eds.) *Communication in Nursing Care*, HM&M Publishers, London.

Macleod Clark, J. and Hockey, L. (1979) *Research for Nursing*, HM&M Publishers, London.

Macleod Clark, J. and Webb, P. (1985) Health education – a basis for professional nursing practice, *Nurse Education Today*, Vol. 5, pp. 210-14.

McEwen, J. (1985) Prevention in a district health authority, *Journal of the Institute of Health Education*, Vol. 23, no. 1, pp. 22-33.

McIntosh, J. (1977) *Communication and Awareness in a Cancer Ward*, Croom Helm, London.

Norell, S.E. (1979) Improving medication compliance: a randomised clinical trial, *British Medical Journal*, Vol. ii, no. 6197, pp. 1031–3.

Paterson, R. and Aitken-Swan, J. (1954) Public opinion on cancer: a survey among women in the Manchester area, *Lancet*, Vol. ii, pp. 857–61.

Pratt, L. (1976) Reshaping the consumer posture in health care. In E. Gallagher, (ed.) *The Doctor–Patient Relationship in the Changing Health Scene*, US Department of Health, Education and Welfare, New York.

Robinson, D. (1971) *The Process of Becoming Ill*, Routledge & Kegan Paul, London.

Seymour, H. (1984) Health education versus health promotion — a practitioner's view, *Health Education Journal*, Vol. 43, nos. 2 & 3, pp. 37–8.

Wakefield, J. (1962) *Cancer and Public Education*, Pitman Medical, London.

Williams, E.M., Cruikshank, A. and Walker, W. (1972) *Public Opinion on Cancer in S.E. Wales*, Tenovus Cancer Information Centre, Cardiff.

Williams, G. (1984) Health promotion – caring concerns or slick salesmanship? *Journal of Medical Ethics*, Vol. 10, Issue 4, pp. 191–5.

Chapter 5

Communication with Patients and Relatives

JILL MACLEOD CLARK PhD, BSc, RGN
Senior Lecturer
Department of Nursing Studies, King's College, University of London
and
SALLY SIMS BNurs, RGN, HVCert, NDNCert
Macmillan Lecturer in Nursing
Department of Nursing Studies, King's College, University of London

Introduction

Communication is an integral part of nursing and the provision of health care, and is central to the theme of this book. Care and support for cancer patients and their families may be communicated verbally or non-verbally, through conversation or silence and through touch or other forms of non-verbal communication, such as eye contact and gestures.

The benefits of effective verbal communication in all areas of patient care have been clearly demonstrated. Studies have shown that information-giving and explanation on admission to hospital (Elms and Leonard, 1966) and prior to diagnostic tests (Johnson *et al.*, 1973; Wilson-Barnett, 1977) and surgical operations (Hayward, 1975; Boore, 1979) have measurable benefits in terms of reducing anxiety, pain and side-effects in the majority of patients. Adequate information and explanation are particularly important to patients with cancer and the beneficial effects of good communication and psychosocial intervention with these patients and their families have been reviewed by Watson (1983). These findings, together with those from research into the benefits of touch for patients (McCorkle, 1974; Lorenson, 1983), readily demonstrate the need for effective verbal and non-verbal communication in patient care.

There is evidence to indicate that patients themselves are well aware that communication is central to their well-being. Patient satisfaction surveys carried out over the past two decades show that patients are frequently dissatisfied with the amount of information they receive and with communication with health care staff in general (McGhee, 1961; Reynolds, 1978). Examination of the Ombudsman's reports over the past six years reveals that poor communication continues to play a significant part in the majority of complaints investigated by the Health Service Commissioner (Vousden, 1987). Cancer patients and their relatives have communication needs throughout the disease process. However, these needs are not always met satisfactorily. Morris *et al.* (1977) found that 33 per cent of the cancer patients they studied were dissatisfied with the information they received compared with only 13 per cent of patients with benign disease. Peck and Boland (1977) found that patients starting radiotherapy had received little preparatory information about their treatment, and Karani and Wiltshaw (1986) found that fifty newly diagnosed patients with ovarian cancer were generally dissatisfied with the quality of the information they had received and had a poor understanding of the wider implications of their treatment, including the more serious and lasting side-effects.

In spite of the fact that the importance and benefit of good communication with patients and relatives are universally recognized, detailed analyses of interactions between patients and nurses in a variety of settings have highlighted the limited verbal communication which often takes place (Altschul, 1972; Ashworth, 1976; Faulkner, 1980; Macleod Clark, 1982). Macleod Clark (1982) found that the pattern of one-to-one communication which emerged from her observations of nurse–patient interaction in surgical wards was one of infrequent and brief interaction, which took place mostly in conjunction with specific nursing tasks. This research also revealed that nurses frequently used blocking tactics to control conversations and, as a consequence, failed to pick up cues about patients' emotional needs. This approach was used with all patients not just those with cancer. The result was a preponderance of superficial interactions similar to those found by Faulkner (1980) in a study of communication between nurses and patients on medical wards.

A study of communication between nurses and dying patients by Drummond-Mills (1983) also revealed a pattern of limited interaction and a failure to assess patients' and relatives' needs for communication and psychological support. Bond (1978), in a study of communication between nurses and cancer patients, found that nurses avoided frank discussions of cancer with their patients and that their interactions were overwhelmingly concerned with physical care and problems associated with ongoing treatment. There were very few examples of discussions about personal, emotional or social issues related to the patient's illness. Bond's findings reinforce those of the earlier studies by Quint (1965), Glaser and Strauss (1965) and McIntosh (1977). These researchers documented the tendency of nurses to avoid involvement with patients and to limit any assessment of their emotional needs by controlling the amount of information that patients were able to give.

These limitations have also been described in studies of interaction between doctors and patients. The conduct of ward rounds has provoked particular criticism. Reynolds (1978) found that the patients disliked the way in which they were excluded from discussion by the doctors, 'who muttered among themselves at the end of the bed, using incomprehensible medical jargon'. The patients also felt that unless they asked questions they would not be given information and those who did ask questions often failed to understand the terms used. This study looked at a variety of patients, some of whom were suffering from cancer. However, research concerned specifically with communicating between doctors and cancer patients has revealed similar problems. McIntosh (1977) found that doctors frequently used tactics of evasion when communicating with cancer patients. Maguire (1976) demonstrated that doctors and nurses tended to avoid patients' social and emotional responses to cancer in outpatient and ward settings. Maguire also drew attention to the fact that patients often do not explicitly report their feelings and anxieties but express them through more subtle cues.

All the research evidence discussed above illustrates vividly the gap that exists between what is theoretically desirable in terms of communication between cancer patients and their nurses and doctors and what tends to happen in reality. Until recently it was commonly assumed that good communicators were born, not made. However, there seems no doubt that in order to become adequately prepared to meet the communication needs of their cancer patients, nurses and doctors should be helped to develop specific interpersonal skills. There is ample evidence to support the view that such training can significantly improve health professionals' communication skills (Ellis, 1980; Maguire *et al.*, 1980a; Maguire, 1984; Macleod Clark *et al.*, 1987).

As knowledge and understanding of the psychological and social consequences of a diagnosis of cancer have grown, it has become evident that the needs of cancer patients and their families for effective communication with nurses and doctors cannot be underestimated. Cancer arouses more fear than other diseases carrying the same or a worse prognosis (McIntosh, 1974). The diagnosis of cancer may elicit anger, anxiety, depression, helplessness (Peck, 1972) and fears associated with death and the unknown (Weisman, 1979). These emotions may become stronger as a result of treatment methods which often produce altered body function and disfigurement (Maguire *et al.*, 1978). Due to the overall intensity of the cancer experience, cancer related concerns may predominate. The knowledge of cancer has been likened to a crisis event (Krouse and Krouse, 1982) and a number of authors have used stress models to describe the experience of cancer (Miller *et al.*, 1976). The diagnosis of cancer affects the family as much as the patient. Family roles and responsibilities may change and added responsibility may heighten the anxiety and stress experienced by family members. Nurses have a vital role to play in the care and support of these patients and their families throughout the disease process. Effective communication is an essential prerequisite if attempts to facilitate coping or adaptation are to succeed and if the cancer patients' communication needs are to be met.

Communication Needs of Cancer Patients and their Families

Cancer patients, in common with all patients, have a potentially wide range of communication needs. These include the need for social contact, practical information, advice, reassurance, information about diagnosis, treatment and prognosis, discussion about feelings and, in some situations, counselling. While not necessarily having *all* these needs, patients with cancer will almost certainly require social interaction, information and opportunities to discuss emotions or feelings.

SOCIAL INTERACTION

Social interaction or social contact is a fundamental human need and it is easy to underestimate or disregard this aspect of communication. For cancer patients and their families normal social interaction can assume a particular importance in that it facilitates coping in times of stress or grief. As Brewin (1977) says: 'To deny the patient with cancer the humour, good fellowship and gossip he could expect if he did not have cancer serves only to increase his sense of isolation'. Patients who are terminally ill may be particularly prone to social isolation (Glaser and Strauss, 1965; Drummond-Mills, 1983).

Social interaction is also important because it provides the foundation for a more substantial and equal relationship between the patient and nurse. Such a relationship is an essential prerequisite for any accurate assessment of a patient's physical and psychological needs. It is also necessary that a warm and trusting relationship has developed between nurse and patient before any deeper communication can comfortably and effectively take place, particularly in relation to discussions of feelings and emotions.

This ideal of meeting the cancer patients' needs for social interaction is not always easy to achieve in practice. As discussed earlier in this chapter, many studies of interactions between nurses and cancer patients have found that these are limited and superficial (Quint, 1965; Bond, 1978). These findings reinforce the importance of nurses developing the ability to use social interaction as a means of developing relationships with their patients. However, many nurses find this process threatening and avoid 'engaging' in this way, because it quickly becomes apparent that what appears to be 'safe' social contact can lead to an exploration of more complex issues. Patients may directly or indirectly ask 'difficult' questions about cancer, terminal illness or death, and nurses may find themselves picking up messages and cues from patients or relatives which they do not feel confident to cope with. Nurses then 'protect' themselves by erecting barriers and maintaining superficiality and, in the process, fail to meet patients' needs.

It is evident, then, that in order to satisfy cancer patients' needs for social interaction, nurses must be skilled communicators and feel comfortable in this role. As skilled communicators they can use the process of social interaction to observe, listen and assess. In this way they will recognize and pick up cues, problems and anxieties from patients and will, in turn, encourage patients to feel able to ask more direct questions and engage in deeper level discussion. Thus it will become possible to begin to meet other important communication needs – information, advice and explanation.

THE NEED FOR INFORMATION, ADVICE AND EXPLANATION

Most patients find that the need for information, advice and explanation is particularly acute prior to definitive diagnosis when anxiety is intensified by waiting for test results (Wilson-Barnett and Carrigy, 1978). The first two to three months following diagnosis have been reported as being the most distressing time for approximately 70 per cent of cancer patients (Weisman, 1979). Cumulative anxiety may result from multiple diagnostic procedures, admission to hospital and treatment, and may be compounded by fears of recurrence and poor survival. Information-giving and advice have been shown to be beneficial throughout the treatment period in terms of reducing physical and psychological discomfort and enhancing feelings of personal control (Maguire *et al*, 1980a; Hames and Stirling, 1987). Towards the end of treatment, anxiety may be associated with the cessation of treatment and concern about recurrence. If the cancer recurs, need for advice and reassurance may be greater than at initial diagnosis. Silberfarb *et al.* (1980) found that the first recurrence was considered to be the most emotionally distressing time for patients with breast cancer.

Discharge from hospital may arouse particular concern, yet evidence suggests that cancer patients and their families are not always made aware of potential problems or how to care for the patient once at home (Googe and Varrichio, 1981; Bond, 1982; Hinds, 1985). Family members are often responsible for the majority of care and support given to the chronically ill cancer patient in the community. It is, therefore, essential that they receive adequate preparation prior to discharge so that they are able to cope with the patient's physical and emotional needs. The onus is often on the relative to approach medical and nursing staff for information while the patient is in hospital (McIntosh, 1977; Bond, 1982). Relatives who may wish to talk to the doctor or nurse but who find themselves too inhibited or uncertain, may not receive the information they require.

Individual preferences for the amount of information desired should be respected. Some patients and relatives prefer not to know or comprehend all of the pertinent facts. For the most part, however, increased knowledge and understanding promote a sense of control with a consequent decrease in anxiety. Patients' and relatives' needs for information and advice should be assessed individually. Accurate assessment of patient information needs can be facilitated by listening attentively, picking up cues, asking questions and using paraphrasing and reflection to clarify responses. Research indicates that a large proportion of cancer patients experience problems of adjustment (Weisman, 1979) and significant psychological morbidity associated with treatment (Devlin *et al.*, 1971, Morris *et al.*, 1977; Maguire *et al.*, 1978; Silberfarb *et al.*, 1980). It has been suggested that many of these problems are exacerbated by a failure to meet the patient's needs for information.

If patients do not receive adequate information about their illness through formal communication networks (the doctor and other health professionals) they may be forced to seek information through other channels, for example by picking up cues (McIntosh, 1974). Relying on cues such as the health carer's manner, the type of examination or treatment and evasion factors in terms of a diagnostic label (Knight and Field, 1981), can cause a great deal of unnecessary anguish. The patient may also automatically assume that the prognosis is bad. The unknown is often a greater source of fear and turmoil than the known (Maslow, 1963). Lack of knowledge and information about diagnosis and treatment can lead to misconceptions or even a lack of concern. If patients do not understand the reasons behind their treatment, they may refuse it.

More attention has been given to the kind of information that cancer patients want and obtain about their condition than to any other illness. Whether or not to tell cancer patients their diagnosis has been the subject of debate and research for decades (Kelly *et al*, 1950; Aitken-Swan and Easson, 1959; McIntosh, 1974). In the majority of studies there has been a tendency for those who actually have cancer to favour being told. However, what constitutes 'telling' is often problematic. Hinton (1974) points out that the question is not only, 'Does the doctor tell?' but 'How much do they discuss?' McIntosh's (1977) study of communication and awareness in a cancer ward found that while, in theory, doctors stressed the individuality of patients and the need to adjust what is communicated according to each patient's needs, in practice they relied on routine ways of handling information which limited the amount of information disclosed. Bond (1983) also found that the management of communication processes involved generalized practices of avoiding words like cancer or malignancy and the use of euphemisms such as 'suspicious cells', 'warts', 'ulcers', as well as sometimes completely denying that the illness was malignant. The routine explanations were aimed at increasing the patient's uncertainty about diagnosis while implying certainty over a good outcome. Communication of this kind is not helpful for patients who cope by seeking information, although for those who cope through denial, it succeeds in perpetuating denial through the maintenance of uncertainty.

Typically, the approach to giving information about diagnosis and prognosis is not managed on an individualized basis because many health carers tend to anticipate a stereotyped negative reaction from the patient. They fail to recognize that the patient can be helped to make a satisfactory adjustment over time (Glaser and Strauss, 1965). Giving information or explanation about diagnosis, treatment or prognosis should not be attempted in one go, when the patient or relative is told everything. Ideally, it should be a careful imparting of honest information as the illness progresses, taking into account the patient's verbal and non-verbal cues which indicate what the patient wants to know.   There is a growing body of opinion that cancer patients have a right to be informed for medico-legal reasons, as well as humanitarian ones (Knight and Field, 1981).

Communication about diagnosis, treatment and prognosis will be influenced by the amount of information shared by all persons involved. McIntosh (1974) points out that relatives are more likely to be told the diagnosis than the patient. This has consequences for the relationship between patient, next of kin and members of the family, especially if the medical staff and family collude not to tell the patient. Glaser and Strauss (1965), in their study of interactions with terminally ill patients, identified four different awareness contexts. These refer to the differing levels of awareness about the patient's impending death, which may exist between the patient and other individuals.

1. *Closed awareness.* The patient does not recognize his or her impending death although everyone else does.
2. *Suspected awareness.* The patient suspects what others know and, therefore, attempts to confirm or invalidate his or her suspicions.
3. *Mutual pretence awareness.* Everyone, including the patient, is aware that the patient is dying but pretends to the other that he or she does not know.
4. *Open awareness.* Everyone, including the patient, is aware that the patient is dying and acts on this knowledge relatively openly.

The concept of awareness contexts has relevance for those involved in cancer care throughout all stages of the disease process, since individuals guide their talk and actions according to who knows what and with what certainty. The patient may move to another awareness context as a result of the deliberate disclosure of information to the patient or by picking up cues and asking questions. How the questions are answered will influence the degree of awareness which is facilitated. The doctor usually has sole responsibility for imparting information about diagnosis and prognosis. However, other health professionals may subsequently discuss what the diagnosis and prognosis mean to the patient. It is, therefore, essential that the nature of what has been disclosed is written in the patient's notes or discussed with other members of the health care team. Unfortunately, in reality, uncertainty often exists about what has been said to whom. This presents problems when patients seek explanations or clarifications about what they have been told (Tait *et al.*, 1980) and when relatives seek information (Bond, 1978).

Webster (1981) points out that nurses may not even know that the patient they are caring for is expected to die. Over 30 per cent of nurses in her study reported that they were not always or ever told which patients were expected to die, and 60 per cent reported that they were not always or ever told whether or not patients had been informed of their poor prognosis. One of the main recommendations in Hitch and Murgatroyd's (1983) survey of communication in cancer care, was for more information to be passed between those involved with a given patient. A suggestion frequently put forward was for information to be recorded routinely in the case notes. Where forms have been incorporated into the patient's notes to record information given about diagnosis and at subsequent interviews, it is felt by those concerned that communication improves (Lyall, 1986). Because of the chronic nature of cancer and the lengthy period that the illness can span, patients and relatives may receive information from numerous doctors and health care professionals. Continuity of communication is essential if conflicting advice and information are to be avoided and confidence in the health care team maintained. In addition, it may be difficult to estimate the impact the information is having on the patient unless what has been said is known.

It is not only the content and continuity of communication which are important but also the way in which the information is communicated. In Gould and Toghill's (1981) study, all but one of the next of kin wished to know the diagnosis but approximately one-third were not satisfied with the way in which the information about the diagnosis (acute leukaemia) and the prognosis had been presented to them. Stedeford (1981) describes how two patients in her study were angry about the thoughtlessness which had led them to learn by accident that the diagnosis was cancer. Information about diagnosis which is disclosed publicly, casually or with insufficient time for discussion may cause additional unnecessary emotional distress.

The manner in which the cancer patient's need for information is handled has critical implications for the way in which the patient and the family will subsequently adjust to and cope with this 'life crisis'. Nurses, therefore, have an immense responsibility to develop the skills which will enable them to assess their patients' needs for knowledge, explanation and information and to recognize conflict and uncertainty when they exist. These skills involve active listening, observation and the use of open questions to check understanding, such as 'What did the doctor tell you?', 'What does that mean to you?', 'How do you think the treatment will affect your life?' Clearly if questions like these are asked then nurses must be prepared to cope with the type of responses which may follow. This means they require the necessary communication skills and confidence to deal with any further information needs that are expressed. Satisfying patients' needs for information will inevitably lead to the development of increasing trust. The nurse must therefore feel comfortable with, and open to, the possibility of meeting patients' needs to discuss their feelings, fears and anxieties related to the diagnosis of cancer.

THE NEED TO DISCUSS FEELINGS, FEARS AND ANXIETIES

Research indicates that cancer patients' needs to express anxiety and fears often go undetected. Maguire *et al.* (1978) found that obvious verbal and non-verbal cues exhibited by women who were distressed while attending a breast clinic went unnoticed in 70 per cent of cases. Ratings of surgeons' verbal behaviour showed that they rarely responded to the cues directly. In another study, Maguire *et al.* (1980b) found that only one in twenty interactions with nurses were concerned with the emotional well-being and psychological reactions of patients following mastectomy. Few interactions involved explicit enquiries by the nurse or disclosures by the patient. Discussion about feelings, fears and anxieties with cancer patients and their families may evoke a range of emotions which can be difficult for carers to handle without appropriate preparation and training (Buckman, 1984). Reactions to the diagnosis of cancer include shock and disbelief, denial, anxiety, anger or guilt and sadness (Peck, 1972; Greer and Silberfarb, 1982).

A recent study (Holmes and Dickerson, 1987) has indicated that cancer patients feel isolated and unable to discuss their anxieties with nursing staff. The main reasons patients gave for this were that nurses appeared too busy and were too young and the patients felt that the nurses would not understand. Other reasons why patients may be reluctant to reveal their problems include fears of an unsympathetic response, doubts that anything can be done to help, fear that an admission of their problems would make them appear silly and unco-operative to others and the desire to protect relatives and staff concerned with their care (Maguire *et al.*, 1978). However, it is important to remember that not all patients with cancer will want to talk about their diagnosis or feelings while in hospital. Dansak and Cordes (1978-79) believe that absence of expected or desired communication about cancer, death or dying does not necessarily mean that the patient is manifesting denial. Other reasons for not communicating include the need for privacy, maintaining a sense of independence, avoiding sadness or guilt or other emotions that are difficult to tolerate and deliberately 'making time' for adjustment. When a clinical label of denial is given to a patient Dansak and Cordes (1978-79) have observed that staff will often begin to reduce communication and time spent with the patient, rather than respecting the patient's wish to cope with the illness in this way and providing continued contact and listening attentively for cues that the patient is ready or wishes to talk about the situation. Patients need to be given a clear indication that it is safe and appropriate to reveal their feelings if that is their wish, and they must be offered a supportive relationship in which to do so.

Quint (1965), McIntosh (1977) and Bond (1978) have shown that the disclosure of feelings, fears and anxieties by cancer patients is sometimes prevented by health carers who erect barriers to communication and use a variety of tactics to avoid communicating at this level. These may be conscious or unconscious mechanisms which ensure that patients will not feel sufficiently comfortable to express their feelings openly. Webster (1981) has identified several tactics which are frequently used by nurses and doctors to avoid and discourage communication with terminally ill patients.

1. *Denial of the seriousness of the patient's illness*
   Patient: 'I don't seem to be getting any better.'
   Health professional: 'Nonsense.'
2. *Abrupt change of conversation*
   Patient: 'Do you think I'll ever get home again?'
   Health professional: 'You like shaving lotions don't you?'
3. *Intense concentration on the physical task in hand*
   Patient: 'Do you think I'll be going home this weekend?'
   Health professional: 'Just a minute I must get this done'(wound dressing).
4. *Pursuing the least threatening aspect of a conversation*
   Patient: 'Not much point booking a holiday now I'm so ill.'
   Health professional: 'Have you had some good holidays?'
5. *Introducing inappropriate humour*
   Patient: 'What a sight I look' (lady with swollen abdomen).
   Health professional: 'Come on it's not that bad – you're only going to have twins now instead of triplets.'

In each of the foregoing examples, a similar process is taking place. The nurse is probably 'hearing' what the patient says but is not actively listening. In other words, the nurse is not listening to the patient's words with the intention of assessing and meeting his or her communication needs. In each of these instances the patient is giving the nurse a cue, a clue that something is worrying him or her and the nurse deals with the situation by avoidance either through failure to pick up the cue (examples 2, 3 and 4) or through the use of false reassurance (examples 1 and 5). These are very effective mechanisms for meeting the nurse's need to be comfortable.

Assessment Skills

In order to begin to meet patients' communication needs nurses must develop and practise a repertoire of skills which allow them to assess patients' needs and then communicate more appropriately. The bases of these skills are now listed.

ACTIVE LISTENING AND OBSERVATION

These are essential in order to recognize cues from the patient or relative.

REINFORCEMENT SKILLS

These are based on behaviours which encourage the patient or relative to continue talking. These include small words, like 'um', 'uh hm', 'yes', 'go on', which encourage without interrupting the flow of the conversation, and non-verbal reinforcers, such as nodding the head, touching a hand, continued eye contact. An additional and very powerful reinforcement skill is embodied in the use of echoing or mirroring back a significant word or phrase. If this approach had been used in example (4) above, the conversation would have looked like this:

Patient: 'Not much point in booking a holiday now I'm so ill.'
Health professional: 'Now you're so ill?'

The patient would then have elaborated on his or her perceptions or feelings and this could have given the nurse valuable extra information on which to base an assessment of the patient's needs.

REFLECTION

Another powerful skill which facilitates the expression and exploration of feelings and emotions is that of 'reflection of feelings'. Here the nurse must incorporate active listening with empathy to get behind patients' words and metaphorically 'step into their shoes'. If this approach had been used in example (1) the conversation might have looked like this:

Patient: 'I don't seem to be getting any better.'
Health professional: 'That must be very disappointing/upsetting for you.'

The patient may well then elaborate his or her feelings assuming that the nurse's attempt to reflect feelings was accurate. It is clear that this form of reinforcement will only be appropriate and successful if the nurse already has a good understanding of the patient.

OPEN QUESTIONS

The use of open questions provides the nurse with perhaps the most useful tool when attempting to assess and meet the communication needs of patients and relatives. Open questions, which are always prefixed by the words *what, where, why, how, which or when*, do not place any constraints or limitations on the way in which a question is answered. They place the emphasis on the patient's perception of the world rather than the nurse's and can be used in a wide variety of situations. An open question could have been used by the nurse in example (1).

Patient: 'I don't seem to be getting any better.'
Health professional: 'What makes you say/think that?'

This approach ensures that the patient elaborates on his or her perceptions of the situation and again gives the nurse valuable information on which to base further communication.

Skilled use of open questions and reinforcing strategies combined with active listening and observation will ensure that the nurse is able to make an accurate assessment of the patient's psychological and physical needs. A careful picture can be built up then of how much the patient and relative understands, what they want to know and believe and how they can be helped to cope with their problems.

Helping Patients and Families to Cope

Once cancer patients and their families have become well informed about the illness and its progress, the need to explore their fears, feelings and anxieties is likely to become more manifest. Most importantly the cancer patient and family will require help to feel in control of, and responsible for, their own lives. In these circumstances the approaches and techniques used in counselling provide a useful way of helping patients and families deal effectively with distress and make decisions.

Counselling is a process through which one person helps another by purposeful conversation in an understanding atmosphere. It seeks to establish a helping relationship in which the counselled can express their thoughts and feelings in such a way as to clarify their own situation, come to terms with some new experience, see their difficulty more objectively and so face their problems with less anxiety and tension. Counselling assists individuals to make their own decisions from the choices available. Nurses take a non-directive role, that is, they facilitate the patient's decision-making rather than imposing their own ideas or solutions.

Using a behavioural intervention model, Weisman and Sobel (1979) describe how counselling techniques can be used to help cancer patients cope by revising and scaling down their problems to a manageable size (Figure 5.1). Patients are encouraged to verbalize their feelings, therefore communication skills discussed previously are essential to the success of this process.

As well as gaining support and help from nurses and other health professionals, there is increasing evidence that some cancer patients can benefit significantly from patient support or self-help groups (Miller and Nygren, 1978; Paulen and Kuenstler, 1978; Fredette and Beattie, 1986). These groups aim to enhance the coping ability of cancer patients and their families by sharing information, clarifying misconceptions, discussing common emotions and identifying resources. This is an interesting development and further research is needed to evaluate systematically the extent to which different types of supportive interactions and counselling in cancer care can meet the communication needs of the patients and their families.

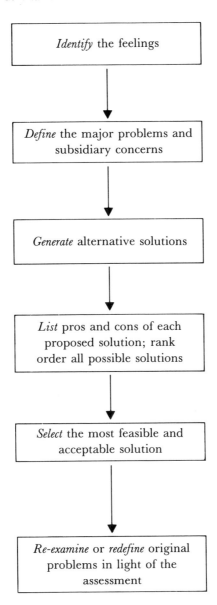

Figure 5.1   Behavioural intervention model.

Conclusion

The research reported in this chapter clearly demonstrates the importance of meeting the communication needs of cancer patients and their families. There is undeniable evidence, however, that much still needs to be done to improve communication in this area. Many important research issues must also be addressed. These include an investigation of:

1. The extent to which communication between cancer patients and health professionals is controlled and, if control exists, whether this is a deliberate or conscious mechanism, who controls the interaction and why.
2. The type of communication skills training which is most successful in assisting health professionals to meet the communication needs of cancer patients and their families.
3. The types of counselling and supportive interventions cancer patients and their relatives find most beneficial.
4. The extent to which problems or barriers to open communication exist between health professionals in cancer care and, if they exist, why and how may they be overcome.

These are all important areas which, through careful research, will enrich understanding of the complex processes of cancer care. However, existing evidence about our current failure to meet the communication needs of cancer patients and their families cannot be ignored. It is essential that every nurse and doctor working in this field is helped to develop and improve his or her communication skills. Moreover, the stress that communicating effectively with these patients and their families imposes on the nurses themselves must be faced.

It is not possible to help patients and relatives communicate their fears and feelings about cancer, death, pain and loss, unless nurses themselves have examined and have the continued opportunity to explore their own feelings about each of these areas. At present there is a dearth of adequate training and support for nurses and other health professionals. Until these issues are addressed and higher priority given to communication skills training, the communication needs of cancer patients and their families will not be adequately met.

References

Aitken-Swan, J. and Easson, E.(1959) Reactions of cancer patients on being told their diagnosis, *British Medical Journal*, Vol. i, pp. 779–83.

Altschul, A. (1972) *Patient Nurse Interaction*, Churchill Livingstone, Edinburgh.

Ashworth, P. (1976) An investigation into the problems of communication between nurses and patients in an intensive care unit. Unpublished MSc. Thesis, University of Manchester.

Bond, S. (1978) Processes of communication about cancer in a radiotherapy department. Unpublished PhD. Thesis, University of Edinburgh.

Bond, S. (1982) Communicating with families of cancer patients (1) Relatives and doctors, *Nursing Times*, 9 June, pp. 962–5.

Bond, S. (1983) Nurse's communication with cancer patients, in J. Wilson-Barnett, (ed.) *Nursing Research: Ten Studies in Patient Care*, J. Wiley, Chichester.

Boore, J. (1979) *Prescription for Recovery*, Royal College of Nursing, London.

Brewin, T. (1977) The cancer patient: communication and morale, *British Medical Journal*, Vol. ii, pp. 1623–7.

Buckman, R. (1984) Breaking bad news: why is it still so difficult? *British Medical Journal*, Vol. 288, pp. 1597–9.

Dansak, D. and Cordes, R. (1978–79) Cancer: denial or suppression? *International Journal of Psychiatry in Medicine*, Vol. 9, pp. 3–4.

Devlin, M. *et al.* (1971) Aftermath of surgery for anorectal cancer, *British Medical Journal*, Vol. iii, pp. 413–18.

Drummond-Mills, W. (1983) Problems related to the nursing management of the dying patient. Unpublished MSc. Thesis, University of Glasgow.

Ellis, R. (1980) Social skills training for the interpersonal professions, in W. Singleton, P. Spurgeon and R. Stammers (eds.) *The Analysis of Social Skill*, Plenum, New York.

Elms, R. and Leonard, R. (1966) Effects of nursing approaches during admission, *Nursing Research*, Vol. 15, pp. 39–48.

Faulkner, A. (1980) The student nurse's role in giving information to patients. Unpublished M.Litt. Thesis, University of Aberdeen.

Fredette, S. and Beattie, H. (1986) Living with cancer, a patient education programme, *Cancer Nursing*, Vol. 9, no. 6, pp. 308–16.

Glaser, B.G. and Strauss, A.L. (1965) *Awareness of Dying*, Weidenfeld and Nicolson, London.

Googe, M. and Varrichio, C. (1981) A pilot investigation of home care health needs of cancer patients and their families, *Oncology Nursing Forum*, Vol. 8, no. 4, pp. 24–8.

Gould, H. and Toghill, P. (1981) How should we talk about acute leukaemia to adult patients and their families? *British Medical Journal*, Vol. 282, pp. 210–12.

Greer, S. and Silberfarb, P. (1982) Psychological concomitants of cancer, current state of research, *Psychological Medicine*, Vol. 12, pp. 563–73.

Hames, A. and Stirling, E. (1987) Choice aids recovery, *Nursing Times*, Vol. 83, no. 8, pp. 49–51.

Hayward, J.C. (1975) *Information: a Prescription Against Pain*, Royal College of Nursing, London.

Hinds, C. (1985) The needs of families who care for patients with cancer at home: are we meeting them? *Journal of Advanced Nursing*, Vol. 10, pp. 575–81.

Hinton, J. (1974) Talking with people about to die, *British Medical Journal*, Vol. iii, pp. 25–7.

Hitch, P. and Murgatroyd, J. (1983) Professional communications in cancer care: a Delphi survey of hospital nurses, *Journal of Advanced Nursing*, Vol. 8, pp. 413–22.

Holmes, S. and Dickerson, J. (1987) The quality of life: design and evaluation of a self-assessment instrument for use with cancer patients, *International Journal of Nursing Studies*, Vol. 24, no. 1, pp. 15–24.

Johnson, J. *et al.* (1973) Psychological preparation for an endoscopic examination, *Gastrointestinal Endoscopy*, Vol. 19, no. 4, pp. 180–2.

Karani, D. and Wiltshaw, E. (1986) How well informed? *Cancer Nursing*, Vol. 9, no. 5, pp. 238–42.

Kelly, W. *et al.* (1950) Do cancer patients want to be told? *Surgery*, Vol. 27, pp. 822–6.

Knight, M. and Field, D. (1981) A silent conspiracy: coping with dying cancer patients in an acute surgical ward, *Journal of Advanced Nursing*, Vol. 6, pp. 221–9.

Krouse, H. and Krouse, J. (1982) Cancer as crisis: the critical elements of adjustment, *Nursing Research*, Vol. 31, no. 2, pp. 96–101.

Lorenson, M. (1983) The effects of touch in patients during a crisis situation in hospital, in J. Wilson-Barnett (ed.) *Nursing research: ten studies in Patient Care*, J. Wiley, Chichester.

Lyall, J. (1986) Cancer: to tell or not to tell? *The Health Service Journal*, 29 May, p. 719.

McCorkle, R. (1974) Effects of touch on seriously ill patients, *Nursing Research*, Vol. 23, pp. 125–32.

McGhee, A. (1961) *The Patient's Attitude to Nursing Care*, Churchill Livingstone, Edinburgh.

McIntosh, J. (1974) Processes of communication information and control associated with cancer: a selective review of the literature, *Social Science and Medicine*, Vol. 8, pp. 167–87.

McIntosh, J. (1977) *Communication and Awareness in a Cancer Ward*, Croom Helm, London.

Macleod Clark, J. (1982) Nurse patient interaction: an analysis of conversation on surgical wards, Unpublished Ph.D. Thesis, University of London.

Macleod Clark, J. (1983) Nurse–patient communication – an analysis of conversations from surgical wards, in J. Wilson-Barnett, (ed.) *Nursing research: ten studies in Patient Care*, J. Wiley, Chichester.

Macleod Clark, J. *et al.* (1987) *Helping Patients and Clients to Stop Smoking*, Health Education Authority research report no. 19, Health Education Authority, London.

Maguire, P. (1976) The psychological effects of cancers and their treatment, in R. Tiffany (ed.) *Oncology for Nurses*, Vol. 2, Allen and Unwin, London, Chap. 1.

Maguire, P. (1984) Communication skills in patient care, in A. Steptoe and A. Mathews, (eds.) *Health Care and Human Behaviour*, Academic Press, London.

Maguire, P. *et al.* (1978) Psychiatric problems in the first year after mastectomy, *British Medical Journal*, Vol. i, pp. 963–5.

Maguire, P. *et al.* (1980a) Planning a caring programme, *Nursing Mirror*, 17 January, pp. 35–7.

Maguire, P. *et al.* (1980b) A conspiracy of pretence, *Nursing Mirror*, 10 January, pp. 17–19.

Maslow, A.H. (1963) The need to know and the fear of knowing, *Journal of General Psychology*, Vol. 68, pp. 111-25.

Miller, C. *et al.* (1976) Assisting the psychosocial problems of cancer patients: review of current literature, *International Journal of Nursing Studies*, Vol. 13, pp. 161-6.

Miller, M.W. and Nygren, C. (1978) Living with cancer - coping behaviours, *Cancer Nursing*, Vol. 1, no. 4, pp. 297-302.

Morris, T. *et al.* (1977) Psychological and social adjustment to mastectomy, *Cancer*, Vol. 40, pp. 2381-7.

Paulen, A. and Kuenstler, T. (1978) Learning to discuss the unmentionable, *Cancer Nursing*, June, pp. 197-9.

Peck, A. (1972) Emotional reactions to having cancer, *American Journal of Roentgenology, Radiation Therapy and Nuclear Medicine*, Vol. 114, pp. 591-9.

Peck, A. and Boland, J. (1977) Emotional reactions to radiation treatment, *Cancer*, Vol. 40, pp. 180-4.

Quint, J.C. (1965) Institutionalised practices of information control, *Psychiatry*, Vol. 28, no. 2, pp. 119-32.

Reynolds, M. (1978) No news is bad news: patients' views about communication in hospital, *British Medical Journal*, Vol. i, pp. 1673-6.

Silberfarb, P. *et al.* (1980) Psychosocial aspects of neoplastic disease functional status of breast cancer patients during different treatment regimens, *American Journal of Psychiatry*, Vol. 137, no. 4, pp. 450-5.

Stedeford, A. (1981) Couples facing death (II) Unsatisfactory communications, *British Medical Journal*, Vol. 283, pp. 1098-101.

Tait, A. *et al.* (1980) Plan into practice, *Nursing Mirror*, Vol. 150, No. 4, pp. 19-21.

Vousden, M. (1987) When the care collapses, *Nursing Times*, Vol. 83, no. 8, pp. 16-17.

Watson, M. (1983) Psychosocial interventions with cancer patients: a review, *Psychological Medicine*, Vol. 13, pp. 839-46,

Webster, M. (1981) Communicating with dying patients, *Nursing Times*, 4 June, pp. 999-1002.

Weisman, A. (1979) *Coping with Cancer*, McGraw Hill, New York.

Weisman, A. and Sobel, H. (1979) Coping with cancer through self instruction: a hypothesis, *Journal of Human Stress*, Vol. 5, pp. 3-8.

Wilson-Barnett, J. (1977) Patients' emotional reactions to hospitalisation, Unpublished Ph.D. Thesis, University of London.

Wilson-Barnett, J. and Carrigy, A. (1978) Factors influencing patients' emotional reactions to hospitalisation, *Journal of Advanced Nursing*, Vol. 3, pp. 221-9.

Chapter 6

Teaching Patients and Relatives

PAT WEBB RGN, RNT, DipN (London), DipSocRes
Senior Nurse – Education
The Royal Marsden Hospital, London and Surrey and Marie Curie
Memorial Foundation, London

Introduction

One of the results of the twentieth century's information explosion is that data are available on every conceivable subject requiring newer and better technology to contain them. The management of health care has been no exception to this general rule. Despite this, patients still lack the information they need to function during their illness, particularly when it is a protracted, life-threatening illness as many of the cancers are. In addition, patients may need new coping mechanisms and skills to deal with their lives following the effects of cancer or its treatments. Those close to them, relatives or friends, feel at a loss to know their role and how best to help and support the sick person. The largest single complaint from patients and relatives within health care services is that they are given insufficient information and support (Health Service Commissioner, 1983, 1984, 1986). This chapter addresses some of the reasons for this, together with the rationale for more specific, focused teaching for patients and relatives and how to achieve it.

Health education is one of the most essential functions of the nurse and yet, paradoxically, it is still poorly understood and greatly undervalued (Macleod Clark and Webb, 1985). While there is a constant and urgent need to continue with primary health education (influencing and motivating behaviour to avoid disease) and secondary health education (slowing down or stopping pathogenesis by early detection and treatment) there is an equally urgent need to provide support and education for those trying to live each day with their illness. Teaching patients and relatives is an integral part of the nurse's health education role.

Patient teaching is by no means the sole property or responsibility of the nurse. All those health care professionals who have contact with patients may be involved in teaching, either intentionally or unwittingly. Much teaching is accomplished unintentionally and sometimes not advantageously. However, the nurse has the most frequent contact with patients whether in hospital or in the home and much of the literature concerned with the teaching of patients and relatives is written by nurses. Patient education is now well established as an ideal although there is considerable variety in the definition of the term and in its implementation.

Communication Patterns

A prerequisite of effective information-giving or teaching is effective communication skills. Considerable discussion has already been given to this in Chapter 5 of this volume. A few points bear repeating or reinforcing in the context of this chapter on teaching patients and relatives. Learning cannot take place where barriers to communication exist.

The management of the nation's health and ill-health is usually in the hands of a vast army of health care professionals and other supportive staff. For the person who is ill, the first point of entry to this bureaucratic organization will be through either the doctor or the nurse in the primary health care setting. It is at this early stage that the first problems may arise in the communication patterns to be established for the rest of that person's 'career' as a patient (Parsons, 1951). It is here that the individual presenting with his or her symptom or suspicion first encounters the established learned roles of *patient* and *care-giver*, a relationship which so often precludes effective communication and, therefore, information-giving and teaching.

Figure 6.1 shows the imbalances that can occur in this relationship and subsequent ones with other health care professionals. The potential patient goes to the professional to seek advice and confirmation, or otherwise, of his or her symptoms or suspicions. The individual lacks the professional's knowledge and becomes dependent immediately on another for accurate information. He or she relies on the expertise of the professional to proceed onwards.

The health care professional has the knowledge-base and education to meet some of the potential patient's expectations. He or she can confirm that suspicions or symptoms are indicative of 'something

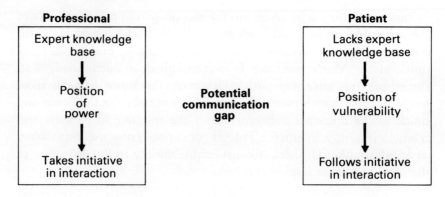

Figure 6.1 Communication problems between patient and professional.

serious' and can begin to categorize these into a prescribed illness.

Yet at this first encounter the seeds of poor understanding may be sown through inadequate communication endorsing misconceptions and assumptions on both sides of the interaction. Freidson (1970) describes this graphically in his classic work on the sociology of applied knowledge. Patients put doctors, and to a certain extent other health professionals, in a position of power. Even though the interaction may be intended to follow a model of guidance from the professional and co-operation from the patient, or potential patient, the professional usually initiates more of the interaction than the patient and the patterns of relative dominance and vulnerability are established (Figure 6.1). This unequal relationship may be compounded further by social inequality and all that this implies. It is this pattern which often goes on to feed the misconceptions and expectations for the rest of the patient's experience and which militates against effective communication and teaching. However, patients may still want the doctor to be the prime source of information provision. McIntosh (1977) discovered in his study on communication patterns in cancer that nurses were not perceived by patients as those who were allowed to give information about diagnosis of cancer. The development of multidisciplinary health care teams in cancer care is increasing all the time. Where these exist, mutual respect for professional credibility of all team members means that anyone may be the prime information-giver.

Patient Education

There is now a body of research demonstrating the value of informing and teaching patients. Some projects demonstrate reduction in distressing symptoms as a result of giving information (Hayward, 1975; Raphael, 1977; Webb, 1983; Wilson-Barnett, 1983). Others are more concerned with the degree of personal control that patients can have, leading to better coping strategies when patient teaching is part of their care (Bowen *et al.*, 1961; Levine and Britten, 1973; Levine *et al.*, 1979).

In the cancer context, the need not only for effective communication but also for active patient teaching is obvious. The impact of cancer on the patient and family is outlined in Chapters 2 and 5. The fear associated with cancer and the threat to life that this implies may predispose patients and their families to profound helplessness where they experience total loss of independence and control of their lives. This often leads to extreme anxiety and depression (Morris *et al.*, 1977; Maguire *et al.*, 1978; Petty and Noyes, 1981).

Blumberg *et al.* (1983) describe cancer patient teaching as sharing many of the challenges associated with patient education for any chronic disease. However, the extra dimensions of cancer compound the problem. These may include misconceptions about the disease, inappropriate attitudes of friends and family, the fear of mutilation and vulnerability caused by the disease and its treatment and the uncertainty associated with outcome. Care-givers are also affected by their own attitudes to cancer (Elkind, 1982) which again serve to reinforce any negative feelings.

Teaching patients and relatives may be seen as an overall philosophy related to any cancer patient or may focus on more specific subgroups with tailor-made frameworks for teaching.

General programmes have been demonstrated in a variety of contributions from the United States of America. Fredette and Beattie (1986) devised a five-session programme using multiple educational strategies to achieve its objectives. The first piloted projects of 1982–83 led to the programme, 'Living with Cancer' being taught subsequently throughout Massachusetts on a regular basis. Similar ventures have been recorded by Blumberg (1982) for the National Cancer Institute Programme in Bethesda, Maryland, and the 'I can cope' programme introduced by Johnson in Minneapolis, Minnesota (1981). A project concentrating on the reinforcement of verbal information-giving and teaching by the use of written booklets has begun as part of an overall strategy for patient education in the United Kingdom (Webb, 1988).

Specific patient teaching for subgroups is more common although many initiatives remain unrecorded. Some examples are documented by Watson (1982) whose aim in teaching adults with cancer is to assist patients to resume self-care and independence. Psychological problems of cancer patients responded to part-teaching and part-counselling in a programme devised by Freidenbergs *et al.* (1980). Materials to assist in teaching adolescent cancer patients were developed by Blumberg (1983) as part of the work of the National Cancer Institute in Maryland. Geriatric oncology and the specific problems of patient teaching relating to the elderly have been addressed by Welch-McCaffrey (1986). Programmes also exist for those with specific cancers (Dropkin, 1981), and for those undergoing specific treatment for cancer (van Scoy-Mosher, 1978; Dodd and Mood, 1981; Israel and Mood, 1982). Much remains to be explored and tested if high-quality teaching for patients and relatives is to be achieved.

Before moving on to describe the types of patient teaching and how they may be implemented, it is important to talk about the relatives.

WHO ARE 'THE RELATIVES'?

Stereotypes abound in our attempts to involve others in the care of patients with cancer. Assumptions are made that a spouse, sibling or parent may be the one closest to the patient and therefore the one who should be included in discussions about a patient's illness and its effects.

This is a very sensitive and important area and one which should be addressed more conscientiously. The traditional family unit is present and strong in many societies whereas it has begun to change significantly in others. In some societies it may still be appropriate to approach the husband or wife, sibling or parent as the assumed next-of-kin and person closest to the patient; in others it may be entirely inappropriate. Close friends or partners of either sex may be the ones that patients want and need at this time. It must be determined at the very beginning what the social needs and norms are for each individual and then to identify those people or that person who is to be closest to the patient during the illness experience.

In addition, a frequent check needs to be made as to whether or not the person with cancer wants information about himself/herself and his or her illness to be shared automatically with the nominated person or people. Frequent checking is essential as things may change over time. Relationships are under a great deal of strain during a serious, chronic illness and it is inappropriate to assume that everything will remain static. Patients should always be asked who they want to be involved in information-giving and teaching and how they want it to be organized. It should never be the case that the patient is excluded from such interactions without first determining the strategy which may, for example, need to be followed when they are in dependent periods of acute illness, when an advocate may be needed.

For the remainder of this chapter, therefore, when the term 'relatives' is used, it indicates whomever the patient has nominated to act in the capacity of helper and supporter as described above.

Teaching Patients and Relatives

There is often an indistinct line between the giving of straight, practical information and the process of teaching. However, the two are different and need to be approached in different ways. The issue of giving information has already been covered in Chapter 5. Inevitably, there is some repetition of principles and reinforcement of ideas in this section on teaching.

The fundamental difference between direct information-giving and teaching is that in the former one does not need necessarily to know the 'why', while in the latter one does. The ultimate aim in teaching is to produce a change in behaviour as a result of the learning that takes place. Learning is a process, therefore, and may take time. In the context of health care and specifically the care of cancer patients, there may be a considerable mixture of both information-giving and teaching. Indeed, the giving of information may sometimes be the first step in establishing a relationship on which future teaching and learning can be based.

WHO DOES THE TEACHING?

Many health professionals may be involved in a patient's care, each of them attempting to give information and/or produce a change in behaviour through teaching. The very fact that many people are involved can lead to considerable confusion for the patient and relatives. Co-ordination of the multidisciplinary team is essential, therefore, with adequate communication occurring at all times. Failure to co-ordinate may result in fragmented care for the patient and frustration for the health carers. Neither is conducive to constructive support for someone in a state of crisis. Professional jealousies, where they exist, must be dealt with at the appropriate level and must not be allowed to burden the patient.

Clearly, a whole range of people may want to be involved in patient teaching: doctors, nurses, the physiotherapist, other therapists, the dietitian, social worker and chaplain. However, before any of this takes place, assessment of the patient is of paramount importance in order to have a base-line from which to work.

PATIENT AND FAMILY ASSESSMENT

Assessment in this context is the use of psychosocial skills to elicit information that will give a view of the patients' world from their own perspective. It is the skill of allowing patients to tell the story of their current illness, or new feature of it, from their perspective while augmenting that, as appropriate, with the wider context that can be given to it by the relatives. Skilled assessment can provide not only factual information about the situation but data on the patients' attitudes, responses and reactions to it.

Although nurses are not the only people who may assess patients, assessment may be seen by them as the first part of planning individualized care using an approach such as the nursing process. The variations are considerable in what kinds of data are collected and how useful they are for subsequent care. In either case, the assessment is the basis on which to plan, implement and evaluate care together with the patient and relatives. It is the beginning of the partnership between patient and health professional to manage the illness and its effects.

Assessment as a base-line is certainly very important but it should not be seen as a static one-off procedure, rather as a dynamic process. Patients may, and frequently do, change the way they view their world. This may happen many times in one day rather than several times in one period of admission to hospital or period of care at home. Reassessment is a necessary prerequisite to dynamic care. The assessment includes identification of learning needs and does, therefore, provide the basis for patient teaching.

The skills for good assessment are outlined in Chapter 5. They are reinforced here because they are fundamental to subsequent care. The aim of assessment is twofold: first, to gain information and second, to try to see the effect a diagnosis of cancer is having on the patient's world. If the assessment is successful, assumptions and misconceptions on behalf of the professional, which can lead to inappropriate care, can be avoided. From the patients' perspective, it allows them to identify their own problems and needs rather than adopting those that health care professionals may suggest are theirs.

Faulkner (1984) has suggested some guidelines for interviewing patients which were used as part of a research-based project to teach assessment skills to student nurses. The following are a variation on a similar theme because the underlying principles of good assessment are the same.

To achieve successful assessment, attempt to:

1. **Use** open questions which will allow people the space to tell their own story from their own perspective. These questions allow people to say what they really feel and discourage them from saying what they think you want them to say.

   Example: 'What do you understand about your current illness?' This is a good way to elicit facts without guiding or leading the client.

   Example: 'How do you feel about that?' This guides, in that it requests responses and feelings, but in no way dictates the subject matter.

2. **Avoid** closed questions. These are questions to which you have to answer 'yes' or 'no';

   Example: 'Do you know where your bladder is?'

3. **Avoid** leading questions as much as possible. These are questions which suggest to the responder how they are to answer.

   Example: 'You know what your bladder does of course, don't you?'

4. **Use** 'echoing' to encourage more information to be given.

   Example:

   Patient:'I have a feeling my cancer has been caused by something I have done in the past.'

   Interviewer: echoes the last few words using a questioning tone, namely 'something you have done in the past?'

5. **Use** reflection (of feelings) so that the interviewer can attempt to put himself/herself in the place of the patient. This requires active listening and empathy.

   Example:

   Patient: 'I just do not understand what is going on. Nobody tells me anything.'

   Interviewer: 'That must be very frustrating for you.'

6. **Avoid** talking all the time. Silence is a powerful tool in all communication. It can also be a very uncomfortable one. It allows the patient space to think and consider the answers and makes for a more relaxed atmosphere.

7. **Watch** for cues. Be aware of the verbal and non-verbal cues that are coming from the patient. For example, an expression on a patient's face may signify extreme anxiety while that person is telling you that he or she is feeling fine.

8. **Create** a relaxed atmosphere and one conducive to conversation. Give thought to the location of the interview, how you introduce yourself, your position in relation to the patient and the way you use encouraging gestures and paralinguistics. Be aware of those things that increase vulnerability in patients and dominance in interviewer and avoid them at all costs.

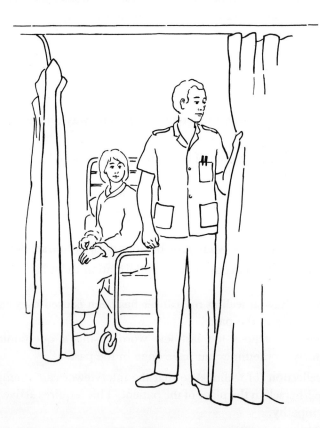

Figure 6.2*a–d*, Communication – things that help and things that hinder.
a, Things that help: creating an illusion of privacy.

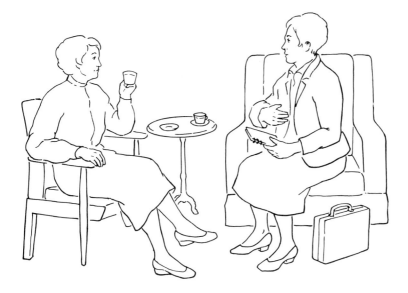

Figure 6.2*b*, Things that help: comfortable relaxed position.

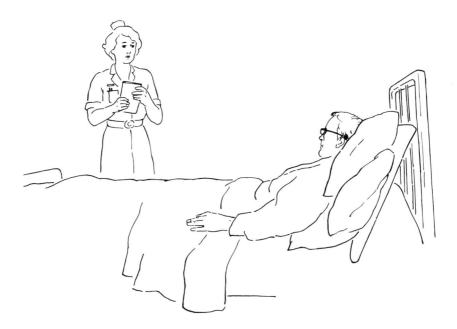

Figure 6.2*c*, Things that hinder: dominant nurse, vulnerable patient.

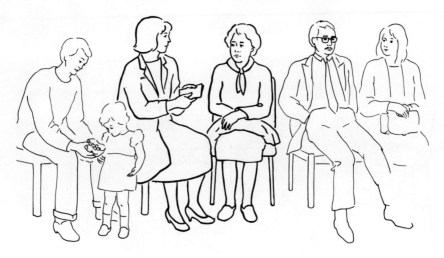

Figure 6.2*d*, Things that hinder: choosing the wrong place to talk.

WHAT KINDS OF TEACHING MAY BE REQUIRED?

A patient is a complex individual whose 'self' is not left behind with the onset of illness, but rather all the facets of 'self' are brought into sharper focus. Some of these facets may be subdued for a while as the diagnosis of cancer is realized. Weisman and Worden (1976), in a paper outlining the impact of a diagnosis of cancer, demonstrated how little new information can be retained when patients are grappling with a threat to life itself. This is an important consideration when determining learning needs and how to meet them. It may prove to be a considerable constraint on chosen techniques. Nurses are particularly bad at taking time to plan appropriate teaching strategies, resulting in unsuccessful responses from patients and learning not taking place at all.

Questions to Ask Yourself about the Patient's Requirements for Learning

1. Is it *conditioning* learning – learning without trying to learn?
2. Is it *psychomotor* learning – is there a skill to be learned?
3. Is it *cognitive* learning – do patients need to know facts, principles, concepts?
4. Is it *attitude modification* – do patients need to develop strategies?

Example. A woman is to undergo surgery for breast cancer followed by a course of radical radiotherapy. The surgery is limited to the removal of the primary tumour only, the radiotherapy providing the largest and most dramatic part of the treatment.

Taking aside the 'self' that will be a very real part of the assessment and will influence the teaching plan, this woman will need a variety of learning opportunities to help her through this experience and her subsequent altered lifestyle.

She will need a considerable amount of *cognitive* learning. She needs to know facts about the extent and effects of lumpectomy and the implications of not having a simple mastectomy. She will need to understand the concept of radiation therapy and how it will affect her systemically and locally, both therapeutically and in the unwanted side-effects it will produce. At some point she will need to understand lymphatic drainage and the problems of lymphoedema that will be experienced following radiotherapy to axillary lymph nodes.

Should she have any local or systemic reaction to radiotherapy, she may need the *conditioning* approach to help her remember to take anti-emetics at an appropriate time before treatment or apply lotion to a skin reaction.

She may need to learn new *psychomotor skills*. Depending on the healing of her wound, she may need to learn the skill of applying a small sterile dressing to the operation site or drainage site.

As a result of lymphoedema following radiotherapy, she may need to learn to use her other hand for some activities or to adapt the use of her affected arm to accommodate the disability. She may be advised and encouraged to self-examine her breasts in the future which requires dextrous skills also.

Such a patient would certainly be confronted with some *attitudinal* and coping problems. Dealing with the diagnosis itself is one area to look at, although emphasis need not be given again to the profound effect of a diagnosis of cancer. In addition, this woman has the potential problems of adapting to an altered body image and to issues of sexuality. She will also have to look for long-term ways of coping with emotional and physical disability or impairment.

This example identifies possible needs for one hypothetical patient. The following guidelines will enable adaptation to any given situation or example.

GUIDELINES FOR TEACHING PATIENTS AND RELATIVES

1. *Establish* the basis from which to continue a partnership with the patient by making a good initial assessment.

2. *Determine* the type of learning needs from the variety of data collected.
3. *Discuss* with patients your assessment and suggestions and determine their response and whom else they would like to be involved in future discussions.
4. *Plan* and *implement* some teaching, giving patients and relatives short-term goals that are achievable.
5. *Evaluate* the effects of teaching and learning together with the patient, and *reassess* needs and how to meet them.
6. *Remember* that everyone learns at his or her own pace. There is no right time for learning to take place.
7. *Be aware* of instability of mood and other psychological states as patients try to make some meaning out of their experience.
8. *Encourage* patients to involve others to help them through this period.

THE ROLE OF THE RELATIVES

Although there has been some discussion of the patient's relatives earlier in the chapter, the role of the relatives has still to be emphasized. An outmoded but none the less true cliché is that 'cancer is a family affair'. The rest of the family or equivalent cannot be excluded from the patient's experience. Such a profound effect on one life inevitably affects all others concerned.

Relatives often find the whole experience confusing and wonder what role they can play. Patients will be trying to grasp what is happening to them and may exclude loved ones from this search for a meaning. Conspiracies of silence may follow where each person is trying to protect the other from what they feel will hurt or harm.

Those professionals working with patients will be able to facilitate close relationships by exploring together with the whole family and by including others in teaching and learning programmes, particularly those which involve coping strategies. It may in fact be impossible to exclude them as their involvement will be integral to the success of the strategy. Cancer is a heavy burden to carry and encouragement to share that burden with those close to the patient can be a very constructive help towards coping.

However, it must be remembered that not all relatives are capable or want to be involved in care. Neither does the patient always want them to be involved. Considerable strains are put on the most stable relationships let alone those that, when put to the test, have no real substance or stability at all.

What Else May Help in Teaching Patients and Relatives?

A key factor in effective communication, information-giving and teaching is the use of more than one medium to present the material and the message.

Written leaflets for patients on aspects of cancer were almost unheard of in the United Kingdom until a few years ago. Thankfully, now there is the beginning of a considerable number and variety of styles of leaflets to help reinforce messages and aid memory. The Royal Marsden Hospital, a national cancer hospital, responded to the direct needs and requests of patients by forming their own interdisciplinary Patient Education Group to produce a series of leaflets, the *Patient Information Series*, to help people to understand better their illness and its effects. Considerable work went into the design of these booklets to make the best resource possible for cancer patients throughout the United Kingdom, where these booklets are now used (Royal Marsden Hospital, 1985).

Cancer help agencies have since developed and they too are now providing some materials of their own as well as establishing a telephone information service for those with still unanswered questions (BACUP and CancerLink)*.

Cancer societies in other developed countries often provide a similar service of information and resources to help professionals in their information-giving and teaching and to provide resources directly to patients. In the past 10 years there has been a considerable increase in the establishment of self-help agencies and groups for cancer patients throughout the Western world in response to an overwhelming need for such services.

Teaching patients and relatives in the context of the group of illnesses corporately called 'cancer' is no longer an optional extra reserved for the few. It is integral to competent professional practice and is, quite rightly, an expectation of every cancer patient. Chronic illness cannot be managed by others; it can only be experienced by those unfortunate enough to have developed it. The professional's role is to support, advise and help throughout this experience by encouraging the development of patients' own resources to learn to cope with their situation and, through understanding, retain control and a degree of independence and quality in their lives.

*BACUP (British Association for Cancer United Patients), 121/123 Charterhouse Street, London.
CancerLink, 17 Brittania Street, London WC1X 9JN.

References

Blumberg, B.D. (1982) N.C.I.'s Coping with Cancer Information and Education Programme — evolution, planning and implementation, *Progress in Clinical and Biological Research*, Vol. 83, pp. 83–90.

Blumberg, B.D. (1983) Meeting the educational needs of adolescents with cancer, *Progress in Clinical and Biological Research*, Vol. 130, pp. 85–9.

Blumberg, B.D., Kerns, P.R. and Lewis, M.J. (1983) Adult cancer patient education: an overview, *Journal of Psychosocial Oncology*, Vol.1, no. 2. pp.   –

Bowen, R.G., Rich, R. and Schlotfeldt, R.M. (1961) Effects of organised instruction for patients with the diagnosis of diabetes mellitus, *Nursing Research*, Vol. 10, pp.151–9.

Dodd, M.J. and Mood, D.W. (1981) Chemotherapy: helping patients to know the drugs they are receiving and their possible side-effects, *Cancer Nursing*, August, pp. 311–8. ·

Dropkin, M.J. (1981) Development of a self-care teaching programme for post-operative head and neck patients, *Cancer Nursing*, April, pp. 103–6.

Elkind, A.K. (1982) Nurses' views about cancer, *Journal of Advanced Nursing*, Vol. 7, pp. 43–50.

Faulkner, A. (1984) *Communication: Recent Advances in Nursing Series*, 7, Churchill Livingstone, London, pp. 137–9.

Fredette, S.L. and Beattie, H.M. (1986) Living with Cancer – a patient education programme, *Cancer Nursing*, Vol. 9, no.6, pp. 308–16.

Freidenbergs, I., Gordon, W., Hibbard, M.R. and Diller, L. (1980) Assessment and treatment of psychosocial problems of the cancer patient: a case study, *Cancer Nursing*, April, pp. 111–19.

Freidson, E. (1970) *Profession of Medicine*, Dodd, Mead and Company, New York.

Hayward, J. (1975) *Information – A prescription against pain*, Series 2, no. 5, Royal College of Nursing, London.

Health Service Commissioner (1983) *Selected Investigations October 1982 – March 1983*, HMSO, London, pp. 11–12.

Health Service Commissioner (1984) *Selected Investigations April – September 1984*, HMSO, London, pp 7–8.

Health Service Commissioner (1986) *Selected Investigations April – October 1986*, HMSO, London, pp. 13–14.

Israel, M.J. and Mood, D.W. (1982) Three media presentations for patients receiving radiation therapy, *Cancer Nursing*, February, pp. 57–63.

Johnson, J. (1981) A patient's structured educational programme to help people to live with cancer, in R. Tiffany (ed.) *Cancer Nursing Update*, Baillière Tindall, London.

Levine, D.M., Green, L.W., Deeds, S.G., Chivalows, J., Russell, R.P. and Finlay, J. (1979) Health education for hypertensive patients, *Journal of the American Medical Association*, Vol. 241, pp. 1700–3.

Levine, P.H. and Britten, A.F.H. (1973) Supervised patient management of haemophilia, *Annals of Internal Medicine*, Vol. 78, pp. 195–201.

McIntosh, J. (1977) *Communication and Awareness in a Cancer Ward*, Croom Helm, London.

Macleod Clark, J. and Webb, P. (1985) Health education — a basis for professional nursing practice, *Nurse Education Today*, Vol. 5, pp. 210–14.

Maguire, G.P., Lec, E.G., Bevington, D.J., Kilchemann, C.S., Crabtree, R.J. and Cornell, C.E. (1978) Psychiatric problems in the first year after mastectomy, *British Medical Journal*, 15 April, no. 6118, pp. 963–5.

Morris, T., Greer, S. and White, P. (1977) Psychological and social adjustment to mastectomy, *Cancer*, Vol. 40, no. 5, pp. 2381–7.

Parsons, T. (1951) *The Social System*, Free Press of Glencoe, New York, pp. 428–47.

Petty, F. and Noyes, R. (1981) Depression secondary to cancer, *Biological Psychiatry*, Vol. 16, no. 12, pp. 1203–21.

Raphael, W. (1977) *Patients and Their Hospitals*, King Edward's Hospital Fund for London.

Royal Marsden Hospital (1985) *Patient Information Series*, Patient Education Group publications, The Royal Marsden Hospital, London and Surrey.

Scoy-Mosher, Van, M.B. (1978) Chemotherapy: a manual for patients and their families, *Cancer Nursing*, Vol. 1, no. 3, pp. 234–40.

Watson, P.M. (1982) Patient education: the adult with cancer, *Nursing Clinics of North America*, Vol. 17, no. 4, pp. 739–52.

Webb, C. (1983) Teaching for recovery from surgery, in J. Wilson-Barnett (ed.) *Patient Teaching. Recent Advances in Nursing 6*, Churchill Livingstone, Edinburgh, pp. 34–55.

Webb, P. (1988) Patient teaching, in A. Faulkner (ed.) *Nursing the Patient with Cancer*, Scutari Press, London (in press).

Weisman, A.D. and Worden, J.W. (1976) The existential plight in cancer: significance of the first 100 days, *International Journal of Psychiatry in Medicine*, Vol. 7, no. 1, pp. 1–15.

Welch-McCaffrey, D. (1986) To teach or not to teach? Overcoming barriers to patient education in geriatric oncology, *Oncology Nursing Forum*, Vol. 13, no. 4, pp. 25–31.

Wilson-Barnett, J. (ed.) (1983) Keeping patients informed, *Nursing*, Vol. 31, pp. 1357–8.

Chapter 7

Spiritual Issues in Cancer Care

ROD COSH BSc

Chaplain's Assistant
The Royal Marsden Hospital, London and Surrey

Introduction

In health care, it is no longer popular to perceive a person simply as a certain 'disorder' lying in a bed. With such innovations as the nursing process and primary nursing, the focus can more clearly be directed at the whole person. Care is not just about dealing with a particular set of physical disorders but is planned for all aspects of the person who is sick. This demands a far more integrated approach to patient care. It means that the nurse in particular not only has to tend to the physical needs of the patient but also has to be at least aware of the other aspects of that person's life. When a person is suffering from a serious, life-threatening illness, including many of the cancers, he or she faces many challenges at many different levels. The sick person not only faces physical distress but may also experience many other stresses.

The spiritual dimension is a fundamental part of every person's life. Every human being has spiritual needs and everbody has a need to fulfil them and the capacity to address them. One definition of the spiritual dimension within life is a desire to contemplate those things which are greater than ourselves; those things which lie beyond our control but which affect us. It is a fundamental human need to ponder the imponderable. From the dawn of time, human beings have desired to be able to put their own existence into some greater perspective and, from this, to attempt to make sense of those most puzzling of circumstances, such as birth, death and, above all, the meaning of life itself.

Religious Needs and Spiritual Needs

It is a common mistake to think that religious needs and spiritual needs are synonymous. Consider this simple analogy: all registered general nurses (RGN) are nurses but not all nurses are RGNs. Similarly, everyone has spiritual needs but not everyone will have a religious component to them. Religious needs are met by formalized religion and many people fulfil their spiritual needs through formalized religion by their adherence to a faith, whether it be Christian, Muslim, Hindu or whatever. In this instance, spiritual needs are fulfilled by a set of basic tenets which are adhered to by a community of faith of which they are a part. Further, these religious needs are strengthened and ratified by communal worship with people of like mind.

THE DECEPTION OF IMMORTALITY

Although the same cannot necessarily be said of many Eastern cultures, in Western society today those people who are actively involved in a religious faith are somewhat of a minority. The majority appear to remain agnostic and for most of their lives they do not see any need to engage actively in any sort of religious praxis. However, this does not deny the fact that we all have *spiritual* needs. Why is it that the majority of people do not seem interested in exploring some of the earth-shattering questions during their lives? In part, this can be answered by the concept of the deception of immortality. For most of our lives the consideration of death is not something very high on our list of priorities. Most people are too busy living to engage in any sort of contemplation of greater things. We may be busy studying or working, building a home, having a family – activities which are not always conducive to considering philosophical dilemmas. Death is something which seems a long way off – so far away, in fact, that the thought of it is pushed far into the recesses of the mind. Death is not something that will happen to us yet; what are the medical profession for, if not to save our lives and keep us living?

It is often only when we, or someone we are close to, is actually faced with a life-threatening disease, that we begin for the first time to come to grips with our own mortality. Only then do we begin to consider those questions which we may ignore when we are healthy and life continues uninterrupted. However, one does not experience different spiritual needs when faced with a serious illness. What *does* alter is the urgency with which these needs are addressed. Someone who is faced with a limited quantity of life may have a lot of unfinished business and, as far as their spiritual needs are concerned, these are suddenly placed into a sharper focus.

SPIRITUAL NEEDS

How, then, may we describe spiritual needs? It may be helpful to consider them in four separate categories:

1. the need for meaning and purpose in life;
2. the need to receive love;
3. the need to give love;
4. the need for hope and creativity.

(Highfield and Carson, 1983)

The Need for Meaning and Purpose in Life

Individuals with a life-threatening illness need to have certain desires fulfilled. They need to be able to make sense of what has gone before; to be able to put their past life into perspective. They need to gain some sort of approval or even ratification of their lives. They need to know that it has been of worth to themselves, their family and friends, perhaps even to the community. All these things help to give perspective to the meaning and purpose of life for them, if not for the significant people around them.

The Need to Receive Love

It follows from this that because we need agreement and approval in life, we also need to know that we are loved. We need to know that others care for us, that others love us and know our worth. When a person is suffering from a serious illness he or she can often feel isolated and need reassurance that, although the person is ill, his or her relationships have not been lost because of that illness.

Isolation may be particularly felt when people have had a change in their body image, either as a result of disease or its treatment. Someone who has undergone disfiguring facial surgery has to be reassured that he or she is still loved by those people who matter to that person, despite a sometimes drastic change in appearance. The same can be said for a woman who has had to undergo radical treatment for breast cancer. Not only has she lost a part of her body but she may also feel that her whole sexual identity has altered; that she is perhaps no longer the person to whom her partner was attracted. Recognition that love is more profound than the changes that have overtaken a person with altered body image, is all important.

The Need to Give Love

If the need to receive love is important then so is the other side of the coin. We need to know that we have been able to give love, to respond to other people's needs, desires and wishes. We need to be reassured that we have been able to love and care for others.

The needs to love and be loved in return are often associated with the word *reconciliation*. An important part of loving others is to be able to come to terms with the fact that there are times when we need to be reconciled to them. We not only need to know that we are forgiven by people whom we have hurt in the past, but also we may find ourselves in the position of having to forgive others. This reconciliation may be needed because of a small issue like an argument or disagreement, or it may be the result of something more major, such as a marital breakdown. Those with faith in God also need to know that they are reconciled to their God whom they believe they will meet when they die.

The Need for Hope and Creativity

Where does the need for hope and creativity fit in to all this? Many people need to be reassured that just as their past life has been of worth, there needs also to be some assurance of a future; the fact that they may shortly experience death does not mean the end of existence. We all need hope and, for many, that lies in the belief that life and death are in some way a continuum.

It might be argued that this is not the case for an atheist, but this is not so. A true atheist is someone who does not believe in the existence of a god and therefore does not believe in any sort of after-life However, this is not to deny the fact that the atheist is a person of faith. Just as Christians put their faith in the existence of God, so atheists put theirs into the non-existence of any sort of superior being. Therefore, at a most cynical level atheists need to have hope that there is nothing after life. Nevertheless, they still need positive and creative hope. Hope that their worth will not be forgotten and that even if they cease to exist, they will be remembered by those whom they affected during their life.

Within these four categories, it is possible to begin to build up a picture of a person's spirituality. That spirituality may be something that fits within the context of a defined religious faith. Alternatively, it may be something different; something which is unique to the individual.

For those committed to a theistic faith, interactions with fellow human beings are not the only part of spirituality. All of the above categories will relate to their relationship with the God in whom they believe. The second and third of these, to give and to receive love, are particularly crucial. We can only begin to make any sense of the senselessness of suffering if we can grasp the truth that God loves us despite everything and that he needs our love. From these concepts one can build hope for the future and take meaning from any sort of relationship with God.

Approaching Spiritual Issues

Well, this is all very interesting and erudite but how can the nurse, for example, assist in this spiritual quest? As has already been mentioned above, the nursing process can be a helpful tool in modern nursing practice. Within this framework for individualized care, adequate assessment is a prerequisite. This assessment should identify patients' needs, including their spiritual ones. However, formal teaching of knowledge and skills to achieve this is often lacking from nurse education programmes at all levels. This often results in entirely inadequate information on which to base a plan of care for the patient. At best, a specific religious affiliation may be documented and at worst, the issues of spirituality may not be addressed at all.

Many nurses do not find it easy to approach spiritual issues with patients. Some would say that it is not the nurse's place to become involved or interfere with this very personal part of their lives. The excuse of privacy is a poor one, however, when you consider how invasive and embarrassing are some procedures and interviews that are regularly carried out for patients by nurses and others; privacy is not an issue that is addressed in many other situations. Nurses have been particularly emphasized because they are usually involved in making a detailed assessment of patients as a prerequisite for planning care. However, all health care professionals have a role to play in considering the spiritual needs of patients along with all their many other needs.

In any interaction, the patient must be given the right and space to make the rules and set the agenda. There should never be an occasion when nurses or others either force a person in their care into a discussion about spiritual issues, or impose their own spiritual values on that patient. The health professional or visiting minister of religion needs to be open, available and ready to listen whenever patients need to talk about these issues. One rule is to avoid proselytization; that is, not trying to convert people but to assist them to fulfil their own spiritual and religious needs. Individuals do not have to deny or ignore their own beliefs and values but rather understand and embrace the patient's own beliefs, whatever they are.

It is all too easy to act out of ignorance or insensitivity when dealing with people whose faith differs from one's own. Until relatively recently there was a dearth of straightforward material about other people's religious or spiritual practices. Now there are some excellent publications (Neuberger, 1987) which can reveal to health care professionals exactly what is expected in most of the world's major religions. Regardless of publications, if anyone is not sure what they should be doing to help someone in this context, it is best to check with the patient or a relative or friend. These issues need to be determined as much as any other, in order to negotiate care.

THE HUB OF THE WHEEL

It may be prudent to call in a chaplain if there appears to be a spiritual problem that the nurse or another health professional cannot help with. There is a growth in the concept of the patient receiving treatment and supportive care from a multidisciplinary team. The co-ordinator of patient care is the nurse who is there with patients through 24 hours of each day. The nurse and patient together may be seen as the hub of the wheel around which other health care professionals circle. This is fast becoming a more popular pattern of care than that of any hierarchical management structure and puts the patient at the centre of things. However, there is a whole range of people in the team to call on and the primary nurse needs to be constantly aware of this and to utilize every resource to the benefit of patients and those close to them.

Nurses often find themselves in a central role with regard to the spiritual needs of a patient, because there may be nobody else within the team who will have the opportunity to get as close to that person as the nurse. It is less likely that others will be so frequently in the position to listen to the outpouring of a troubled soul while completing the most demeaning of tasks. Even if nurses cannot answer the ultimately imponderable questions that are being posed, they should at least be sensitive to know that someone is trying to work them out, and acknowledge them.

It is the role of the nurse as a carer and sometimes an advocate to give the person enough confidence to be able to share these things. Honest replies are always required of honest questions and this may sometimes mean an admission of lack of knowledge or resource to answer. We all crave answers to questions about life, some of which are unlikely to be answered.

Pain

Pain is a sponge-like word that soaks up many meanings. For each of us, pain is peculiarly personal. If a person cuts his or her hand then the ensuing pain experienced is totally subjective; only that person can experience it. The perception of pain is physiopathological (Bonica, 1953) but the reaction to any perceived pain is a complex physiopsychological process which involves the incorporation of the highest cognitive functions (Meier, 1981). The reaction to pain is the sum of what the individual feels, thinks and does about the pain he or she perceives. Just as we are all unique individuals, each of our reactions to a painful stimulus will be similarly unique. The pattern of reaction will depend on such diverse things as past experiences, attitudes, emotional status, mood, will and the presence or absence of anxiety. Thus, to the observer, pain is an abstract concept which may be used to describe a multitude of states.

There are many different definitions of pain, all pertinent to workers in differing fields. It may be defined as a harmful stimulus which signals current or impending tissue damage. It may be a pattern of responses which operate to protect the organism or a personal, private sensation of hurt. Whatever definition of pain is used it must always be remembered that what may be abstract to the observer is a concrete entity to the person suffering it (Anderson, 1981).

PSYCHOSOMATIC

A word that seems to have come into common coinage in recent years is psychosomatic. Although a very useful word, meaning 'of mind and body as a unit', it is often misused to the extent that it may be used in a derogatory way for any ailment which has no obvious aetiology. This word is unfortunately sometimes used for those suffering pain and may reflect the health professionals' inadequacy to assess and treat the pain or, worse still, it may reflect the lack of credence given to the pain on behalf of the health professional. Pain is a response to objective stimuli which may be physical, such as those experienced from the effects of cancer, or may be due to social problems or family tensions. To the individual suffering them they are all just as real as each other.

There can be very little place in the caring professions for the sort of insensitive judgements and comments such as, 'You cannot be in pain'. It may be that a person is not in the sort of pain that the carer initially thought and attempted to control. However, it does not automatically follow that to have administered is to have alleviated. Relief of pain is a subtle art. It may not simply rely on titration of analgesia and an appropriate combination of drugs but also on a careful assessment of the source of the pain and subsequent management of it with all its component parts.

PAIN IS A DIRECT RESPONSE TO DIS-EASE

Pain may be defined as a direct response to dis-ease. If a person is not at ease with himself/herself then he or she is likely to experience some sort of pain. It is easy to see this when considering physical pain because there is an organic source to it. However, there is also social pain for someone who is likely to be evicted from their home for some reason as a result of being ill for some time. This is likely to cause them a great deal of stress and dis-ease. Similarly, if someone is about to undergo a disfiguring surgical procedure, he or she is likely to experience psychological pain among other traumas. The same may be said when considering unfulfilled spiritual needs.

SPIRITUAL PAIN

If the sort of spiritual needs that have been mentioned are left unresolved then a person is not at ease with himself/herself either; the person is dis-eased spiritually and continues to experience pain. It may be helpful to illustrate this by describing a real patient's situation.

> Mrs A., a 45-year-old mother of two with carcinoma of the cervix, was admitted into hospital for surgery. She was convinced that God had given her cancer because she had done something wicked in her life. The only thing that she was puzzled about was exactly what that wicked thing was. By her own admission she had led a relatively normal and good life. No one could persuade her that God was unlikely

to send this sort of retribution on her and she remained convinced that her cancer was her fault and that she was being punished. Immediately prior to the operation she sent for the chaplain who had been visiting her previously and announced with a certain amount of triumph that she had discovered the reason why God had given her cancer. She said, 'The reason is that I have had sex with my husband, and if God cures me of this illness I have promised him that I will never have sex with my husband again'.

Fortunately, this type of extreme case does not occur very frequently. However, it is an example of spiritual pain. Mrs A. had lost sight of the possibility that she could be loved. She believed that the husband (who in fact did love her very much) was the very vehicle by which God had reaped his retribution. Consequently, any need to love either God or her husband was rendered meaningless. In turn, this meant that she had lost any perspective of hope either in the short term, for this meant bargaining cure against a normal marital relationship, or in the long term that God could love her. She had lost any meaning and purpose in her life, for that would have validated the very things that God was condemning her for: that is, her relationship with her husband and her two children, the fruit of their union.

Often the difficulty in identifying spiritual pain lies in a person's inability to articulate the problem. People who are suffering from a serious illness may be faced with questions that have never arisen for them before – questions about death and dying. Perhaps they feel they have to begin to contemplate the meaning of life itself, in order that they can place their own life into context. Not only is it difficult to suddenly spring these questions on ourselves, but there may also be no definitive answers to them.

The sort of questions which are posed frequently are: 'Why is this happening to me?' or 'How can there be a God if he lets people suffer in this way?' Such questions, along with expressions indicating doubts about their own self-worth, or their feeling of isolation can all be expressions of spiritual pain. There may be no definitive answers to these questions but the reassurance that these are not abnormal sentiments and that they are worth asking, is an all important response for the carer to make. All this spiritual caring must be done with patience. One thing must never be forgotten: pain is an all-consuming experience and must be acknowledged as such. Because of this, any logical or philosophical approach to pain and suffering is contra-indicated. What is far more pertinent is that the carer should be able to reassure the person who is suffering that they are still human and that they are still of worth, despite all that they are experiencing.

Elizabeth Kubler-Ross

In 1969 a book by Dr Elizabeth Kubler-Ross was published entitled *On Death and Dying*. It has subsequently become regarded as a classic text on the subject because it describes most perceptively some of the changes in society's attitudes and those of dying patients and their relatives. One of the things that Kubler-Ross is most famous for is her identification of various stages through which a person may pass following a confirmed diagnosis of an incurable illness. These stages of denial, anger, bargaining, depression, anticipatory grief and acceptance are described in full in Chapter 14.

An important fact that must always be remembered when considering the stages identified by Kubler-Ross is that they may lead to acceptance of the situation but do not always occur in the same order as stated. It is naïve to think that one can mentally or even. literally tick the phases off as they occur. The danger of this sort of approach to Kubler-Ross's work is that patients' progress may be incorrectly anticipated. Having been angry on one occasion there may be an expectation that the person would no longer deny his or her prognosis. Not all people pass through the stages in the recognized order. Some people remain in one or other of the stages and some may not ever reach that final stage; all patients do not come to terms with their own mortality. These stages are not universal truths but merely observations.

Accepting this, the role of the carer is to be aware that a patient may be in one or other of these states and may need help to progress through them. However, this help to progress should never be perceived as a race to get the person to the acceptance winning post, prior to death. Some people have spent a lot of their life being angry or depressed. The fact that they are dying will not necessarily change the way they have always lived or their attitudes to life, nor is it appropriate that others try to change them. If somebody wants to die in an angry state, that is his or her right. What is an acceptable state for one person to die in, is not necessarily so for another. In the same way as religious values cannot be forced onto another person, so values and attitudes to dying cannot be either prescribed or enforced. The health professional, however, can support patients in the way they themselves are coping with the fact of dying.

The Waiting Room

A further problem with the dying process and with the way in which we approach supporting it, can be seen in some patients who perhaps go through all the stages described by Kubler-Ross and eventually come to terms with their own death. They are in a state of acceptance and once in this state they are ready to die. They then realize that physically they are not going to die at that time. They are in a sort of 'waiting room', having moved completely through the stages but not to the expected end. This is a stage which perhaps was not identified definitively by Kubler-Ross and is perhaps even more distressing for some people than not reaching a stage of acceptance at all. Some may remain in this state for several days or even weeks and it may eventually lead to clinical depression caused in part by unfulfilled expectation.

It may be helpful to illustrate this with an example. A man with carcinoma of the lung who, three months earlier had accepted his prognosis and was ready to die and was looking forward to meeting the God in whom he had always had a profound belief, was found at home in bed in a fetal position. He was very angry at God for not 'taking him' when he had expected him to do so. This anger and resentment, coupled with depression, made the waiting almost intolerable for him. Unfortunately, this is not as rare an occurrence as many believe and needs to be recognized so that support can be given during this time, both to patients and those close to them who are inevitably affected by this state of affairs.

The timing of the inevitablility of death and of death itself is crucial. Further, the state of acceptance for some people can only be one in which a dying person can reside for a limited time. Something positive has to be offered to those who have reached a state of acceptance but are perhaps in danger of losing its fragile tranquillity. For just as in a doctor's waiting room there are magazines to read while you wait, there has to be something positive offered to the patient who is in that 'waiting room' prior to death.

A Good Death?

In some environments, it is common to talk about 'a good death' or 'a bad death'. What people seem to mean by this is that a good death occurs when someone dies in full acceptance, at peace with the world and his or her creator and within the bosom of the family. Conversely, a bad death may be seen as one where somebody dies outside of a state of acceptance and alone. There is no such thing as a good or a bad death for the patient. However, it may be that the affect of the death on the carer could be termed in this way. Although it is inappropriate to discard the carer's feelings and role in symptom control and support for the dying patient and his or her family, it is not possible to control the way a person dies. We have to accept the fact that just as death is a mystery so is God's reconciling involvement with that person. No one living can know definitively what is a good death or a bad death. Those who have seen many deaths can probably relate episodes of people dying in a peaceful fashion, apparently completely resolved and at one with the world and their possible future. At the same time they can probably also remember times when people have died in apparently uncomfortable or distressing circumstances. However, the fact is that death has occured and there is no way to determine objectively what was good or bad about it.

Many people do not articulate a fear of death so much as a fear of *dying*. 'Will it hurt?', 'Will I be in pain?', 'How will I know when it's happening?', are some of the questions frequently asked by people facing their own death. The main role of the carer is not to try to dispute that some of these feelings may be present, but that the patient will not be alone when feeling them. Isolation is probably the most profound fear experienced. This sort of reassurance can often assist the dying person in facing what is to be.

The 'Ontological Problem' of Suffering, or The Problem of Doers Being in a Busy Place

We must now look at a further complication for those involved in caring for the spiritual needs of people who are suffering. Most of our lives are taken up by doing things. We go to work or school; we actively do things around the house or garden. Some philosophers have suggested that human beings can be defined as the sum of their roles. However, to suggest that this is the total human condition is almost inferring that we are no more than automatons who execute certain tasks in response to certain stimuli. This seems to be tantamount to a denial of any spiritual basis to our being. Because of our preoccupation with doing, admission to hospital with an illness is particularly disruptive to the usual pattern of life. Not only is that alien environment frightening and bewildering with its highly technological atmosphere, it also requires that lifestyles are changed by confining a person to a bed for much of the time and restricts activity and indepencence. Above all, other people have to be relied on to do things for us, rather than we ourselves doing them. Patients spend a large amount of time simply waiting for things to be done either for them or to them, instead of being their usual busy selves. This can be an exceedingly uncomfortable experience, particularly for those who have led a very active life. To suddenly be without any *raison d'être*, any way of validating their being by doing, can be very disruptive and uncomfortable.

The initial response to a loss of action, a loss of the freedom to do things for oneself, can often be one of isolation and perhaps even panic. This compounds any spiritual problems that the individual may already be experiencing. It may be more appropriate for carers just to be with a patient rather than necessarily being busied by tasks, only making the patient feel yet more discomfort. Carers also find inactivity discomforting for the same reasons. Sitting quietly with someone without forcing conversation is an art in itself and can be difficult for both parties; if used well, it can also be extremely therapeutic.

Some Religious Issues from a Christian Perspective – Pondering the Imponderable

Suffering is a mystery. Together with illness it has always been among the greatest problems that trouble the human spirit. So often people suffering ask the question, 'Why does God do this to me?' To say that God has caused the suffering infers some kind of judgement on that person. If it is accepted that God is a loving God then it is unlikely that he who loves will inflict suffering on his beloved. Suffering is pure and unadulterated evil. One only has to see the expression of pain on the face of a seriously ill person to observe the way in which he or she changes and degenerates, to confirm these feelings. However, this does not mean to say that those who experience suffering are evil themselves. Suffering is essentially evil just as rain is essentially wet and, like the rain, suffering falls on people with very little discrimination.

A further question may be: 'If this God that we believe in is so good, so loving, then why does he not simply take all the evil suffering away?' Here, perhaps, is one of the most difficult questions to answer.

One philosophical approach is to say that love is a costly process. If we enter into a loving relationship with someone then that love, if it is to be profound, must have an element of freedom. If we say we love someone but are unable even to allow that person out of our sight then the relationship becomes stifling. So it is the same with God. His relationship with us is not one of God simply pulling the strings that keep us close to him. He loves us sufficiently to give us free will – the freedom to accept him and his love or to reject it. Because love is a costly process, a process of giving freedom, then God who is a God of love cannot be all powerful. This striking proposition in no way denies God's omnipotence or omniscience but it does acknowledge that the costliness of love ensures that we are not manipulated like pawns in a celestial chess game.

What many people seek when they ask these sorts of questions is the miraculous cure – God intervening with a thunderbolt from heaven to make it all right. It must never be denied that miracles can and do happen. They are, of course, not beyond the providence of God. However, if we continually insist on looking for the ice-cream van down the street we may miss the meal laid out at home. The miraculous is among us here and now; day by day throughout hospitals the miraculous is being performed by God. Instead of using the thunderbolt or the primaeval flash of lightning, God used his best creation – his people. Doctors, nurses and others in the multidisciplinary team respond to the needs of patients to care and help and promote cure.

Cure is an awkward word. It simply means to get better, perhaps to be restored to one's former self. But there is no such thing as being restored totally to one's former self. Because life is an ongoing process, the best that can even be hoped for is to be returned to the health that we would expect at that time in our lives. None of us can turn the clock back, nor can we deny entropy.

Cure seems to be bound up with the physical restoration of health. Perhaps a more useful word is 'heal'. Healing does not just talk about curing or simply getting better but describes a state of wholeness. This healing process may include curing the physical disease but it has to be admitted that this can only be a small part of the process. Healing is about being a whole person, a complete person within the limitations of our humanness. Those limitations may include an illness. To say that a person cannot be whole in the sight of God when he or she is ill, infers not only that a congenitally blind person is unloved by God but also that God can only accept us as physically or mentally complete.

Wholeness and healing are all about being open to the will of God and accepting the infinite love he has to offer. It must be remembered that even God experienced human suffering on the cross. So the lover knows from first-hand experience the condition of the beloved. Put into the context of the eternal, healing does not have to necessarily take place in this life. Although death may be seen as a failure of the curing process, there is a real possibility that the healing process may be fulfilled after life. For it is God's involvement with his creation that brings about healing and wholeness.

The Sacraments of the Sick

From this, springs our sacramental theology. Many nurses feel awkward about staying with patients while they are receiving the sacraments. This is a constant sadness for many chaplains. Apart from the Sacrament of Reconciliation (confession), it seems illogical that those who have cared most for a particular patient should not be present when that person receives communion or is anointed with the oil of the sick. For the Christian, the three most commonly used sacraments in hospital are Holy Communion, Anointing and the Sacrament of Reconciliation. Perhaps the best and shortest definition of a sacrament is 'an outward and visible sign of an inward and invisible grace' (*Book of Common Prayer, 1662*). What is meant by that is that God takes ordinary things like bread and wine, oil and ourselves and shows us something of his true nature by transforming them. He takes bread and wine and through them gives us Christ his Son whose body and blood were broken and poured out for us. The same can be said for the oil which, blessed by God, gives the strength of the Holy Spirit to those who need it and are anointed (*The Holy Bible*, 1952a).

In the Sacrament of Reconciliation the elements that God takes and makes holy are not at first so obvious. Although this sacrament is by definition of a penitential nature, it must be recognized that reconciliation is a celebration. It is a reminder to those who take part in it that God is a God of love and however far we move from his love, we can always return. In many ways it is an enactment of the parable of the prodigal son (*The Holy Bible*, 1952b); it did not matter how much the prodigal son turned his back on his father, his father was always there waiting for him to come back. So in this sacrament God does not take inanimate elements and transform them. He takes our very beings and transforms them by reassuring us of his continual love for us.

We cannot admit to having all the answers, for as St Paul says, 'For now we see in a mirror dimly' (*The Holy Bible*, 1952c). But that image which we perceive, however darkly, is our hope – hope that all will be revealed in its true and radiant light when everything is accomplished.

Conclusion

In this chapter an attempt has been made to approach some of the spiritual issues involved in cancer care. Many of them have only been touched on briefly so that others may be encouraged to consider them when dealing with patients. As has already been suggested, spiritual needs are not just the needs of the sick or dying but they are with us throughout our lives. However, they may become more apparent or focused during such periods of our lives. We who may not be in such a phase would do well to be sensitive and approachable to those who are.

References and Further Reading

Ainsworth-Smith, J. and Speck, P. (1982) *Letting go*, Society for the Propagation of Christian Knowledge (SPCK), London.

Anderson, L.P.(1981) The relationship between perception of pain, cognitive behavioural variables and coping strategies in chronic pain patients. Unpublished Ph.D. thesis, University of Houston.

Aulton, N. (1986) *Pain — an Exploration*, Darton, Longman and Todd, London

Bonica, J.J. (1953) *The Management of Pain*, Lea & Febiger, Philadelphia.

The Book of Common Prayer of the Church of England (1662) The Catechism, W.M. Collins, Glasgow, (1964 edn.).

Church Information Office (1983) Our Ministry and Other Faiths, CIO Publishing, London.

Fish, S. and Shelley, J.A. (1978) *Spiritual Care*, Inter Varsity Press, London.

Gunstone, J. (1987) *Prayers of Healing*, Highland Books, New York.

Highfield, M.F. and Carson, C. (1983) Spiritual needs of patients: are they recognised? *Cancer Nursing*, Vol. 6, p. 3.

The Holy Bible, Revised Standard Version (1952a) The Letter of James, chap. 5, verses 13–16, Thomas Nelson, London.

The Holy Bible, Revised Standard Version (1952b) The Gospel of Luke, chap. 15, verses 11–32, Thomas Nelson, London.

The Holy Bible, Revised Standard Version (1952c) The First Letter of Paul to the Corinthians, chap. 13, verse 12, Thomas Nelson, London.

Kubler-Ross, E. (1969) *On Death and Dying*, Tavistock, London.

Lewis, C.S. (1961) *A Grief Observed*, Faber, London

Maddox, M. (1981) *The Christian Healing Ministry*, Society for the Propagation of Christian Knowledge (SPCK), London.

Meier, L. (1981) Chronic pain, suffering and spirituality: the relationship between chronic pain, suffering and different religious approaches. Unpublished Ph.D. thesis, University of South Carolina.

Neuberger, J. (1987) *Caring for People of Different Faiths*, The Lisa Sainsbury Foundation, UK.

Wald, F.S. (1968) In quest of the spiritual component of care for the teminally ill, Proceedings of a colloquium, Yale University.

Chapter 8

Sexuality and Cancer

CHRISTINE WEBB BA, MSc, PhD, RGN, RSCN,
RNT
Principal Lecturer in Nursing
Bristol Polytechnic
and
JOANNE O'NEILL Msc, BNurs, RGN, HVCert, DNCert
Part-time Clinical Lecturer, Department of Nursing
University of Manchester

Defining Sexuality

What is sexuality? Most of us may think we know the answer to this question, but would find it difficult to give an exact definition of the multiplicity of ideas which the concept of sexuality brings into our minds. Specialist writers seem to share this difficulty, for they often avoid saying precisely what is sexuality. Instead they talk of what is involved in sexuality and what factors influence its expression. Those who do venture a definition may do so in a way that is vague and general, leaving their readers still asking 'Yes, but what *is* sexuality?' Hogan (1980) for example, writes that

> Sexuality is intrinsic to our being – a basic need and an aspect of humanness that cannot be divorced from life events. It influences our thoughts, action, and interaction and is involved in aspects of physical and mental health. As a basic need, it is one of the essential focuses of health care.

A more precise attempt at definition is that of Woods (1984) who states:

> Human sexuality is a highly complex phenomenon. Sexuality pervades human beings, influencing their self-images, and feelings. It influences

their relationships with others. In addition, sexuality involves the biologic basis for experiencing sexual pleasure, giving and receiving sensual pleasure, and is a powerful force in a person's ability to bond to another person.

Woods' definition clearly has affinities with conceptual frameworks of nursing, which view humans as biopsychosocial beings. Some of these frameworks explicitly incorporate sexuality in their assessment schemes, and Roper's 'Activities of Living' framework is one of these (Roper *et al.*, 1980). It sees the expression of sexuality as an activity of living. Others do not have specific categories referring to sexuality but their assessment schemes offer the possibility of incorporating sexuality under one or more headings. For example, in the approach of Roy (1980), a nurse assessing a client using the physiological, self-concept, interdependence and role function modes could include information about sexuality under all four headings. With Orem's (1980) framework, information related to sexuality could be placed under various headings but perhaps her unfortunately named category of 'being normal' is particularly relevant.

If there is little consensus on a precise definition of sexuality, there is at least agreement that it is part of a person's total personality and has biological, psychological and social aspects. Although a holistic perspective is recommended, it may be helpful to look separately at these different aspects in order to be a little clearer about what is involved in sexuality.

The biological aspects of sexuality are its foundations in the anatomy and physiology of the reproductive systems of women and men, and include physical appearance, physical aspects of sexual activity, menstruation and contraception. There is little agreement about how influential these biological aspects are in forming a person (Webb, 1985). A biological determinist view, which sees biology as playing the major role in influencing human behaviour, is contradicted by evidence from psychological and sociological research. It seems more likely that biology is a base on which personality is built but that other foundations are equally – if not more – influential. The fact that children whose sex is misdetermined at birth have great difficulty in changing once their true sex is discovered, is evidence that cultural influences can override biology (Archer and Lloyd, 1982).

Psychological aspects of sexuality include body image or the mental photograph of themselves that people carry around in their heads. Self-concept is another aspect of one's self-picture, representing a definition of the self as a person – personality rather than physical self.

Self-esteem emerges from the kind of body image and self-concept a person has. People who feel good about their bodies and are happy with the kind of person they are have positive self-esteem. However, those who are unhappy with their bodies or their personalities have negative self-esteem. These self-definitions do not simply grow out of people's own views of themselves. Rather, they are strongly influenced by social factors, including how people in their culture generally define good or healthy individuals. Closer to home, self-definition depends greatly on how family, friends and associates react to a person – both with overt and covert messages about whether they like and approve of a person or not. The views and judgements of these other people are based on the norms and values of the culture and they are likely to incorporate stereotypes of appropriate behaviour for men and women. These stereotypes, known as sex-role stereotypes, are based on ideas about the kinds of clothes, hairstyles, jobs and other roles to which men and women are best suited. These socially prescribed roles are called 'gender roles'. Other aspects of sexuality which are socially influenced include 'gender identity' – whether people see themselves as women or men – and 'gender preferences' – whether people are attracted to and prefer to have sexual relationships with people of the same sex, of different sex, or both.

Sexuality, then, is a complex concept and it is perhaps not surprising that writers on the subject have found difficulty in producing a precise definition. Breaking down sexuality into its component parts means sacrificing a holistic approach but does allow us to be clearer about exactly what is involved. Before going on to see how sexuality may be affected by ill-health in general and by cancer in particular, it may be of interest to return to a holistic view and let Stuart and Sundeen (1979) have the last word on definition: 'Sexuality is an integral part of the whole person. Human beings are sexual in every way, all the time. To a large extent human sexuality determines who we are. It is a factor in the uniqueness of every person.'

Sexuality and Ill-health

Ill-health affects sexuality in many ways, even when the illness concerned is a relatively trivial and transitory nuisance, such as a common cold. If the condition is a serious, life-threatening or chronic one then the effects will be all the greater.

Any illness saps a person's physical and mental energy, and

tiredness and lack of interest in activities of all kinds are likely to ensue. Moods can rapidly be affected, with anxiety about health leading to depression and introspection about physical and psychological health. A person who feels physically and/or mentally ill is obliged or feels able to take less interest in his or her appearance and to withdraw from activities of all kinds, ranging from work, home and leisure to sexual activities. A downward spiral can easily be set in motion whereby lassitude and disinterest feed on themselves and the person becomes even more withdrawn and socially isolated. This results in a poor body image, damaged self-concept and a fall in self-esteem.

Linking this with the earlier discussion of sexuality, it is possible to see how the various aspects of sexuality may be affected by illness. A person who is ill is likely to be less able to participate in sexual activity. Pain, breathlessness, nausea or other symptoms may inhibit activity and a woman's menstrual cycle may be disrupted. Men may lose the ability to have or sustain an erection. Treatment for the illness may, in either the short or long term, add to these difficulties. A surgical operation causes pain, weakness and decreased activity levels for varying lengths of time. Drug treatments may cause debilitating side-effects.

Psychologically, altered mood states may affect desire and ability to participate in sexual activity. Sick people may feel that they are unattractive as sexual partners or social companions and may decide that it is better to isolate themselves from the possibility of rejection by avoiding company. Part of their feelings may be due to an alteration in body image, whether as the result of a visible change, such as a scar or removal of a body part, or as a more hidden and less obvious change which makes them feel less whole and complete in their body integrity. These feelings and their accompanying fall in self-esteem can add to depression, loss of libido and all the other physical accompaniments of depression such as altered sleep, reduced activity and changes in bowel functions. Thus the vicious spiral takes another downward turn.

Socially, the person may fall short of his or her own or other people's expectations of appropriate and healthy ways of behaving. If a women is unable to care for her family or a man is unable to support his family financially, other people may intentionally or inadvertently convey judgements of inadequacy towards that person. Giving social support is an important means of conveying to people that they are cared for, respected and loved (Cobb, 1976). When someone is ill, family and friends may not feel able to give the support they know is needed because they are over-committed, do not know how best to help or even because they are repelled by some aspect of the illness and cannot cope with being near the patient. Social isolation increases, offers of support are not taken up, and self-esteem falls further.

Sexuality in all its facets, then, can be seriously affected by ill-health and people with, or being treated for, cancer are particularly vulnerable.

Sexuality and Cancer

These general repercussions of illness on sexuality are likely to be all the greater when the disease concerned is a life-threatening condition such as cancer, and receiving such a diagnosis may lead people to reassess their priorities in life (Anderson, 1985). For some this may mean that questions of sexuality assume less importance in favour of coping with the cancer itself and its implications for the patient, family and friends. This does not mean that desire for physical closeness and capacity for sexual response disappear but simply that other concerns take precedence. Derogatis and Kourlesis (1981) consider that, despite the fact that a person is ill, sexuality remains of major importance for many patients and may even assume greater importance than previously. They consider that cancer patients are the victims of myths and negative attitudes about illness precluding sexuality and elderly people losing interest in sex. Because many cancer patients are in the older age-groups they will be subject to both myths. Definitions of quality of life for cancer patients should incorporate the realization that 'Sexual intimacy is one of the most rewarding and sought after experiences life has to offer: its importance is not diminished by the unfortunate experience of developing cancer' (Derogatis and Kourlesis, 1981).

Physical effects of cancer can interfere with sexual activity if a patient is suffering from pain, nausea or excessive fatigue and treatments can have a similar result. Radical surgery may involve loss of essential autonomic innervation or functional organs, as in the cases of abdomino-perineal resection of the rectum, total pelvic exenteration and radical vulvectomy. Radiotherapy can result in temporary or permanent sexual dysfunction due to premature menopause, scarring, drying of vaginal secretions and dyspareunia in the case of carcinoma of the cervix, and erectile failure for men with prostatic cancer. Hormone treatments can also interfere with physical acts of sex, causing lowered libido and erectile and ejaculatory difficulties for men and premature menopause for women (Shipes and Lehr, 1982; Anderson, 1985; Walbroehl, 1985). However, Goldberg and Cullen (1985) report that sexual problems are not necessarily associated with the site of the cancer and can arise when the site is not gynaecological or genito-urinary.

Psychological effects may follow from disruption or loss of phyiscal capacity for sexual activity or may arise from knowledge of the diagnosis and its implications. They may also occur as a result of treatment. A person who is unable to have sexual relations may become depressed and suffer from feelings of inadequacy as a sexual partner. Relationships with intimate contacts may thereby be prejudiced at a time when social support is so vital (Goldberg and Cullen, 1985).

Resumption of sexual activity has been found to be related to the kind of treatment carried out, with less sexual dysfunction occurring after lumpectomy for breast disease than after more radical surgery (Beckman *et al.*, 1983). Lumpectomy survivors report less alteration in body image and sexual desire, greater comfort with nudity and less change in frequency of sexual intercourse. Ovarian preservation in the surgical treatment of cervical carcinoma in premenopausal women may have advantages but vaginal shortening can contribute to coital discomfort. Radiotherapy, however, can both destroy ovarian function and cause vaginal atrophy and stenosis. Ellis and Grayhack (1963) compared patients with cancer of the colon and rectum treated with and without stoma formation, with patients treated similarly for inflammatory bowel disease. No significant differences were found according to whether or not the patient had a stoma but the wider excision needed by cancer patients led to greater nerve damage and more sexual dysfunction. De Haes and van Knippenberg (1985) also report better sexual function after sphincter-saving resection rather than abdomino-perineal resection and after limb-sparing surgery and radiotherapy rather than amputation.

Anderson (1985) concludes that different sites and different treatments lead to different effects on patients' sexuality and, therefore, the implications for care and treatment must be carefully considered.

Body image disturbances related to cancer may be linked with the mutilating effects of surgery or with side-effects of other treatments (Derogatis and Kourlesis, 1981). Breast cancer is perhaps most widely acknowledged to provoke threats of this kind and has been the subject of research involving follow-up by nurses who were able to detect psychological complications and refer patients for help by experts

(Maguire *et al.*, 1983). Ganz (1985) reports that, in a study of 84 patients being treated for cancer in a variety of sites including the lung, prostate, oesophagus and colon, only 6 per cent reported no problem with body image. Psychological problems of this type were also found to lower tolerance to the side-effects of treatments. Patients report feelings of self-disgust, guilt, shame, loss of autonomy, anger, resentment and feelings of being crippled by a damaged body image (Lamont *et al.*, 1978). Alopecia can have a profound effect on body image and self-esteem, and Baxley *et al.* (1984) report that alopecia is more damaging to men than women. Loss of body hair from any site can have this effect, making people feel like babies. Men who had undergone amputation were reported by Reinstein *et al.* (cited in Walbroehl, 1985), to experience greater decreases in sexual activity than women; this may be due to associations of manliness with being physically strong and active. Younger people may be more severely disturbed by altered body image according to Walbroehl (1985), because they have not had as much time as older people to become sure of their self-image. They are also less likely to have a permanent partner to offer support.

Social support is a vital factor in mediating the effect of illness (Cobb, 1976) but not all relatives and friends of cancer patients are able to be supportive (Anderson, 1985). Myths and attitudes exist in society about cancer being transmissible, particularly by sexual activity when a genital site is involved (Lamont *et al.*, 1978), and these may lead associates to withdraw from the patient. It is widely agreed, however, that the quality of sexual relationships after a diagnosis of cancer has been made, is more strongly related to the previous quality of the relationship than to any other factors (Lamont *et al.*, 1978; Wabrek and Gunn, 1984). Partners may not want to have sex with cancer patients for fear of hurting them physically, but this can give patients feelings of self-disgust, undesirability or 'emasculation' (Derogatis and Kourlesis, 1981).

Ganz (1985) reports severe disruptions in interpersonal interactions in the patients studied, with 70 per cent saying they had difficulty communicating with their spouse, 85 per cent having problems interacting with family and friends, and 80 per cent having difficulties in the area of sexuality with their spouse. For single people the latter figure was 91 per cent. Ganz concludes:

> This is of critical importance because spouses, family and friends provide the major source of support for patients in reducing the negative impact of the illness. These findings highlight the need to develop programmes that

include family members and that teach strategies to reduce stress and communicate effectively in dealing with illness-related issues.

Lamont *et al.* (1978) agree that the most important factor in total sexual rehabilitation for cancer patients is an educated and informed partner.

Information is also a form of social support and cancer patients, like many others, report great inadequacies in the quantity and quality of information they receive from health care staff. Baxley *et al.* (1984) report that many of their patients had not been warned to expect alopecia and thus had not had an opportunity to prepare themselves either psychologically or by obtaining a wig or other form of head covering. A poor correlation between patient's and physician's assessment of overall quality of life was reported by Presant (1984) in a review of a number of studies using a quality of life questionnaire. This provides further evidence of lack of communication between doctors and patients. Williams *et al.* (1986) report that nurses, too, did not seem aware of the sexual needs of cancer patients and 67 per cent of those studied were uncomfortable discussing sexual issues with patients. The majority of nurse respondents also did not feel that sexual counselling was part of their role. It appears that information-giving by health professionals is not likely to meet patients' expectations in a specialty where social support is particularly needed.

Sexuality, Cancer and Nursing Care

The potential role of nurses in relation to sexuality and cancer is clearly enormous and offers great rewards in terms of quality of life for patients. As with any nursing care, the first stage of the process is to carry out a baseline assessment and several writers offer suggestions of the form this might take.

McPhetridge (1968) proposes a concise format consisting of four questions:

1. Has having cancer (or its treatment) interfered with your being a mother (wife, husband, father)?
2. Has your cancer (or its treatment) changed the way you see yourself as a man (woman)?
3. Has your cancer (or its treatment) caused any change in your sexual functioning (sex life)?

4. Do you expect your sexual functioning (sex life) to be changed in any way after you leave the hospital?

This format has the advantages of conciseness and the fact that it includes biological, psychological and social components of sexuality. However, it omits the areas of friendships, social life and work and would need to be supplemented in these areas. Additionally, MacElveen-Hoehn and McCorkle (1985) suggest probing further when any problem is identified, by asking:

1. For a description of the problem by the person:
   Tell me about what is happening.
2. For a history of the problem:
   When did this begin?
   What else was happening to you around that time?
   How often does it occur?
   Does it seem to be changing in any way?
3. The cause of the problem:
   Why do you think this is happening?
   What do you think is causing this?
4. About previous treatment attempts:
   What have you tried to do about this so far?
   How much has it helped?

Additional assessment questions suggested by Webb (1985) include:

Most of us have some religious or other beliefs about relationships, marriage, families, and so on. What beliefs like this are important to you?

People often hear stories or half-truths about sexual matters. Have you heard anything like this?

Do you have any worries about your health/illness/treatment and its effects on your personal life or your sex life?

People often have questions they would like to ask about the sexual side of life. Is there anything you would like to ask?

These latter questions fit the thinking of Hogan (1980) who writes both of the importance of taking into account patients' cultural and religious beliefs in relation to sexuality and of using a form of questioning which is non-threatening and does not imply value judgements on the part of the nurse about approved or disapproved beliefs and practices.

PLANNING CARE FOR PATIENTS WITH PROBLEMS LINKED
WITH SEXUALITY

In order to show how knowledge of sexuality can be combined with
other areas of nursing theory in planning care for cancer patients, it is
useful to look at some of the examples of patient problems. Because of
the very individual nature of sexuality it is unrealistic to talk in terms
of standard care plans, but an attempt has been made to consider some
of the factors most commonly associated with disturbances in
sexuality. Because of the complex biopsychosocial nature of sexuality,
patient problems in this area are rarely simple and it is understandable
that many nurses have difficulty with this aspect of care. Unfortunately, this is not the only reason why sexuality is a neglected area.
Assessment of sexuality requires getting to know the patient as a
person and many nurses hesitate to take on this commitment. All skills
improve with practice and the handling of problems related to
sexuality is no exception. If sexuality were to become as much a
regular aspect of nursing as wound care or nutrition, nurses'
confidence and skill in handling problems would improve.

The personal nature of sexuality makes some people argue that
inquiry into this area is an invasion of privacy. But it is precisely
because patients may find this a difficult topic to speak about, that the
nurses should indicate that sexuality is a legitimate subject for
discussion. Patients are not expected to work out for themselves how
to care for the obvious physical concomitants of cancer treatment such
as a surgical wound or an intravenous infusion. It is unfair,
therefore, to deny them help and information in adjusting and
responding to changes in sexuality.

To illustrate how sexuality may be affected when people have
cancer, and how care planning can attempt to respond to their needs,
three patient studies are discussed. The studies have been chosen to
show how different types of malignant disease may affect people in
varying age-groups and how body image changes and doubts about
self-worth, as well as biological and social sex-related roles, may be
involved.

Rose – an Adolescent with Body Image Disturbance

The period of adolescence is a difficult time even in the best
circumstances. It is a time of physical and emotional growth towards
maturity and independence, and the biological and psychosocial
development which takes place helps to shape the young person's

sexual identity. An adolescent with cancer must achieve the developmental tasks of this period while facing a potentially life-threatening illness and unpleasant treatment. Despite the difficulties of coping with long-term cancer treatment at this crucial period of life, it is encouraging to note that chronic disease does not inevitably lead to pyschological disturbances. Usual patterns of development most often prevail in spite of the stress imposed by the disease (Kellerman *et al.*, 1980).

Adolescent's images of their own body change rapidly as their bodies mature physiologically (Schonfeld, 1963). Cancer therapy results in undesirable changes that cause further stress and a poor body image. In particular, amputation of all or part of a limb is devastating and may result in withdrawal from peers, cessation of education and general isolation (Klopovich and Clancy, 1985).

Rose was a 17-year-old schoolgirl who had osteosarcoma of the knee for which she had had an amputation at mid-thigh. Surgery had been performed at her local hospital and she had been referred to an oncology unit for chemotherapy. Although she was only a couple of years younger than many of the student nurses on the ward, they reported that they found her difficult to talk to or to get to know. She appeared withdrawn, spending most of her time reading and did not communicate with other patients. It seemed that she had a very fatalistic attitude to her illness and was lying there waiting for the next piece of bad news; she showed no anger or denial, simply a resigned acceptance. It was thought at first that this behaviour was a reaction to her diagnosis but discussion revealed a further complicating aspect.

Rose had a photograph on her locker of a recent fancy dress ball at her school where she had dressed as a bride. She referred to this photograph, saying that marriage would never happen for her now in real life as nobody would want a disfigured girl with only one leg. Rose did not appear to view her cancer as a threat to survival but she felt condemned to a future without sexual love. She felt that her family would still care for her but she had never had a regular boyfriend and, because of her amputation, she was sure that no boy could find her attractive. These feelings led her to avoid any acknowledgement of her change in appearance and she was unable to touch or look at the affected limb. Rose's care plan is shown in Table 8.1.

Joe – a Young Adult with Disturbance in Reproductive Function

While most aspects of sexuality are of concern to people of all age-groups, fertility is likely to be of particular importance to young adults of parenting age. The ability to produce children is an integral part of

Table 8.1   *Care plan for Rose – an adolescent with body image disturbance*

Problem	Goal	Nursing Intervention
Difficulty in adjusting body image to accommodate to loss of leg	*Long term* Body image changes to accept loss of original limb and addition of artificial limb *Short term* Rose is able to look at and touch the limb stump	Refer to artificial limb centre for appointment at six weeks post-op., for fitting of temporary prosthesis. Give information about stages involved in fitting the artificial limb. Explain how appearance and function of final prosthesis will differ from the temporary one. Support Rose in her preferred method of familiarization with the amputated limb, e.g. viewing stump and touching it when bandages are changed or when getting dressed either alone or with a nurse or relative Refer to physiotherapist for teaching of exercises to strengthen remaining muscle and prepare stump for fitting of prosthesis Using Rose's own magazines, discuss how current fashions can be worn to disguise the artificial limb and make the most of her other attractive physical features

| Loss of self-esteem, and feeling unattractive and unlovable | Is able to voice positive attitudes towards herself, indicating that she feels attractive.
Is able to identify the positive characteristics she could contribute to a relationship. | Prepare Rose for other physical changes associated with treatment, e.g. hair loss. Demonstrate how hats, scarves and wigs can be used to minimize changes. Help her to express her feelings about these side-effects. Emphasize that they are temporary and that she will return to normal when treatment ends

Ask Rose to identify the characteristics in others that she finds attractive. Focus on intellectual and psychological aspects. Discuss the factors needed for the maintenance of long-term relationships Encourage her to realize that physical attributes are only one aspect among many. |

sexuality, but the psychological effect of the loss of this ability has not been well studied in cancer patients. It is only because of recent advances in treatment and improved survival rates that cancer patients are now seen to have a choice regarding parenthood. Ironically, it is the intensive nature of these life-saving treatments which causes problems with fertility. In cancers such as Hodgkin's disease, where prognosis has been good for some years, effects of treatments on fertility have been relatively well studied (Chapman *et al.*, 1979; Horning *et al.*, 1981). In other cancers, where long-term survival is a recent phenomenon, much less is known about the effect of the cancer and its treatment on gonadal function or its genetic implications. Until more is known about the effects on fertility of cancer therapy for various tumour types and involving treatment combinations, definitive patient guidelines cannot be provided.

Surgery, radiotherapy and chemotherapy have all demonstrated the ability to produce temporary or permanent sterility in humans. In radiotherapy and chemotherapy this occurs either through gonadal toxicity or by damage to the hypothalamic-pituitary region, which then disrupts gonadotrophic regulation of ovarian and testicular function.

Preliminary studies suggest that sterility induced by chemotherapy may be affected by age, total drug dose, duration of treatment, amount of time since cessation of treatment and single-agent versus combination drug regimens (Waxman, 1983).

Radiation therapy which includes the ovaries in the treatment field produces temporary sterility above a dosage of around 4 Gy. Radiation therapy in the region of the testes may produce temporary sterility below a dosage threshold in the vicinity of 5 Gy and permanent sterility above that dosage.

Surgical removal of both gonads or the organs of reproduction because of tumour involvement or the removal of both gonads in hormone-dependent cancers obviously precludes subsequent reproduction. Removal of a single gonad in the presence of a normal contralateral ovary or testis should, however, leave fertility intact.

Joe was a 28-year-old solicitor in remission from acute myeloid leukaemia and was being prepared for a bone marrow transplant. He was not married but had lived with his girlfriend, an accountant, for three years. One morning he came up to the ward after visiting the outpatients clinic. Although he was normally cheerful and outgoing, on this occasion he appeared anxious and upset and asked to speak to the ward sister.

Joe had discussed the possibility of bone marrow transplant with the consultant at two previous appointments and the consultant had tried to explain what the procedure involved. Joe said that he realized it was 'kill or cure' but he saw it as his only chance of long-term survival and was willing to take the risk. That day for the first time as far as Joe could remember, the consultant had mentioned that one side-effect of total body irradiation was infertility. Joe was horrified. During treatment he had had to cope with many assaults on his self-image. Normally a very fit, athletic young man, he had found the muscle wasting and hair loss particularly distressing but during remission he had worked hard to get himself fit again. Joe had always wanted children and this desire had become stronger when he was faced with his own mortality. Now to lose irreversibly his fertility seemed a high price to pay for survival. From Joe's account it seemed that the consultant had discussed the possibility of banking sperm but Joe had been too upset and confused to understand what he was saying. He had come to the ward to speak to the sister, hoping that she would be able to explain more to him. The care plan she negotiated with him is shown in Table 8.2.

Mrs. Short – an Older Adult with Progressive Disease and Inability to Fulfil Expected Roles

Denial, fear, anxiety, hopelessness, anger, hostility, resentment, guilt, shame, loneliness, sadness, depression and despair are all common psychological responses to advanced cancer (McCorkle and Benoliel, 1983). In addition to the early grief response following diagnosis and initial treatment, a patient with progressive disease has to cope with the repeated losses associated with metastases and the unyielding deterioration of the body. Symptoms associated with advanced disease include pain, nausea and vomiting, anorexia, diarrhoea, weakness, fatigue, debilitation, muscle atrophy, neurological impairment and alopecia. All of these threaten the person's self-concept and can lead to fears of rejection and abandonment by others. These fears are often reinforced by avoidance and withdrawal demonstrated by family, friends and carers who are unable to cope with the patient's deteriorating condition. People with cancer may be concerned not only about their own ability to cope but also about how well those close to them will adjust to the changes.

Mrs Short was a 60-year-old woman with advanced metastatic malignant melanoma. She was being cared for at home by her 63-year-old husband with help from their three daughters. The daughters were

Table 8.2   *Care plan for Joe – a young adult with disturbance in reproductive function*

Problem	Goal	Nursing Intervention
Shock and distress at prospect of loss of fertility after bone marrow transplant	If he decides to go ahead with transplant, will indicate that he is prepared to accept its implications for fertility	Make it clear that all areas discussed can be covered again in a later interview either with Joe alone or with his girlfriend also. Let him know that he does not have to remember everything at once
Unaware of methods of preserving possible fertility	Understands the possibilities and limitations of sperm banking	Explain how sperm bank works and sperm is collected. Stress that pregnancy cannot be guaranteed as it depends on: present sperm count, which may be depressed following recent chemotherapy, fertility status of his partner, and success of artifical insemination procedure Explain difference between fertility and sexual function. Ability to have an erection, ejaculate and have orgasm should not be changed by total body irradiation, although worry about loss of fertility may affect performance

all married and the youngest had very recently had a baby girl. This baby was Mrs Short's first grandchild and her birth seemed to precipitate very conflicting emotions in her. She expressed great joy at the new life and continuation of the family, but she was also deeply saddened because she would not see her grand-daughter grow up. For some time Mrs Short had been dependent on her husband to help her with hygiene and dressing. He also did the housework and one of her daughters provided the meals.

Five days after the birth of her grandchild, Mrs Short became very tearful, lost all interest in her appearance and made no effort at all to care for herself. She said that she felt useless as a wife because she was unable to look after her husband and, in addition, she was a failure as a mother and grandmother because she was unable to support her daughter in the difficult period of adjustment to motherhood. Her care plan is shown in Table 8.3.

Table 8.3 *Care plan for Mrs Short – an older patient with progressive disease and inability to fulfil expected roles*

Problem	Goal	Nursing Intervention
Depression because of inability to fulfil expected roles of wife, mother and grandparent	Is able to accept modified roles based on emotional and psychological support rather than physical contributions	Ask Mrs Short to identify ways her family have helped support her during her illness. Focus on any psychological or emotional support she mentions. By demonstrating how important these factors are to her, help her to see that others may find such support valuable too Ask Mrs Short to list the characteristics of the wife and mother roles other than physical carer. Discuss ways she can carry out these aspects of the roles

Conclusion

In choosing examples of patients for this chapter, a decision was made to avoid malignancies and treatments most obviously associated with disturbances in sexuality. It was felt that problems associated with tumours of the reproductive organs or secondary sexual organs would be covered in the relevant chapters. It is hoped that the patient studies and accompanying discussion demonstrate that aspects of sexuality such as body image, reproductive function and role function are important issues for many patients and not just for those with gynaecological or genito-urinary malignancies.

In conclusion, it is hoped that this chapter will serve as a reminder that we are all sexual beings at every age, in all states of health and illness and in every aspect of our lives. Facilitating the expression of sexuality in all its facets can add to the quality of life for cancer patients and therefore this should be a fundamental part of nursing care. For, as Shipes and Lehr (1982) remind us, those we care for are 'not cancer patients, but people who happen to have cancer'.

References

Anderson, B.L. (1985) Sexual functioning morbidity among cancer survivors, *Cancer*, Vol. 55, no. 8, pp. 1835–42.

Archer, J. and Lloyd, B. (1982) *Sex and Gender*, Penguin, Harmondsworth.

Baxley, K.O., Erdman L.K. and Henry. E.B. (1984) Alopecia and body image, *Cancer Nursing*, Vol. 7, no. 6, pp. 499–504.

Beckman, J., Johansen, L., Richardt, C. and Blickert-Toft, M. (1983) Psychological reactions in younger women operated on for breast cancer, *Danish Medical Bulletin*, Vol. 30, pp. 10–13.

Chapman, R., Sutcliffe, S. and Malpas, J. (1979) Cytotoxic induced ovarian failure in women with Hodgkin's disease. I. Hormone failure, *Journal of the American Medical Association*, Vol. 242, pp. 1877–81.

Cobb, S. (1976) Social support as a moderator of life stress, *Psychosomatic Medicine*, Vol. 38, pp. 300–14.

Derogatis, L.R. and Kourlesis, S.M. (1981) An approach to evaluation of sexual problems in the cancer patient, *Cancer Journal for Physicians*, Vol. 31, no. 1, pp. 46–50.

Ellis, W.J. and Grayhack, J.T. (1963) Sexual function in ageing males after orchiectomy and oestrogen therapy, *Journal of Urology*, Vol. 98, pp. 895–9.

Ganz, P.A. (1985) Psychosexual impact of cancer on the elderly, *Journal of the American Geriatric Society*, Vol. 33, no. 6, pp. 429–35.

Goldberg, R.J. and Cullen, L.E. (1985) Factors in the psychosocial adjustment to cancer. A review of the evidence, *Social Science and Medicine*, Vol. 20, no. 8, pp. 803–7.

Haes, J.C. de and Knippenberg, F. van (1985) Quality of life and cancer patients. A review of the literature, *Social Science and Medicine*, Vol. 20, no. 8, pp. 809–17.

Hogan, R.M. (1980) *Human Sexuality. A Nursing Perspective*, Appleton-Century-Crofts, New York, p. 20.

Horning, S., Hoppe, R., Kaplan, H. and Rosenbert, S. (1981) Female reproductive potential after treatment for Hodgkin's disease, *New England Journal of Medicine*, Vol. 304, pp. 1377–88.

Kellerman, J., Zeller, L. and Ellenberg, L. (1980) Psychological effects of illness in adolescence: anxiety, self-esteem and perception of control, *Journal of Paediatrics*, Vol. 97, pp. 126–31.

Klopovich, P. and Clancy, B. (1985) Sexuality and the adolescent with cancer, *Seminars in Oncology Nursing*, Vol. 1, pp. 42–8.

Lamont, J.A., Petrillo, A.D. and Sargeant, E.J. (1978) Psychosexual rehabilitation and exenterative surgery, *Gynaecological Oncology*, Vol. 6, pp. 236–42.

MacElveen-Hoehn, P. and McCorkle, R. (1985) Understanding sexuality in progressive cancer, *Seminars in Oncology Nursing*, Vol. 1, no. 1, pp. 56–62.

McCorkle, R. and Benoliel, J. (1983) Symptom distress, current concerns and mood disturbances after diagnosis of life-threatening disease, *Social Science and Medicine*, Vol. 17, pp. 431–38.

McPhetridge, L.M. (1968) Nursing history: one means to personalised care, *American Journal of Nursing*, Vol. 68, no. 1, pp. 68–75.

Maguire, P., Brooke, M., Tait, A., Thomas, C. and Sellwood, R. (1983) The effect of counselling on physical disability and social recovery after mastectomy, *Clinical Oncology*, Vol. 9, pp. 319–24.

Orem, D.E. (1980) *Nursing: concepts of practice* (2nd edn), McGraw-Hill, New York.

Presant, C.A. (1984) Quality of life in cancer patients, *American Journal of Clinical Oncology*, Vol. 7, no. 5, pp. 571–3.

Roper, N., Logan, W. and Tierney, A. (1980) *Elements of Nursing*, Churchill Livingstone, Edinburgh.

Roy, C. (1980) The Roy adaptation model. In J. Riehl and C. Roy (eds.) *Conceptual Models for Nursing Practice*, Appleton-Century-Crofts, New York.

Schonfeld, W. (1963) Body image in adolescents: a psychiatric concept for the paediatrician, *Paediatrics*, Vol. 31, p. 845.

Shipes, E. and Lehr, S. (1982) Sexuality and the male cancer patient, *Cancer Nursing*, Vol. 5, no. 5, pp. 375–81.

Stuart, G.W. and Sundeen, S.J. (eds) (1979) *Principles and Practice of Psychiatric Nursing*, Mosby, St Louis, p. 405.

Wabrek, A.J. and Gunn, J.L. (1984) Sexual and psychological implications of gynaecologic malignancy, *JOGN Nursing*, Vol. 13, no. 6, pp. 371–5.

Walbroehl, G.S. (1985) Sexuality in cancer patients, *American Family Physician*, Vol. 1, pp. 153–8.

Waxman, J. (1983) Chemotherapy and the adult gonad: a review, *Journal of the Royal Society of Medicine*, Vol. 76, pp. 144–8.

Webb, C. (1985) *Sexuality, Nursing and Health,*, Wiley, Chichester.

Williams, H.A. *et al.* (1986) Nurses' attitudes towards sexuality in cancer patients, *Oncology Nursing Forum*, Vol. 13, no. 2, pp. 39–43.

Woods, N.F. (1984) *Human Sexuality in Health and Illness*, Mosby, St Louis, p. 8.

Chapter 9

Nutrition in Cancer Care

MAUREEN HUNTER BSc(Hons), SRD
Chief Dietician

and

ELIZABETH M. H. JANES BSc(Hons), RGN, SRD
Senior Dietician
The Royal Marsden Hospital, London and Surrey

Introduction

To many people the word 'cancer' is synonymous with malnutrition, but as Maurice Shils (1979) has pointed out, 'malnutrition is not an obligatory response of the host to cancer'. Although anorexia and weight loss are commonly presenting symptoms in patients with cancer there are now many ways of restoring nutritional status. Indeed this should be considered a major component of treatment in addition to antineoplastic therapy.

The consequences of progressive undernutrition are serious and may complicate or interrupt curative therapies. Nutritional problems caused by the disease are often exacerbated by cancer treatment and contribute to the familiar picture of cachexia. It is extremely likely that a proportion of patients treated for cancer die of the complications of malnutrition rather than of the disease itself.

In this chapter the nutritional requirements and problems of patients with cancer are discussed and ways in which nutritional support can be provided described. Particular attention is drawn to those suffering from tumours of the head and neck, children with cancer, those undergoing treatment for leukaemia and those with advanced disease receiving palliative care. Current ideas on alternative homeopathic diets are also considered.

Nutrient Requirements

The effects of cancer and its treatment often alter the nutrient requirements of the body. This alteration can be due to physiological changes in the gut or disturbances in metabolism.

PHYSIOLOGICAL CHANGES

Impaired Digestion

Impaired digestion of food can occur as a result of reduced enzyme secretion from the stomach, pancreas or small intestine or reduced bile flow into the duodenum. Consequently, valuable nutrients are lost to the body and the patient is likely to become malnourished.

Digestive enzyme secretion may be reduced because of cancer itself or because of the effects of treatment. Total gastrectomy results in a deficiency of intrinsic factor normally secreted by the parietal cells of the stomach. This is needed for absorption of vitamin B_{12} in the ileum. Parenteral replacement of this vitamin is, therefore, essential although body stores will last for several months.

Tumours involving the biliary system or pancreas may obstruct the flow of conjugated bile salts from the liver. Bile is essential for the emulsification of dietary fat and its absence produces steatorrhoea.

Drugs may also impair digestion. Asparaginase reduces pancreatic exocrine function thereby impairing the digestion of protein, and fat. Streptozocin can induce hypoglycaemia and abnormal glucose tolerance by its effect on the pancreatic islet cells.

A depletion in intestinal enzymes can occur as a result of reduced food intake. This is caused by atrophy of the intestinal mucosa. Such an effect will reduce the body's ability to digest protein, fat and carbohydrate.

Impaired Absorption

Reduced absorption of nutrients can result from the effects of surgery, radiotherapy and chemotherapy.

Surgery to the oesophagus can lead to fat malabsorption if the vagus nerve is damaged, and gastrectomy may impair the absorption of fat, iron and vitamins (especially vitamin B_{12}) and calcium. The degree of malabsorption varies and is mild compared with that caused by gut resection, but it can be a contributory factor to weight loss.

'Coeliac syndrome' may be seen in patients with lymphomatous involvement of the small intestine or its mesenteric lymphatics. It has been suggested that this is due to generalized villous atrophy and obstruction of lymph channels. The clinical symptoms include steatorrhoea with enteropathy. There may also be impaired absorption of fat-soluble vitamins and folic acid.

Mucosal atrophy giving rise to malabsorption may be caused by poor food intake. It occurs because of decreased cell proliferation related to the comparative inactivity of the gut.

Changes in the intestinal mucosa also occur following treatment with certain cytotoxic agents, for example 5-fluorouracil, high-dose melphalan and methotrexate. Malabsorption may similarly result from treatment with these drugs.

Radiotherapy involving the gastrointestinal tract, particularly the small and large bowel, commonly causes enteritis and diarrhoea during the acute phase of treatment. In most cases this problem subsides but occasionally secondary radiation-induced enteritis arises due to the laying down of fibrous and scar tissue. This can be very severe and debilitating and without nutritional intervention leads to progressive malnutrition. Bowel resection may cause malabsorption but this will depend on the site and extent of the surgery. Removal of more than 60 cm of ileum and the ileocaecal valve results in increased levels of faecal fat and reduced absorption of vitamin B_{12}. Conversely, up to 2.4 m of jejunum can be removed with no effect on absorption. If, however, the jejunum and ileum are resected there will be malabsorption of all nutrients.

Patients who suffer from diarrhoea or steatorrhoea for any of the above reasons will require nutritional advice and support in order to achieve a satisfactory nutritional status. This may involve the use of high-energy supplements, extra protein, vitamins and minerals. For patients with severe fat intolerance medium chain triglycerides can be beneficial in increasing energy intake. These are fat molecules that can be absorbed directly into the lymphatic system without being digested. Suitable proprietary products containing these can be prescribed. They are best used under the direction of a dietitian.

If a modified normal diet proves to be unsatisfactory a variety of elemental products are available that require no further digestion and are easily absorbed. Parenteral nutrition (the infusion of nutrients into the body through a vein) may be required if it is impossible to maintain adequate nutritional support from the gut.

Metabolic Changes

Investigations into the energy metabolism of patients with cancer has revealed that the basal metabolic rate is frequently elevated despite a reduced food intake. In other words, there is a failure in the normal mechanism of adaptation to starvation. Theologides (1979) has suggested that this is due to lack of feedback regulation brought about by tumour by-products, which interfere with enzyme activity. The degree of metabolic chaos seems to be related to the type and size of the tumour. Some patients with cancer have a degree of glucose intolerance and a reduced sensitivity to insulin. Free fatty acids are mobilized from adipose stores to provide energy and intravenously infused lipids have been shown to be removed from the bloodstream more rapidly than usual. Anaerobic conversion of glucose to lactic acid by tumour cells provides energy for their growth but this is an inefficient use of glucose as it produces only two molecules of adenosine triphosphate (ATP) per molecule of glucose metabolized. (Aerobic metabolism yields thirty molecules of ATP per molecule of glucose.) Gluconeogenesis (synthesis of glucose) in the liver and renal cortex is increased, thereby producing glucose by conversion of amino acids and lactate in enzyme pathways known as the Cori cycle. In many cancer patients there is a reduction in skeletal muscle mass and hypo-albuminaemia is common but it is not known whether this is due to decreased protein synthesis or increased catabolism.

Biochemical studies have shown that patients with cancer in certain sites may have evidence of vitamin deficiency (Dickerson and Basu, 1977). Plasma levels of vitamin A have been found to be lowered in patients with oat and squamous cell carcinomas of the lung. The significance of these findings is not yet known. Ascorbic acid deficiency has been found in women with bony metastases from breast cancer but it is not known whether vitamin C replacement therapy is beneficial.

Although some homeopathic diets advocate the use of mega-doses of some vitamins there is no documentary evidence that this is of value.

It is likely that a proportion of patients with cancer may be deficient in some vitamins because of poor food intake. Vitamin replacement should be considered in these individuals but they should not be handed out like sweets as a general panacea of ills.

Calculation of Nutrient Requirements

Individual requirements for each nutrient vary enormously and are difficult to calculate accurately. Except for critically ill patients being nursed in an intensive care unit, an approximate estimation of requirements is adequate. Energy and protein needs can be assessed on the basis of actual body weight using the figures given in Table 9.1.

Table 9.1   *Energy and nitrogen requirements in different clinical conditions (modified from Elwyn, 1980)*

	Normal	*Intermediate*	*Severely hyper-metabolic*
Energy (per kg body weight)	30 kcal 125 kJ	35–40 kcal 150–170 kJ	40–60 kcal 179–250 kJ
Nitrogen (per kg body weight)	0.16 g	0.2–0.3 g	0.3–0.5 g
Protein (per kg body weight)*	1.0 g	1.3–1.9 g	1.0–3.1 g

* Calculated from nitrogen requirements using a factor of 6.25 and rounded to one decimal place.

Source: Kettlewell, M. (1982) in Andrew Grant and Elizabeth Todd (eds.) *Enteral and Parenteral Nutrition,* Blackwell Scientific, Oxford. With kind permission.

The majority of patients with cancer fall into the intermediate category but a proportion may be severely hypermetabolic, particularly if they are undergoing extensive surgery combined with radiotherapy and/or chemotherapy.

Regular assessment of nutritional status and dietary intake will indicate the effectiveness of these estimates. Modifications can then be made for individuals, as appropriate.

Vitamins, Electrolytes and Trace Elements

The requirement for these nutrients varies considerably depending on age and sex, illness and treatment. Tables 9.2 and 9.3 indicate the suggested range of daily requirements of electrolytes, trace elements

Table 9.2   *Suggested daily requirements for electrolytes and trace elements*

	Allowances/kg body weight in normal diet	Allowances/kg body weight in parenteral nutrition	Authors
Sodium	1.0–1.4 mmol/kg/day	2–3 mmol/kg/day with fat in diet (4.3 mmol/kg bw/day without fat) (1.0–1.4 mmol/kg bw/day with fat)	Dudrick *et al.*, 1969 (Wilmore *et al.*, 1969) (Grotte *et al.*, 1976)
Potassium	0.7–0.9 mmol/kg/day	7 mmol/g N (2 mmol/kg/day with fat) (3.9 mmol/kg/day without fat)	Lee, 1974 (Grotte, 1971) (Wilmore *et al.*, 1969)
Calcium		0.11 mmol/kg (0.5 mmol/kg)	(Grotte, 1971)
Magnesium	0.04 mmol/kg/24 h	0.04 mmol/kg (1 mmol/kg)	Wretlind, 1972 (Wilmore *et al.*, 1969)
Iron	0.25–1.0 mol/kg	1 mol/kg (2 mol/kg)	Shils, 1972 (Fomon, 1967)

(continued over.)

Table 9.2 *(continued.)*

	Allowances/kg body weight in normal diet	*Allowances/kg body weight in parenteral nutrition*	*Authors*
Manganese	0.1 mol/kg	0.6 mol/kg (0.7 mol/kg)	(Wilmore et al., 1969)
Zinc	0.7 mol/kg	0.7 mol/kg (0.6 mol/kg)	Jacobson and Wester, 1977 (Wilmore et al., 1969), RDA, 1968
Copper	0.07 mol/kg	0.07 mol/kg (0.34 mol/kg)	Shils, 1972 (Wilmore et al., 1969)
Iodine	0.015 mol/kg (0.04 mol/kg)	0.015 mol/kg (0.04 mol/kg)	
Phosphorus	0.15 mmol/kg	0.15 mmol/kg (1.5 mmol/kg) Should correspond to calcium intake	Recommended dietary allowance, 1968 (Ricour et al., 1975)

Allowances in parentheses are for neonates and infants

Source: Moghissi, K. and Boore, J. (1983) *Parenteral and Enteral Nutrition for Nurses*, Heinemann Medical, London. With kind permission.

Table 9.3   *Suggested allowances for vitamins in total parenteral nutrition*

Vitamins	Recommended daily allowance in adults	Allowance/kg body weight in complete intravenous nutrition
Thiamine	0.9–1.2 mg	0.02 mg
Riboflavin	1.3–1.7 mg	0.03 mg
Nicotinic acid	15–18 mg	0.2 mg
Folic acid	10–30 mg	3 μg
Vitamin B$_{12}$	about 3 mg	0.03 μg
Ascorbic acid	25–30 mg	0.5 mg
Vitamin A (retinol)	750 μg	10 μg
Vitamin D (cholecalciferol)	2.5 mg	0.04 mg
Vitamin K	about 2 mg	2 μg

Source: Moghissi, K. and Boore, J. (1983) *Parenteral and Enteral Nutrition for Nurses,* Heinemann Medical, London. With kind permission.

and vitamins. The changes in micronutrient metabolism that occur in patients with cancer have been reviewed extensively by Hoffman (1985) and readers are referred to this review for further information.

The Team Approach

Doctors, nurses and dietitians are continually confronted with the problem of the cancer patient who does not eat properly. It is the responsiblity of the whole health care team to provide the patient with adequate nutrition in an acceptable form, and to do everything possible to encourage the patient to eat. This can only be accomplished successfully if all members of the team understand the problems arising from not doing so. Figure 9.1 shows the members of the health care team involved in encouraging the nutritional support of the cancer patient.

No one discipline can be solely responsible for nutritional support of the cancer patient. The most important member of this team is, of course, the patient. The patient must be directly involved throughout and his or her individual nutritional needs and food preferences met at all times.

The nutritional problems most commonly associated with cancer patients are given in Table 9.4, together with some methods of

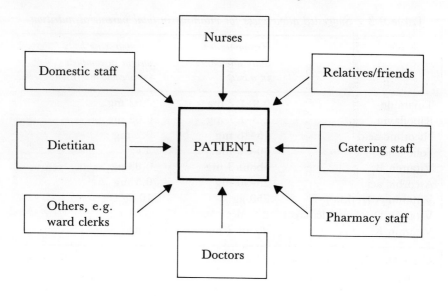

Figure 9.1   Members of the health care team involved in nutritional support of the cancer patient.

overcoming such problems. Some of the most useful methods are now discussed in more detail.

Methods of Overcoming Some Nutritional Problems Associated with Cancer

SMALL FREQUENT MEALS

This is the most useful way of overcoming eating difficulties experienced by cancer patients. Patients often find that taking small amounts of food regularly is an acceptable way of meeting their nutritional requirements. This method of feeding usually involves three small meals a day with light snacks or nourishing drinks in between meals. In order to encourage the patient to eat, a wide choice of food needs to be available to suit every taste. For patients in hospital, this requires close liaison between the nurse, dietitian and catering manager. Flexible menu planning is essential and the role of the catering manager in feeding cancer patients in hospital should not be underestimated. Relatives and friends should be encouraged to bring items of favourite food such as cakes, biscuits and fruit to tempt the patient to eat.

Table 9.4 *Summary of nutritional problems associated with cancer and its treatment*

Problem	Cause	Suggested Dietary Advice
Loss of appetite	Disease state Chemotherapy Radiotherapy	Small nourishing meals In-between meal snacks and/or nourishing drinks Energy/protein supplements, appetite stimulants, e.g. alcohol, steroids
Severe loss of appetite	As above	Supplementary nasogastric feeding may be necessary
Feeling of fullness	Disease state Radiotherapy to upper abdomen Prolonged poor food intake	Small, frequent meals Use nourishing drinks Give drinks separate from meals (half hour before or after)
Tiredness/Weakness	Disease state Treatment in general	Use of convenience foods Use of nourishing drinks Use of help services, e.g. 'Meals on Wheels'
Nausea	Disease state Chemotherapy Radiotherapy to upper GI tract	Small, frequent meals Avoidance of cooking smells Short walk before meals, if possible Dry meals Drinks separate from meals Plain biscuits, dry toast Cold foods Reduce very sweet or very fatty foods Fizzy drinks may help

(continued over leaf.)

Table 9.4   *(continued.)*

Problem	Cause	Suggested Dietary Advice
Severe vomiting	As above	Total parenteral nutrition may be necessary
Difficulties in chewing or swallowing	Carcinoma oesophagus Oral surgery Oesophageal tubes Radiotherapy to mouth/throat	Small, frequent meals of soft liquid diet Nourishing drinks Fizzy drinks may clear oesophageal tubes
Severe difficulties in chewing or swallowing	As above	Tube feeding
Sore mouth/throat	Radiotherapy to mouth/throat Some chemotherapy regimens	Small frequent meals of soft, moist foods Nourishing drinks No salty or spicy foods Cold food/drinks may be soothing No very hot foods No rough or very dry foods Use a drinking straw if necessary
Dry mouth	Radiotherapy to mouth/throat	Frequent drinks Ice cubes to suck Fruit drops, boiled sweets Good appropriate mouth care No dry foods Artificial saliva may be useful

Taste changes metallic taste	Some chemotherapy regimens	Avoidance of foods which accentuate unpleasant taste	
loss of taste	As above plus radiotherapy to mouth/throat	Emphasize the smell of food Strong flavours such as herbs, spices Concentrate on food familiar to and liked by the patient	
Abdominal pain or cramps	Radiotherapy to lower abdomen Subacute obstruction	Try low-fibre diet	
Diarrhoea	Radiotherapy to lower abdomen Some chemotherapy regimens	Low-fibre diet with high fluid intake Suggest use of antidiarrhoea agents	
Intermittent constipation	Some chemotherapy regimens	High-fibre diet Plenty of fluids	
Severe constipation	As above Use of narcotic drugs in pain relief	Suggest possible use of laxatives	
Malabsorption	Radiotherapy or surgery to lower GI tract Fistula	Low-fat diet Low-fibre diet Lactose-free diet Chemical defined fluid diet, e.g. Vivonex, Flexical, Nutranel, etc. Total parenteral nutrition	As appropriate for the type of malabsorption problem

NOURISHING DRINKS

Often patients with eating difficulties arising from their disease or treatment find it easier to drink than to eat. For this reason, nourishing drinks can be used to great advantage, either as a meal replacement or in addition to meals. Energy and/or protein supplements can be added to drinks to further increase their nutritional value.

Nourishing drinks may be home-made such as milk shakes, egg nogs, hot milky drinks or fortified soups. Table 9.5 shows a list of nourishing drinks commercially available in the United Kingdom.

Table 9.5   *Commercially available nourishing drinks**

Complan	(Boots Company)
Build-Up	(Carnation)
Fortisip	(Cow and Gate Ltd)
Fortimel	(Cow and Gate Ltd)
Enteral 250	(Scientific Hospital Supplies)
Fresubin	(Fresenius Ltd)
Ensure	(Abbotts)
Liquisorb	(Merck)

* All come in a variety of flavours and most, except Complan and Build-Up, are prescribable. Current prescribing literature should be checked for details.

ENERGY AND PROTEIN SUPPLEMENTS

Table 9.6 shows ways of adding extra protein and energy to meals using normal foods. Commercial energy and protein supplements are now available and can be added to food or drink to increase its nutritional value. Energy supplements are available either as liquids or as powders. The liquids can either be drunk as they are, diluted or made into ice lollipops or jellies. The powders, which are tasteless, can be added to drinks, soups and puddings. Protein supplements can also be added to drinks, soups and puddings. One of the easiest protein supplements to use is dried milk powder. The commercial protein supplements available in the UK are powders and can be used in the same way as dried milk powder. It must be remembered, however, that commercial energy and protein supplements or nourishing drinks should only be used under dietetic supervision.

Table 9.6   *Adding extra protein and energy to foods*

Normal foods
Use fortified milk (milk + skimmed milk powder added)
Use milk to make up condensed and packet soups
Use milk to make jelly
Beat eggs and/or milk into creamed potato
Add grated cheese to soups, sauces and creamed potato
Add butter to vegetables, potatoes and pasta
Add cream, ice cream or evaporated milk to desserts
Add sugar or honey to cereal or drinks
Add sugar or syrup to ice cream and puddings
Use fried foods if tolerated

Energy supplements
Liquids: Hycal (Beechams)
            Fortical (Cow and Gate Ltd)
            Maxijul Liquid (Scientific Hospital Supplies)

Powders: Polycal (Cow and Gate Ltd)
            Polycose (Abbotts)
            Maxijul (Scienfitic Hospital Supplies)
            Caloreen (Roussel Ltd)

Protein supplements
Powders: Maxipro (Scientific Hospital Supplies)
            Protifar (Cow and Gate Ltd)

SOFTER DIETS

It may be necessary for patients with chewing and swallowing problems to have a soft or semi-solid diet. A soft diet is like a normal meal but is composed of foods which are soft in consistency. The diet must be tailored to suit the patient's needs and preferences. It should consist of as wide a range of foods as possible to prevent flavour and texture fatigue. Examples of soft meals are shown in Table 9.7. Nourishing drinks may be used to supplement a soft diet.

LIQUID/LIQUIDIZED DIET

Patients with severe chewing or swallowing problems may only be able to tolerate liquids and liquidized meals. This diet needs careful

Table 9.7 *Some suggestions for soft meals*

Tinned soup with fortified milk added
Macaroni cheese
Cauliflower cheese
Chopped or minced chicken in cream sauce
Creamed chicken or ham
Minced roast meat and gravy
Casseroles
Poached or flaked fish in sauce
Omelette or scrambled egg
Baby foods
Mousse
Egg custard/crème caramel
Milk jelly
Fruit fools
Souffles
Ice cream
Yoghurts
Milk puddings
Custard
Tinned fruit
Mashed fruit and cream

---

planning if it is to be successful. It is difficult to provide adequate nutrition on a liquid diet. Patients need to take an average of 250 ml of nourishing fluids every two hours to maintain adequate nutritional requirements.

Liquidized or puréed meals may also be useful. Most foods liquidize satisfactorily but attractive presentation is important. If possible, patients should choose their meals in the normal way and then these should be liquidized to the required consistency in the ward kitchen. In this way, both patient and nursing staff can identify the individual components of the meal. Nourishing drinks are likely to be needed between liquidized meals to maintain adequate intake.

It is not uncommon for eating difficulties in cancer patients to be so severe that the above methods alone do not meet the patients' requirements. In these circumstances, tube feeding may be appropriate or, failing all else, total parenteral nutrition (TPN) by the intravenous route.

TUBE FEEDING

This may be by the nasogastric route, by gastrostomy or by jejunostomy tube. A nasogastric tube is the most common and may be used for short-term supplementary feeding, or short-term total nutrition as in patients with anorexia or swallowing difficulties. Long-term nasogastric feeding is suitable for a patient who has undergone radical head and neck surgery.

Nasogastric tubes differ in many ways, including their material, size and length. In general, fine-bore tubes are preferable as these pass easily and cause little discomfort to the patient. PVC tubes are suitable for short-term feeding of up to two weeks' duration. For long-term feeding, Silicone tubes are preferable both for durability and for patient comfort.

Although some hospitals still prepare their own standard formula feeds, most now use one of the many commercially available, ready-to-use nasogastric feeds. The advantages of such feeds are:

1. They have an exact, constant composition.
2. They can be prepared at ward level.
3. They allow patients to manage nasogastric feeds at home.
4. Some are flavoured so they can be used as nourishing drinks as well as nasogastric feeds.

Most of the commercially available feeds provide 1 kcal/ml of feed. A day's supply of 2 litres provides 2,000 kcal and covers the recommended daily intake of all nutrients.

The recommended daily amount of 2 litres may be given in several ways according to the condition of the patient.

1. By gravity drip from a delivery system recommended by dietetic or medical staff with the feed being delivered continuously throughout the day.
2. By gravity drip with the feed given intermittently. For example, 500 ml feed delivered over two hours then a break for two hours and so on four times a day.
3. By a feeding pump with accurate amounts of feed delivered hourly throughout a 16-hour or 24-hour day.
4. Overnight feeding – a prescribed volume of feed may be given overnight only. The patient eats normally during the day.
5. In some cases, bolus feeding by means of a large syringe is still used although the above methods are preferable. They are better tolerated by the patient and require less nursing time.

It is advisable to start on half-strength feed for the first few days of nasogastric feeding before going on to full strength. Ideally, nasogastric feeding should be tailed off gradually as the patient's oral intake increases and should not be stopped until oral feeding is well established.

TOTAL PARENTERAL NUTRITION

Total parenteral nutrition (TPN) or intravenous feeding should only be used when the gastrointestinal tract is either inaccessible or not functioning, otherwise oral or tube feeding is best. Total parenteral nutrition is costly and may predispose patients to complications if not accurately maintained. Many hospitals can now prepare their own TPN regimens as a result of advances in sterile production techniques in pharmacy departments. Those that cannot, rely on ready prepared TPN regimens available from the major pharmaceutical companies.

It is now common to have standard TPN regimens in most hospitals prepared by nutrition teams who specialize in TPN and tube feeding. Standard TPN regimens vary but most consist of one or more of the following:

1. a 3-litre bag containing all nutrients;
2. a 2- or 2.5-litre bag containing all nutrients except the fat emulsion which is supplied in a 500-ml bottle and given separately;
3. separate bottles of feeding solutions which need to be given in combination through a 'Y' connector.

Most TPN is given via a central feeding catheter and care of the catheter using aseptic technique is vital in order to minimize the risk of infection. Accurate monitoring of the patient's daily weight and biochemistry profile is essential to reduce complications.

Feeding for the Child with Cancer

In general the nutritional problems faced by the child with cancer are similar to those experienced by adults. The approaches used to overcome such difficulties are explored elsewhere in this chapter. However, there are some important differences concerning paediatric malnutrition and its correction, which are dealt with here.

The incidence of protein energy malnutrition (PEM) in children presenting with cancer is high. It occurs in 17 per cent of children with newly diagnosed localized tumours and in 37 per cent of those with metastases. Approximately one in two children with cancer will exhibit symptoms of malnutrition (Donaldson, 1982). A survey of 277 children with benign and malignant tumours revealed that 32 per cent scored inadequately in at least one of three anthropometric measurements (anthropometry refers to measurements of the human body such as height, weight and skinfold thickness), indicating a degree of malnutrition (Carter *et al.,* 1983).

Children who are particularly at risk of PEM at presentation are those with advanced tumours, for example:

1. stages II, III and IV – Wilm's tumour;
2. stages III and IV – Ewing's sarcoma;
3. stages III and IV – neuroblastoma;
4. relapsed solid tumours or leukaemias.

The consequences of PEM in the child are severe, especially when compounded by the side-effects of aggressive antineoplastic therapy which makes great metabolic demands on the child. Failure in growth, intestinal malabsorption, reduced immunocompetence, apathy and lack of well-being clearly compromise a child's ability to survive cancer treatment. It is, therefore, essential that children are monitored carefully for signs of malnutrition and that appropriate intervention is made as soon as nutritional difficulties become apparent. A 'wait and see' policy may put a child at unnecessary risk. Once malnutrition has occurred it requires intensive nutritional support to restore the status quo. Useful parameters to measure in children are listed below, but most of these will usually be measured and monitored by the dietitian and paediatrician. Other health professionals, however, can alert those with specialist expertise to (2), (3) and (4). Early referral is all important in these circumstances. The parameters are:

1. dietary history;
2. weight for age;
3. height for age;
4. weight/height ratio;
5. subscapular skinfold thickness;
6. serum proteins, e.g. albumin, transferrin, fibronectin.*

---

*Fibronectin is a high molecular weight glycoprotein found in plasma. It is a useful indicator of malnutrition. Decreased levels may play a direct role in predisposing malnourished patients to infection (Coates *et al.,* 1986).

Even in well-nourished children the aim of nutritional support is to promote weight gain and growth rather than weight maintenance (as is often the case in adults). A child who fails to gain weight may in fact be malnourished even if they are not actually losing weight.

The methods of nutritional support available for use in children are the same as those for adults, in other words oral, nasogastric and parenteral feeding.

ORAL FEEDING

Oral feeding in a nauseated or anorexic child is even more difficult than in adults. It is the best method to use in children who are in an adequate nutritional state but only if they are able to consume sufficient nutrients, which is often not the case. A study of children with advanced neuroblastoma revealed that adequately nourished children who were randomized to received a closely supervised oral diet failed to gain weight and showed evidence of decreasing subscapular and triceps skinfolds. Nourished and malnourished children who received total parenteral nutrition made significant gains during a four-week period of intensive nutritional support. These gains were maintained with intensive oral nutrition during a six-week follow-up period (Rickard *et al.,* 1985). Useful points to remember about oral feeding in children are given in Table 9.8.

Table 9.8   *Points to remember about oral feeding in children with cancer*

---

(1) Try to create a safe undisturbed time for eating.
(2) Involve parents and children in 'creative cooking activities'.
(3) Offer a flexible individualized menu.
(4) Only offer favourite foods to tempt children during *vomiting-free* periods in order to avoid 'learned food aversions'.
(5) Sit with the child during a meal to offer help and encouragement – or parents may eat *with* the child.
(6) Monitor quality and quantity of consumed food constantly to assess nutrient intake.
(7) Position children comfortably 10 minutes before a meal.

Note: Oral feeding may be considered suitable in the following groups:

    (a) nourished children with less advanced disease;
    (b) children with good prognosis acute lymphoblastic leukaemia (ALL);
    (c) children with advanced disease in remission once PEM has been corrected.

NASOGASTRIC FEEDING

Nasogastric feeding is a useful method of feeding some children. It may distress toddlers and preschool children but older children accept it more readily. Very soft, fine polyurethane tubes are now available and these can be used with great benefit.

PARENTERAL NUTRITION

For those children who are already malnourished or who are likely to become so, the most effective way of feeding them is by parenteral nutrition using a central venous catheter. Although this carries with it an additional risk of infection, meticulous catheter care will prevent most problems.

Nutritional support for children with cancer should be considered a major part of therapy. The value of such intervention lies in its ability to prevent or correct the adverse effects of PEM. This can contribute significantly to tolerance of therapy and increased energy and well-being for the child. If this is achieved, nutritional support has reached its goal even if the overall prognosis is unchanged.

Nutrition in Patients with Leukaemia

The special nutritional problems faced by patients with leukaemia are related to the disturbances in bone marrow function and the intensive therapies used to achieve remission of the disease.

Neutropaenia may lead to oral infections which can interfere with eating. *Anaemia* renders the patient easily tired and breathless and this can reduce the desire or ability to eat normally. *Thrombocytopaenia* increases the risk of nosebleeds and bleeding gums which make food consumption difficult or cause vomiting if large amounts of blood have been swallowed. In addition, leukaemia can also cause malaise and anorexia coupled with an increased basal metabolic rate. If left unchecked these problems can lead rapidly to weight loss and severe malnutrition.

Chemotherapy used to try to induce remission in patients with leukaemia often exacerbates existing problems of anorexia, nausea and vomiting. Most of the treatment protocols used in the treatment of the leukaemias include at least one drug that induces such side-effects.

For patients with acute myeloblastic leukaemia (AML) who

undergo bone marrow transplantation, there are further nutritional problems to endure. Priming chemotherapy may include melphalan and/or cylophosphamide, both of which can cause severe nausea and vomiting, oral ulceration and diarrhoea. (Priming chemotherapy is carried out when high doses of alkylating agents such as melphalan and/or cyclophosphamide are to be used. A low priming dose is given a week before high-dose treatment commences. This priming has the effect of reducing the toxicity of the chemotherapy, especially to the bone marrow.)

Total body irradiation, which immediately follows priming chemotherapy, compromises nutritional status in several ways. It causes severe nausea and vomiting (maximal at three to four days post-irradiation) and malabsorption (due to damage to the intestinal villi). Damage to the salivary glands impairs the quality of saliva, which becomes viscous and loses its cleansing properties. In some cases patients experience a very dry mouth (xerostomia) which makes eating difficult. Cranial irradiation induces radiation sickness because of its effect on the vomiting centre. Sedation has been found to be as effective as anti-emetics in treating this problem. Somnolence syndrome occurs about six weeks or later after toal body irradiation. A very sleepy patient is unlikely to have a sufficient food intake.

Compounding all this is the need for the severely neutropaenic patient to consume a sterile diet in order to prevent a gastrointestinal infection. It is therefore extremely important that the diet offered is as varied as possible within the limits imposed by the microbiologists. Table 9.9 summarizes this diet. The details of such a food regimen will vary in different hospitals according to circumstances but the principles are the same. An aseptic technique for preparation and serving of this food is essential. Local policies for staff training and the protocols used need to be formulated and maintained.

When patients go home after a bone marrow transplant, they are advised to avoid take-away meals, delicatessen foods, ice cream from ice-cream vans and damaged fruit. These foods, due to the increased handling and extended storage time they often receive, could have higher numbers of pathogens present, which while rarely causing illness in healthy persons could be potentially risky for a severely immunosuppressed person. It is usually not necessary to continue such precautions for more than six months.

Unfortunately, in some cases, bone marrow transplantation can lead to a graft-versus-host reaction (GVHR). The severity of this rejection reaction (which occurs if the immunocompetent cells of the marrow attack the body) varies and may affect the skin, gut or liver.

Table 9.9 *Foods allowed for neutropaenic patients in protective isolation*

Foods allowed	Foods to avoid
Freshly cooked food (preferably using a prolonged slow method) e.g. stewing braising roasting boiling	Raw food Delicatessen foods, e.g. cheese cold meats 'take-away' foods
Tinned foods (reputable brands, undamaged tins)	Fresh salad Raw vegetables Raw fruit
Freshly opened pasteurized milk	
Cooked cheese	
Plain pasteurized yoghurt	Fruit yoghurt
Cooked eggs*	
Sugar, jam, salt (individual portions)	
Pepper – gamma irradiated	
Tea, coffee made with boiling water	
High-sugar cordials (well-known brands) e.g. Ribena Roses' Lime Cordial Robinsons' Orange and Lemon Barley water Individual bottles of Lucozade	Cheap cordial brands
Butter — autoclaved	
Bread — fresh (handling avoided)	

* This is controversial. Eggs may be contaminated but their food value and palatability are excellent.

When the gut is affected by GVHR, there are major nutritional implications because of the severe malabsorption and stomatitis that occur.

Nutritional support for patients with leukaemia is vital because of the severe and long-term problems they encounter. They should be closely monitored, particulary in terms of their food intake. Although regular recording of body weight and monitoring of blood proteins can be used to evaluate nutritional status in these patients, the frequency and nature of intravenous infusions can complicate the picture. These parameters alone should not therefore be relied on as indicators of nutritional status. Careful observation and recording of food and fluid intake are essential as well.

Well-motivated patients can benefit from dietetic advice and the sensible use of special products such as glucose polymers, and high protein and energy supplements such as Build-Up, Complan and Fortify. For many others, however, it is impossible to achieve an adequate oral intake of nutrients and for such patients alternative methods of feeding should be considered.

Nasogastric feeding is not widely used among patients with leukaemia. This may be because of the nausea and vomiting encountered or because they are at a greater risk of nose bleeds, or if the gut is damaged by total body irradiation (TBI). It has also been suggested that the presence of a nasogastric tube may provide an additional route for infection. Nevertheless, selective nasogastric feeding via a soft, fine-bore tube can be a safe and effective way of providing partial or complete nutritional support if managed carefully.

Parenteral nutrition is also a good method of feeding leukaemia patients, particularly as many of them already have a central venous catheter in place to give their chemotherapy. Ideally a double- or triple-lumen catheter should be used for the several intravenous infusions because of the risk of contamination when a single-lumen line is used for multiple access. The advantages of using parenteral nutrition in patients with leukaemia is that it circumvents any problems of gut dysfunction. There is, however, a greater risk of infection so meticulous care of central catheters is vital. There is also the potential for fluid overload because patients may already be receiving blood, platelet and antibiotic infusions. Care should be taken that nutritional fluids do not take second place in the intravenous regimen.

The patient with leukaemia faces serious nutritional problems as a result of intensive chemotherapy and in some cases total body irradiation. In order to prevent malnutrition and its consequences, nutritional support must be instigated as soon as the normal oral diet becomes inadequate. Medical, nursing and dietetic staff should all be closely involved in this aspect of care.

Nutrition in Patients with Advanced Cancer

The aim of feeding patients is to maintain or restore health. When advanced disease makes this no longer possible, is there still a place for nutritional support? In certain cases the answer is undoubtedly 'yes', but the decision to continue feeding should depend on several factors and be a joint one made by the patient and health professionals together. If the patient is encouraged to contribute to the decision-making process, the utmost care will have been taken to look at all the factors on which such a decision rests. Such factors may be:

1. The potential *benefits* for the patient to continue feeding
   (a) enjoyment of the flavour of food helps to maintain positive psychological status and self-esteem;
   (b) contributes towards the reduction of dehydration.
2. The potential *disadvantages* for the patient to continue feeding
   (a) causes physical or psychological distress;
   (b) length of prognosis.

A high proportion of patients who are receiving symptomatic treatment alone can, and do, benefit from talking with a sympathetic dietitian. Simple dietary manipulation and the use of small, attractive portions of palatable, high-calorie foods and fluids can be a real morale booster. Of particular value in nauseated patients, especially those with liver disease, are low-fat foods and cool, carbonated glucose drinks. Skimmed milk may also be acceptable even if full-cream milk is not. Skimmed milk can be flavoured and made into a milk lollipop which is often more palatable.

Nasogastric feeding should not be dismissed automatically as being too invasive. For the individual with complete dysphagia, this method of feeding can literally be a lifeline and enable good quality of life until the disease becomes so extensive that feeding is discontinued. It could be used just in the night, allowing the patient to be freely mobile during the day. The tube could be removed for special occasions as required, providing the patient can tolerate repeated intubation. The nasogastric tubes now available are much more comfortable and easy to use. Most people are well able to cope with this kind of feeding which can be continued at home.

Parenteral nutrition is the last option to consider but in almost all cases it would be inappropriate unless the patient's prognosis is fairly long and he or she is capable of managing safely at home.

The use of corticosteroids is of value to stimulate the appetite in those with anorexia. A study at St Christopher's Hospice in London (Walsh *et al.*, 1983) showed that patients receiving this kind of medication had the highest energy intakes among a group of patients with advanced cancer. Similarly, small amounts of alcohol served as an aperitif can improve appetite and can be an enjoyable way of consuming extra calories.

It is all too easy to adopt the attitude that nutritional support is of little significance in this group of patients. For some people this may be true but not for others. In all cases the decision not to provide nutritional care should be a positive one. Failure to feed a patient should not arise through neglect, apathy or ignorance.

Eating is a basic requirement for life and is of great social importance. Patients should therefore be encouraged and helped to eat for as long as it is appropriate.

'Alternative' Diets

An alternative diet is usually considered to be any unorthodox or unconventional modification of a normal diet which is claimed to treat or cure cancer. These diets may be used in conjuction with, or instead of, conventional anti-cancer therapies. Most derive from the United States of America or the Far East and are increasing in popularity among cancer patients in the United Kingdom. They have generally been received with great scepticism by both the medical and dietetic professions.

The most popular regimens are:

1. the Bristol Diet – originating from the Bristol Cancer Help Centre;
2. the Macrobiotic Diet as formulated by Michio Kushi at the Kushi Institute, Boston, Massachusetts, USA;
3. the Gerson Therapy, originated by Max Gerson in Germany and now practised by Charlotte Gerson at the Gerson Therapy Centre, Tijuana, Mexico.

All the regimens share the same common philosophy, that is, that diet can be used to correct physical and emotional illness. Most also share the same common principles:

1. they are usually strict vegetarian or vegan diets;
2. they involve eating large amounts of raw foods;
3. they are sugar free;
4. they are low in salt;
5. they are virtually fat free;
6. they often involve taking large quantities of juices;
7. they often involve taking large doses of vitamins and minerals.

Most alternative diets are suggested for all illnesses and not just cancer. It is clear that some think that these regimens are of benefit to some cancer patients. The reason for this is unclear, but seems to be associated with the fact that patients feel involved in, and have some control over, one particular aspect of their treatment and care. Most dietary regimens are closely linked with several other therapies, such as relaxation or visualization techniques. The combination of therapies adds to their popularity and many people claim to feel better as a result of them.

However, in the authors' view the disadvantages of the dietary regimens for cancer patients outweigh any advantages for the following reasons:

1. Most are high in bulk and low in energy – the exact opposite to the nutritional needs of most cancer patients.
2. Patients experiencing loss of appetite or eating difficulties find it almost impossible to eat a high-fibre, mostly raw food, diet.
3. Often patients undertake such regimens as a last resort when they are already weak and malnourished. Such diets further exacerbate these problems.
4. The high dose of vitamins and minerals often recommended may be harmful.
5. Most regimens are costly to follow and difficult to prepare.

For these reasons, patients following or contemplating following such regimens should be referred to a dietitian for nutritional assessment and advice. It is sometimes possible to accommodate particular aspects of such diets into a properly planned nutritional profile for patients, providing it does them no harm and does not conflict with treatment regimens. The dietitian is the best person to give advice on these matters.

References and Further Reading

Boisaubin, E.V. (1984) Ethical issues in the nutritional support of the terminal patient, *Journal of the American Medical Association,* Vol. 84, no. 5, pp. 529–31.

Carter, P., Carr, D., Eys, J. van and Coody, D. (1983) Nutritional parameters in children with cancer, *Journal of the American Dietary Association,* Vol. 2, pp. 616–22.

Coates, T.D., Rickard, K.A., Grosfield, J.L. and Weetman, R.M. (1986) Nutritional support of children with neoplastic diseases, *Surgical Clinics of North America,* Vol. 66, no. 6, pp. 1197-212.

Dickerson, J.W.T. and Basu, T.K. (1977) Specific vitamin deficiencies in patients with cancer and receiving chemotherapy, in M. Winick, (ed.) *Nutrition and Cancer,* Wiley, New York.

Donaldson, S.S. (1982) Effects of therapy in nutritional status of the paediatric cancer patients, *Cancer Research,* Vol. 42, p. 729.

Hoffman, F.A. (1985) Micronutrient requirements of cancer patients, *Cancer,* Vol. 55, p. 295.

Kettlewell, M. (1982) Meeting patients' needs, in A. Grant and E. Todd (eds.) *Enteral and Parenteral Nutrition,* Blackwell Scientific Publications, Oxford, p. 11.

Moghissi, K. and Boore, J. (1983) *Parenteral and Enteral Nutrition for Nurses,* Heinemann Medical, London, pp. 96–7.

Rickard, K.A., Loghman, E.S., Grosfeld, J.L., Detamore, C.M. *et al.* (1985) Short and long term effectiveness of enteral and parenteral nutrition in reversing or preventing protein energy malnutrition in advanced neuroblastoma — a prospective randomised study, *Cancer,* Vol. 56, p. 2881.

Shils, M. (1979) Principles of nutritional therapy, *Cancer,* Vol. 43, pp. 2093-102.

Theologides, A. (1979) Cancer cachexia, *Cancer,* Vol. 43, pp. 2004–12.

Walsh, T.D., Bowman, K.B. and Jackson, G.P. (1983) Dietary intake in advanced cancer patients, *Human Nutrition: Applied Nutrition,* Vol. 37A, pp. 41–5.

Chapter 10

Living with Cancer – Complementary Care

PAT WEBB RGN, RNT, DipN(London), DipSocRes
Senior Nurse – Education
The Royal Marsden Hospital, London and Surrey and Marie Curie Memorial Foundation, London

Introduction

Advances in diagnosing and treating cancer have increased the possibility of cure for patients while significant advances in research and education in palliative care have led to an increased awareness of good symptom control to help patients dying from cancer. These two extremes of the spectrum – active treatment following a diagnosis of cancer and palliation of symptoms for the dying – exclude a very large percentage of cancer patients who are trying to come to terms with living with a chronic, life-threatening illness.

Medical research continues to improve treatment to cure cancer and to develop new strategies for the control of some of the symptoms associated with cancer. Health care professionals have begun to adopt different strategies in their care for cancer patients by reconsidering the impact of this disease and the long-term consequences on them and their families. Skills and attitudes not learnt in initial educational programmes leading to a professional qualification, are now being sought so that the multidisciplinary group working with patients can provide a more comprehensive support service.

Living with cancer implies the intention to continue with a life that has structure and purpose, despite the effects of a chronic, life-threatening illness. It implies a dynamic process not a static situation. It implies positive, creative and enjoyable life given the constraints on that life that cancer may bring. The resourcefulness of individuals continues to be amazing, and cancer patients are certainly a case in point. Most people know of those who have fought and won against all apparent odds. However, maintaining a positive attitude and enjoying the life that is left come easier to some than to others. This is not just the case in illness; it is a facet of human character and personality. Any discussion of human behaviour during illness must be placed in the context of human behaviour generally. Some will be like the patient remembered by many for her contribution at an international nursing conference. Mara Flaherty (1981) closed her memorable paper as follows:

> There are no simple solutions for the problems of all people with cancer. But there are options we can explore, approaches we can try and steps we can take to help ourselves ... please give us the power and sense of control over our lives that knowledge can bring. Together we – nurses and patients – can pool our skills and keep cancer in its place.

Others will need a great deal of support and encouragement to realize their potential to help themselves and adapt to changes that chronic illness can bring.

This chapter is about some of the complementary aspects of care that can be exploited to help and support cancer patients and their families. There may be some overlap with other chapters in this volume but this only serves to reinforce the message. The emphasis throughout is on the particular problem of maintaining support when active periods of treatment have ceased and when the role of 'patient' may no longer be used, even though the dependence and vulnerability associated with it may still be present. Consideration is given to the role of patients and their families, of health professionals and of other professional and non-professional groups. Those whose job is to care and support are considered together with those who volunteer to do so.

This chapter is not about alternative or complementary *medicine*, although there is some discussion about the reasons why alternatives or complements to existing health care services may be sought.

Coping with Cancer

An experience of illness – a deviation from normal, healthy function – demands an adaptation response from the individual. Normal life as we know it has been interrupted, temporarily or permanently, and adjustments need to be made to our perceptions and expectations of life.

Adaptation to illness consists of two major strategies: first, to cope with the illness itself; second, to cope with essential changes in lifestyle as a result of its effects. These are not just problems for patients but inevitably affect those close to them – family and/or friends. Weisman (1976) defines coping as '. . . a reward, quiescence and equilibrium ... If a person cannot cope effectively, then varying degrees of turmoil, anguish, frustration, despair and suffering result.' Developing coping strategies to deal with illness is, therefore, essential.

Chronic illness is characterized by its permanence even though there may be periods of quiescence interrupted by exacerbations of acute symptoms. The impact of chronic illness extends over long periods of time and places great demands on the individual and family alike. Relationships are tested and unexpected breakdowns occur where stability and permanence were previously 'guaranteed'.

FEAR AND STIGMA

To these general problems cancer adds the fear and stigma that are still associated with malignant disease (Wakefield, 1976). The threat to life itself is uppermost in most people's minds when presented with a diagnosis of cancer (Weisman and Worden, 1976). Weisman (1976) further identifies emotional distress and incapacity to cope as frequent indicators of vulnerability in cancer patients. Others, too, have documented the stresses and subsequent psychological morbidity associated with some cancers (Morris *et al.*, 1977; Maguire *et al.*, 1978, 1982; Petty and Noyes, 1981; Pruyn, 1982; Denton and Baum, 1983). Anecdotal accounts from patients who have suffered profound body image change in addition to the other stresses of a cancer diagnosis (Piff, 1985) augment these findings.

Uncertainty is a very real problem for most cancer patients: not only uncertainty about the response of cancer to prescribed treatment, but also that associated with the outcome of treatment and of remission or recurrence of the disease. Mishel (1984) describes the negative contribution that uncertainty makes to illness leading to greater isolation, vulnerability and subsequent psychological morbidity. In his classic work on the communication patterns between cancer patients and health professionals, McIntosh (1977) documents the conflicting signs given by professionals during periods of progress and regression of cancer, leaving patients unable to make any plans for an uncertain future.

Research has progressed in the more qualitative aspects of care for cancer patients. Objective measurements are constantly being devised and tested so that physicians and others can determine the impact a diagnosis of cancer has on an individual's quality of life (Spitzer *et al.*, 1981; Selby *et al.*, 1984).

Why do People Seek Complements or Alternatives to Treatment and Care?

The impact of a diagnosis of cancer has been briefly explored in this chapter and in more detail in others. Coping with this crisis demands a great deal from individuals with cancer as well as the resources of those close to them. If patients have close family members or friends with whom to share this experience then the stresses associated with it also seem to be shared and patients cope better (Weisman, 1976; Wortman and Dunkel-Schetter, 1979; van den Borne *et al.*, 1987).

Having sought professional help from medicine to cure or control the physical effects of cancer, patients reasonably want to discover what else or who else could help them. As cancer is a threat to life itself, it is to be expected that many patients do not want to omit anybody or anything that may contribute to their recovery. The search for meaning as to why they have the cancer and attempts to become involved themselves in regaining health are also understandable.

For some of the cancers, cure is now possible. For others, intermittent treatment may be required as the cancer recurs. In between treatments, however, patients may return to their roles as 'well members of the public'. Some patients need regular symptom control for cancer and may never move back to being 'well'.

In each of these cases, many patients may feel that there must be someone or something else that can help them – irrespective of, or in addition to, the care offered by health professionals. The latter are perceived by patients as busy people dealing with issues of life and death who usually do not have time to deal with all the extra things that patients may want or need (Webb, 1987). Patients often look elsewhere for others to help them. They may seek ways of supplementing medical and nursing care by exploring and experimenting with different diets, looking for methods to reduce stress or finding methods to comfort or support. Much of this may be help received from others but some will also be concerned with self-help.

Augmenting existing orthodox medicine and care is one area which can be considered within the limits of this chapter. Suggestions can be made in the light of others' experience as to what may reasonably be offered as part of the 'holistic' care of oncology patients. The other more controversial area is that of patients seeking alternatives to existing *medical* treatment for cancer. In 1983, an independent consumer organization in Belgium reported the comments of 3,000 people about their experiences of orthodox and alternative medicine. The report was published in *Test Achats*, (the Belgian equivalent of the UK's *Which?*, a well-respected consumer organization publication) and reproduced for wider readership in the *Journal of the College of Health* (1984). The report began by defining the two terms 'orthodox medicine' and 'alternative medicine'. *Orthodox medicine* was defined as medicine practised by doctors, the most used medicine and the only type officially recognized. *Alternative medicine* was described as consisting of various therapies whose practitioners are not necessarily doctors. It has no official recognition and the people who practise it cannot be paid under the social security system. Similarly, reimbursement for medicines prescribed by them is not provided by the State. These are useful definitions and are probably similar to those used by others for the same reasons. The conclusions of the report are many but one which sounded very familiar was that whatever the medicine, the satisfaction felt by the patient was greater if the time given to consultation was 15–30 minutes as opposed to 5–10 minutes.

A discussion on alternative medicine is not within the limit of this chapter. The reader's attention is drawn in particular to two recent papers which put forward the arguments on these issues in a very articulate and balanced way (Jarvis, 1986; Brigden, 1987). The controversies surrounding this matter will undoubtedly continue for some time.

Some health professionals have reacted to these trends in a responsible and mature way by seeking to research some areas of alternative medicine, using quantitative and qualitative methods to determine objectively their value. Those whose roles emphasize care and support rather than treatment have also been looking at ways to enable patients to live more positive and comfortable lives during an experience of cancer – however long or short that experience may be. Many health professionals believe that the extra support that patients seek outside traditional health care should, in fact, be provided within it, despite a severe lack of resources. Others believe it inevitable that people will always look for more and better care and support and will tend to do so outside traditional facilities. It is likely that there will continue to be disagreement about this. Meanwhile, there are some areas identified below to which health professionals can direct patients and their families, and others they may want to pursue themselves through extra education and training. As with any extension of a professional's role, they will need to feel assured that the extra techniques and skills are of value. In addition, they will need to be competent themselves in the skills and be able to convince other professionals in their peer-group, including their professional organization, that such skills will certainly do patients no harm while offering considerable benefit. Finally, some may look to an extended role, one which is not necessarily included in an employment contract. These issues will vary considerably depending on the way in which health and illness are managed in different countries and how the role of health professionals is seen and controlled.

What Kinds of Areas May Be Complements to Existing Care?

It has to be said that some of the items described below may already be included in some health professionals' practice. Others will never have considered them to be within their limit. They are all areas that, in the author's experience, patients have sought regularly and found to be of help.

STRESS REDUCTION

The term 'stress reduction' here is not meant as a definition from psychological medicine although it may have some affinity with it. It is the term used by patients who are trying to manage nervousness, anxiety and anticipatory symptoms, for example the anticipatory nausea and vomiting common in patients undergoing intermittent treatment with cytotoxic drugs (Rhodes *et al.*, 1984). Some have called it 'tension-reducing strategies' (Friedman, 1980) using the examples of negative strategies such as smoking, drinking and overeating, to be replaced by the less destructive and more positive ones of relaxation training, meditation, diversion and support groups.

Some nurses have looked at the reduction of stress in patients in a variety of settings. Wilson-Barnett (1978) researched methods of stress reduction in some patients undergoing distressing investigations. In a separate paper, she lists some of the stressors that many people are subjected to in their lives and that are certainly included in most patient's experiences. They are the stressors of unexpected events, unpleasant symptoms, loss of function, loneliness, unfamiliar surroundings and relationships, altered status and role (Wilson-Barnett, 1984). The impact of cancer often increases these stresses to unbearable limits.

Much research has been completed into methods of stress reduction. Some examples are given although an extensive literature exists for those wishing to pursue the matter further.

Relaxation

Benson *et al*. (1974) describe the possible therapeutic benefits and side-effects of the relaxation response. Taylor *et al*. (1977) have looked more specifically at the relative benefits of relaxation therapy in controlling hypertension and its sequelae. In the cancer context, Kaempfer (1982) reviews stress management techniques as possible symptom management strategies in cancer therapy. When she wrote that paper, she warned that a review of the reported uses of these techniques with cancer patients yielded only a small number of studies, few of which involved systematic research. Her view, then, was that more research was needed with cancer patients and more information required on the nature of the stress response, especially that which accompanies a major illness, such as cancer, with all its complexities. Flaherty and Fitzpatrick (1978) and Wells (1982) have researched the effect of relaxation on postoperative pain and discomfort. A consistent finding was that of self-reported distress being significantly lower in the experimental groups of their studies. Similarly, both studies identified the need for more systematic research into these areas as small numbers were used in their projects. Snyder (1984) concludes her paper on progressive relaxation as a nursing intervention by listing some helpful guidelines to use in determining suitable patients who may benefit from practising relaxation techniques. However, she balances this with precautions for its use, again emphasizing the need for more systematic research.

Donovan (1980) found the use of relaxation together with guided imagery a useful technique for patients with phantom limb pain, for reduction of needle phobia in patients receiving intravenous drugs, including cytotoxic chemotherapy, and for reducing anticipatory anxiety for distressing or painful investigation for cancer. Others (Klisch, 1980) have documented some studies using the visualization techniques made popular by the Simontons from 1971 onwards (Simonton *et al*., 1978). These techniques have been used in conjunction with relaxation therapy quite extensively in some oncology centres and private clinics in the United States of America. Rowden (1984) and Cobb (1984) describe the use of relaxation techniques with, respectively, breast cancer patients and a variety of cancer patients.

Clearly, progressive muscle relaxation as described by Snyder (1984) has been seen to be of benefit to some cancer patients in reducing stress. The request for help in learning to relax is increasing in many nurses' experience, and nurses themselves are increasingly interested in learning and using the techniques. Health food stores and book stores have 'stress-reduction' audio cassettes on sale and organizations concerned with stress reduction in any country appear to be producing similar resources of their own. Nurses working in oncology units have given anecdotal accounts of the increased awareness of patients of this technique and requests for help to learn more about it. More systematic research needs to be done to document adequately the relative advantages and disadvantages of using this technique. Sims (1987) has produced a helpful selective literature review of relaxation training as a technique for helping patients to cope with the whole experience of cancer. Meanwhile those who care for patients throughout the 24-hour period – nurses and some therapists – may want to explore the literature in more detail, establish some research of their own, identify those people to whom cancer patients may be referred should they reveal an interest in relaxation therapy and even consider some education themselves to understand better the techniques. Until the picture is much clearer, the teaching of relaxation needs to be monitored by those with the expertise to do so.

Meditation, Hypnosis and Psychotherapy

Clearly this is an area to be restricted to those with specific skills, namely those with backgrounds in psychological medicine. However, a very brief review of some of the literature may encourage others caring for patients to be aware of the potential therapeutic benefits and unwanted effects and limitations of these techniques. It may further encourage more co-operation between departments of psychological medicine and those who work daily with cancer patients.

Barber (1978) describes the use of hypnosis in the management of cancer pain and concludes his paper with one particular case study of a woman with incurable, extensive cancer. He emphasizes the value of hypnosis in allowing patients to take an active role in controlling their own comfort. In a small study of twenty-seven children in a Denver hospital in the United States of America there were claims of increased quality of life for children with cancer who learned self-hypnosis (La Baw *et al.*, 1975). Increased quality of life was defined by a reduction in insomnia, anorexia and increased tolerance to distressing investigation and treatment.

Radical treatment for cancer, including the unwanted side-effects that it may bring, is the subject of a paper by Dempster *et al.* (1976). They describe the role of supportive hypnotherapy during the extensive treatment protocols available for cancer patients which clearly have increased considerably since this paper was written. A more recent paper by Redd *et al.* (1982) documents a small study of just six patients who participated in a study on hypnosis to attempt to help them deal with anticipatory nausea and vomiting prior to cytotoxic chemotherapy. The benefits to each of the patients are explained and again, emphasis is given to the issue of self-control during a period of illness when much of the control is taken away from the individual as more and more invasive treatment is administered.

In 1983 in the United Kingdom, the British Holistic Medical Association (BHMA) was launched. Dr Pietroni, a senior lecturer in general practice at a London hospital and one of the founder members of the association, claimed that therapies such as relaxation, yoga and acupuncture can reduce significantly drug prescriptions as well as increasing well-being in patients going to their general practitioner with symptoms of stress (Lyall, 1983). However, in the same article it was made clear that the six founder doctors of the association wanted to establish systematic and credible research into these areas as part of the work of the BHMA.

Massage and Touch

This is an area where nurses and physiotherapists have expertise and many oncology units may already be incorporating these into their total care for cancer patients.

McCorkle (1974) described the effect of touch on seriously ill patients as a technique in non-verbal communication so easily lost with high-technology medicine. Her findings could certainly be applied to some categories of cancer patients and certainly to the dying. More detail of non-verbal communication is given in Chapter 5. Barnett (1972), in her paper on the concepts of touch, concludes with a list of proposals for further research into the area. Massage has been used by physiotherapists in many therapeutic interventions but it has a brief documented history in the care of cancer patients. Probably one of the most recent publications is that of a pilot-study by Sims (1986) on the use of slow stroke back massage for cancer patients. Some benefits were seen for patients involved in this small pilot study and recommendations were made for further research to be conducted in this area.

There are other interventions which may be seen as stress reducers and, like those mentioned above, some may perceive them as legitimate therapies to be used as part of the total care of cancer patients, while others may perceive them as falling in with the realm of alternative medicine. Whatever the individual reader's perception, it is hoped that he or she will become informed about techniques that cancer patients are themselves seeking, search the literature extensively and, where appropriate, initiate research to measure objectively the effects of their use. In doing all this, the messages of caution contained within this section also need to be firmly noted.

DIET AND NUTRITIONAL ADVICE

The subject of diet is adequately dealt with in Chapter 9. This area clearly falls within the remit of the dietitian but other members of the health care team need to be aware of its importance and their contribution to it. Patients may be seeking advice about the many alternative diets that claim to alter the course of cancer and others which claim to make patients feel better while dealing with the effects of their illness. Some diets are certainly harmful and have been documented by Hunter and Janes in their own investigation into the wide range of nutritional advice given to cancer patients (see Chapter 9).

INITIATING A NEW SKILL OR LIFESTYLE – COPING STRATEGIES

This topic has also been addressed in several chapters in this volume. The issue of helping patients and those close to them to come to terms with their illness and its effects may not yet be seen by all as an essential and integral part of their care. It may not be within the expertise of many who are involved with cancer patients and, in these circumstances, firm links need to be made with a network of those who can help and to whom patients may be referred. The establishment of the network may, therefore, be the most useful function the health professional can perform in this particular instance.

DIVERSIONAL THERAPY AND MUSIC THERAPY

Music therapy can be seen as an example of diversion but it may also be used therapeutically in other ways. Diversional therapy for cancer patients may be subject to different definitions. Occupational therapists may well see this as coming firmly within their remit, while other health professionals, non-health professionals and non-professional groups may also feel they have a part to play. Again, it is mentioned here to draw attention to the potential benefits of diversion for cancer patients.

Diversion can range from interventions for occupation provided by a rehabilitation unit or occupational therapy department, through a whole range of facilities provided by the creative arts, to the hospital radio station provided for patients. It is an area open for the imaginative and enterprising carer to fill. Rowden and Jones (1983) write of some of the aspects of a diversional programme for cancer patients at The Royal Marsden Hospital and illustrate its use with a case study of a 16-year-old male.

The effect of music in hospitals is described by Sackett and Fitzgerald (1980). Their experience is based on work for those suffering from physical and mental disturbance. Music was seen to be beneficial particularly to those suffering from anxiety and depression. Clearly, there could be positive benefits for many cancer patients in this respect. Rowden (1984) has again reported on the use of music in oncology and outlines the benefits to patients. Cook (1986) looks particularly at the role of the nurse in her article on music as an intervention in the oncology setting.

National voluntary associations are also involved in this kind of therapy for those with mental illness or handicap. Diversional and music therapy for those with mental illness or handicap has a much longer history. Individuals or national voluntary organizations may want to exploit this expertise and apply the existing body of knowledge to the benefit of cancer patients.

What Can Be Done to Complement Existing Care?

An exhaustive list is impractical but a few further suggestions may stimulate individual initiatives.

HELP AGENCIES

In most developed countries there are some voluntary organizations concerned with helping cancer patients. Some of these are partly funded by government or by cancer centres and others are self-funding using voluntary donations from the public. All those involved in caring for cancer patients should be aware of the local and national agencies that can offer help. Details of these can then be displayed helpfully on notice-boards or in hospital booklets provided especially for patients. The range of services offered by these organizations may extend from information about cancer, its treatment and outcome to financial benefits that may be available for some patients to help them through this time when financial burdens are often increased. Some organizations provide a network of support groups while others may be involved in public and professional education.

Other help agencies, not specifically for cancer, should also be exploited as, although cancer patients may be unique in many respects, they also share a great deal with other chronic illness sufferers. There are so many examples that could be given in this context, including organizations to help the disabled, for example the Disabled Living Foundation (United Kingdom); organizations involved in some adaptation to lifestyle, for example the Relaxation for Living organization (United Kingdom); and those concerned with counselling and support. It is so helpful if those health professionals working with cancer patients have available the details of every possible help agency so that they can direct enquirers to them.

MUTUAL SUPPORT BY CANCER PATIENTS

Sometimes there are schemes where help can be given by fellow patients. For example, a patient who has had breast cancer in the past may volunteer to help a new breast cancer patient through her experience. Mutual support by cancer patients has become much more popular and van den Borne *et al.* (1987) describe one such scheme in Holland with lymphoma and breast cancer patients.

The disadvantages and limitations of these schemes can be as numerous as the advantages in that careful selection and training of volunteers are absolute prerequisites. However, there has been considerable success in schemes like those mentioned earlier, throughout the developed world.

SELF-HELP

The development of self-help groups and individual strategies for cancer patients has been considerable over the last 15 years. This appears to be an international trend as more and more cancer patients attempt to find ways to retain control during the sometimes bizarre experience that is cancer. A detailed review of the literature is impossible in this chapter, but a few references are given to guide the reader.

Kempson (1984) describes the proliferation of consumer health information services across the professional disciplines – health education, community work, nursing, librarianship and citizens' advice. She mentions the hospital-based services for cancer patients as well as some of the more general health issues and how these are catered for. Directories are available listing all self-help and other help organizations (Knight, 1980), and some are written exclusively for cancer patients and their relatives (CancerLink).

The mutual aid and self-help movement has been a source of interest to the Policy Studies Institute who conducted a study to research this whole area (Richardson and Goodman, 1983). The Canadian Council on Social Development has written a useful guide for self-help groups which can be applied to the cancer setting as to any other (Hill, 1984). There are many more examples available.

All health care professionals working with cancer patients have a dual responsibility. The first is certainly their own competent professional practice and all this implies. The second is to be aware of, and to make known to others, the vast array of individuals and agencies who may complement the care they give, if only patients are made aware of them. This may take time and effort in the first instance and may require health professionals to do some of their own research into the helpfulness and availability of some of these services. However, patients deserve and are demanding more ways to help themselves and be supported by others during an experience of cancer. The least the health care professional can do is to enable that to happen.

References

Barber, J. (1978) Hypnosis as a psychological technique in the management of cancer pain, *Cancer Nursing*, Vol. 1, no. 5, pp. 361–3.

Barnett, K. (1972) A theoretical construct of the concepts of touch as they relate to nursing, *Nursing Research*, Vol. 21, no. 2, pp. 102–9.

Benson, H. *et al.* (1974) The relaxation response, *Psychiatry*, Vol. 37, pp. 37–46.

Brigden, M.L. (1987) Unorthodox therapy and your cancer patient, *Postgraduate Medicine*, Vol. 81, no. 1, pp. 271–80.

Borne, H.W. van den *et al.* (1987) Effects of contacts between cancer patients on their psychosocial problems, *Patient Education and Counselling*, Vol. 9, pp. 33–51.

CancerLink, 17 Britannia Street, London, WC1X 9JN.

Cobb, S.C. (1984) Teaching relaxation techniques to cancer patients, *Cancer Nursing*, April, Vol. 7, no. 2, pp. 157–61.

Cook, J.D. (1986) Music as an intervention in the oncology setting, *Cancer Nursing*, Vol. 9, no. 1, pp. 23–8.

Dempster, C.R. *et al.* (1976) Supportive hypnotherapy during the radical treatment of malignancies, *International Journal of Clinical and Experimental Hypnosis*, Vol. XXIV, no. 1, pp. 1–9.

Denton, S. and Baum, M. (1983) Psychosocial aspects of breast cancer, in A.G. Margolese (ed). *Breast Cancer*, Churchill Livingstone, Edinburgh, pp. 173–85.

Donovan, M.I. (1980) Relaxation with guided imagery: a useful technique, *Cancer Nursing*, February, Vol. 3, no. 1, pp. 27–32.

Dwyer, J.C. (1986) Nutrition education of the cancer patient and family — myths and realities, *Cancer*, Vol. 15 (suppl.), pp. 1887–96.

Flaherty, G.G. and Fitzpatrick, J.J. (1978) Relaxation technique to increase comfort level of postoperative patients, *Nursing Research*, Vol. 27, no. 6, pp. 353–5.

Flaherty, M. (1981) Living with cancer, in R. Tiffany (ed.) *Cancer Nursing Update*, Baillière Tindall, London, pp. 40–2.

Friedman, B.D. (1980) Coping with cancer: a guide for health care professionals, *Cancer Nursing*, Vol. 3, no. 1, April, pp. 105–9.

Hill, K. (1984) *Helping You Helps Me: A Guide Book for Self-help Groups*, Canadian Council on Social Development, Ontario.

Jarvis, W. (1986) Helping your patients deal with questionable cancer treatments, *Ca - A Cancer Journal for Clinicians*, Vol. 36, no. 5, pp. 293–301.

Johnson, J. (1981) A patient's structured educational programme to help people learn to live with cancer, in R. Tiffany (ed.) *Cancer Nursing Update*, Baillière Tindall, London, pp. 38–40

Journal of the College of Health (1984) Attitudes to medicine, *Self Health - Journal of the College of Health*, no. 5, pp. 7–9.

Kaempfer, S.H. (1982) Relaxation training reconsidered, *Oncology Nursing Forum*, Vol. 9, no. 2, pp. 15–17.

Kempson, E. (1984) Consumer health information services, *Health Libraries Review*, Vol. 1, pp. 127–44.

Klisch, M.L. (1980) The Simonton method of visualization: nursing implications and a patient's perspective, *Cancer Nursing*, Vol. 3, no. 4, August, pp. 295–300.

Knight, S. (1980) *Help! I Need Somebody*, Henry Kimpton, London.

La Baw, W. *et al.* (1975) The use of self-hypnosis by children with cancer, *American Journal of Clinical Hypnosis*, Vol. 17, no. 4, pp. 233–9.

Lyall, J. (1983) Yoga can reduce need for drugs, lecturer says, *The Times* (London), 24 September, p. 12.

McCorkle, R. (1974) Effects of touch on seriously ill patients, *Nursing Research*, Vol. 23, no. 2, pp. 125–32.

McIntosh, J. (1977) *Communication and Awareness in a Cancer Ward*, Croom Helm, London.

Maguire, G.P. *et al.* (1978) Psychiatric problems in the first year after mastectomy, *British Medical Journal*, Vol. i, no. 6118, pp. 963–5.

Maguire, P. (1985) *Towards More Effective Psychological Intervention in Patients with Cancer*, Cancer Care Medical Education Series Ltd, pp. 12–15.

Maguire, P. *et al.* (1980a) A conspiracy of pretence, *Nursing Mirror,* Vol. 281, pp. 17–19.

Maguire, P. *et al.* (1980b) Effect of counselling on the psychiatric morbidity associated with mastectomy, *British Medical Journal*, Vol. 281, pp. 1454–55.

Maguire, P. *et al.* (1982) Cost of counselling women who undergo mastectomy, *British Medical Journal*, Vol. 284, pp. 1933–5.

Mishel, M.H. (1984) Perceived uncertainty and stress in illness, *Research in Nursing and Health*, Vol. 7, pp. 163–71.

Morris, T. *et al.* (1977) Psychological and social adjustment to mastectomy, a two-year follow up study, *Cancer*, Vol. 40, no. 5, pp. 2381–7.

Petty, F. and Noyes, R. (1981) Depression secondary to cancer, *Biological Psychiatry*, Vol. 16, no. 12, pp. 1203–21.

Piff, C. (1985) *Let's Face It*, Victor Gollancz, London.

Pruyn, J.F.A. (1982) Coping with stress in cancer patients, *Patient Education and Counselling*, Vol. 5, no. 2, pp. 57–62.

Redd, W.H. *et al.* (1982) Hypnotic control of anticipatory emesis in patients receiving cancer chemotherapy, *Journal of Consulting and Clinical Psychology*, Vol. 50, no. 1, pp. 14–19.

Rhodes, V.A. *et al.* (1984) Development of reliable and valid measures of nausea and vomiting, *Cancer Nursing*, Vol. 7, no. 1, pp. 33–41.

Richardson, A. and Goodman, M. (1983) *Self-help and Social Care*, Policy Studies Institute, London.

Rowden, L. (1984) Relaxation and visualisation techniques in patients with breast cancer, *Nursing Times*, Vol. 80, no. 37, pp. 42–4.

Rowden, R. (1984) Music pulled them through, *Nursing Mirror*, Vol. 159, no. 9, pp. 32–4.

Rowden, R. and Jones, L. (1983) A diversional programme for patients with cancer, *Nursing Times*, Vol. 80, no. 11, pp. 25–9.

Sackett, J. and Fitzgerald, V. (1980) Music in hospitals, *Nursing Times*, Vol. 76. no. 42, pp. 1845–8.

Selby, P.J. *et al.* (1984) The development of a method for assessing the quality of life of cancer patients, *British Journal of Cancer*, Vol. 50, pp. 13–22.

Simonton, O.C., Matthews-Simonton, S. and Creighton, I.L. (1978) *Getting Well Again*, Bantam Books, New York.

Sims, S. (1986) Slow stroke back massage for cancer patients, *Nursing Times*, Vol. 82, no. 47, pp. 47–50.

Sims, S. (1987) Relaxation training as a technique for helping patients cope with the experience of cancer: a selective review of the literature, *Journal of Advanced Nursing*, Vol. 12, no. 5, pp. 583–91.

Snyder, M. (1984) Progressive relaxation as a nursing intervention: an analysis, *Advances in Nursing Science*, Vol. 6, no. 3, pp. 47–58.

Spitzer, W.O. *et al.* (1981) Measuring the quality of life of cancer patients, *Journal of Chronic Disease*, Vol. 34, pp. 585–97.

Taylor, B. *et al.* (1977) Relaxation therapy and high blood pressure, *Archives of General Psychiatry*, Vol. 34, pp. 339–42.

Wakefield, J. (ed.) (1976) *Public Education About Cancer*, Union Internationale contre le Cancer (UICC), Geneva, pp. 71–93.

Webb, P.A. (1987) Patient education, *Nursing*, no. 20, pp. 748–50.

Weisman, A.D. (1976) Early diagnosis of vulnerability in cancer patients, *American Journal of the Medical Sciences*, Vol. 271, no. 2, pp. 187–96.

Weisman, A.D. and Worden, J.W. (1976) The existential plight in cancer: significance of the first 100 days, *International Journal of Psychiatry in Medicine*, Vol. 7, no. 1, pp. 1–15.

Wells, N. (1982) The effect of relaxation on postoperative muscle tension and pain, *Nursing Research*, Vol. 31, no. 4, pp. 236–8.

Wilson-Barnett, J. (1978) Patients emotional responses to barium X-rays, *Journal of Advanced Nursing*, Vol. 3, pp. 37–46.

Wilson-Barnett, J. (1984) Prevention and alleviation of stress in patients, *Nursing*, Vol. 10, pp. 432–8.

Worden, J.W. and Weisman, A.D. (1977) The fallacy in post-mastectomy depression, *American Journal of the Medical Sciences*, Vol. 273, no. 2, pp. 169–75.

Wortman, C.B. and Dunkel-Schetter, C. (1979) Interpersonal relationships and cancer: a theoretical analysis, *Journal of Social Issues*, Vol. 35, no. 1, pp. 120–55.

Chapter 11

Living with Cancer – Rehabilitation

DIANA STUMM BS, RPT
Staff Physical Therapist
Home Care Services, Stanford University Hospital, California

Introduction

Experiencing a life-threatening illness can be one of the most devastating events of a person's life. It can also have unexpected rewards. Unquestionably, having cancer changes the course of an individual's life but change can be the opportunity for growth, and growth is the ultimate human experience. The discovery of being able to direct and control that change can be the unanticipated gift of illness.

These concepts are usually the furthest thing from a person's mind on learning that he or she has cancer. The immediate reaction to the diagnosis alone is overwhelming fear, anger and resentment. These feelings can quickly escalate into depression and isolation. The diagnostic process, which usually involves time-consuming tests, anxiety-producing delays and painful or frightening procedures, easily leaves the patient confused and immobilized by fear. In addition, there can be enormous financial consequences. One day, you are in control of your life; the next day, chaos has taken over.

Those health care specialists who work closely with cancer patients bear a unique and important responsibility in that they are presented with the opportunity to guide and support patients in participating in their own recovery. The concepts of recovery and rehabilitation are relatively new in cancer treatment. Traditionally, cancer management has involved diagnosis and treatment and the care that goes with this, but there has been relatively little comprehensive planning for a full rehabilitation programme for patients. In reality, significant philosophical and priority gaps exist between this traditional model and the newer ideas of incorporating facilities for rehabilitation, which have been available for other chronic illness groups for some time. When all members of the team caring for cancer patients emphasize recovery and rehabilitation with positive language and attitudes, then patients themselves are encouraged to get back in control of their lives with support from the health carers.

As treatment begins, patients may anticipate disability. If intervention does not occur to assist them to participate actively in their own rehabilitation, they may soon begin to act like disabled people. As soon as they understand that disability is as much an attitude as a physical state, valuable time can be saved. Members of the health care team need to communicate messages of ability and restoration to the patient. It is up to those team members in the supportive and care-giving roles, namely therapists and nurses, to enter the picture early and to stress coping ability with positive attitudes. If patients constantly hear about what *they can* do, rather than what they cannot do, their self-esteem need not be seriously damaged. From the very beginning of treatment, doctors, therapists and nurses together need to demonstrate to patients alternative methods of doing simple tasks to enable self-care. The desired focus is on the accomplishment, however small it may seem, not on the inconvenience.

Assessment of Patients' Needs

Physical rehabilitation techniques need to be introduced into the patient's programme early in the treatment process. The following seven conditions are indications for referring the patient to physical and occupational therapists. They may be the result of the disease process itself, or of conventional cancer treatment, namely surgery, radiation and chemotherapy.

AMPUTATION OF A BODY PART

When any body part is lost, physical therapy involves preparing patients for a prosthetic device where this is available, and then training them in its use. Skin must be toughened, contractures stretched, and muscles strengthened and re-educated for their new roles. When a lower extremity prosthesis is involved gait training challenges both therapist and patient and inevitably results in creating a special relationship between them. The surgical removal of any body part, such as a breast, a portion of the jaw or a muscle group, will affect function of the adjacent joint. Lymph node dissection, usually in the axilla or groin, can cause scarring and shortening of tissue at the joint. The patient needs to learn to stretch the shortened tissue and strengthen the muscles which operate that joint.

The psychological impact of the amputation of any body part is often immeasurable. It is certainly of equal importance to the functional loss. Understandably, body image is distorted. One of the most effective methods for restoring one's sense of wholeness is through touch. Touch is the language of acceptance. Therapists include touch very early as they work on the amputated area as part of the natural course of stretching soft tissue and teaching the patient to 'communicate' with damaged muscles. If the therapist has the skill to teach the patient and family members the nurturing aspects of touch, serious psychological reactions of rejection can be avoided.

LOSS OF MUSCLE STRENGTH

Whenever muscles are directly affected by surgery or radiation, they lose strength and endurance. Even muscles adjacent to the treated area are often involved. If a muscle is too weak to perform, it may well react by cramping. The pain of muscle spasm can be very sharp and immobilizing, and consequently frightens the patient into believing the problem is more serious than it is. Information is the best tool in this situation and time taken to explain to patients that muscles spasm, when they are deprived of oxygen, is time well spent. Weak muscles are particularly susceptible to oxygen deprivation, which results in the formation of an enzyme called lactic acid. When muscles are engorged with waste products, the necessary amounts of muscle oxygen and glucose are not achieved and weakness continues. Patients can be taught to contract and relax muscles alternately. Smooth, rhythmical contractions flush the muscles and circulate fresh blood. Simple isometrics, such as pressing one hand or arm against the other, or crossing the ankles and doing a simultaneous push–pull action, accomplishes all of these goals and gives the patient a quick sense of being in control. Short exercise sessions performed regularly, such as five to ten repetitions of each movement two or three times a day, are the ideal.

Patients who experience loss of strength as a result of chemotherapy can be helped in much the same way as patients with any form of generalized weakness. Care must be taken to ration the patient's energy. Progressive walking, stationary cycling and swimming are the most simple and efficient methods to restore energy and strength.

Occasionally motor nerves which supply muscles are invaded directly by the cancer or are sacrificed during surgical excision of a tumour. A significant number of women who undergo axillary dissection for breast cancer experience temporary paralysis of the serratus anterior muscle. Fortunately, almost all patients have full recovery as the long thoracic nerve is not damaged directly but denervates in reaction to the adjacent vascular trauma. When damage is permanent, therapists can teach patients to compensate by learning to re-educate adjacent muscles. Temporary denervation is resolved with the passing of time.

Teaching patients to regain lost strength and endurance through repetition of active movements is essential to restoring muscle power. As safe ambulation and physical independence are dependent on muscle power, attention to this area must be an early priority. Because nurses are usually attending patients from the early stages of treatment they are the key people in the referral network. Whether patients are in hospital or are outpatients, the nurses are in a position to spot signs of weakness and physical debilitation which can be referred to the appropriate therapist.

LOSS OF JOINT MOBILITY

Post-surgical adhesions, post-radiation fibrosis and muscle contractures are the chief causes of reduced joint mobility. Early referral to physiotherapy can sometimes mean the difference between a temporary versus a permanent joint contracture. The softer and less mature the scar tissue, the more easily it is stretched. Post-mastectomy patients are an excellent example of patients susceptible to joint mobility problems. The shoulder joint itself is not directly involved in the surgery, but can lose function quickly if the patient is not directed to stretch adhered chest wall skin and a tight pectoralis major muscle. Even those patients who are treated with axillary dissection, lumpectomy and radiotherapy have mobility problems. The axillary incision is particularly troublesome as the skin can heal in a puckered fashion and the damaged lymphatic vessels may adhere to the axillary fold and act as bow-strings. Some women with axillary incisions may have more difficulty than those with standard radical mastectomy chest wall incisions. Unquestionably, radiotherapy complicates the picture, by adding radiation fibrosis thus making the tissue less elastic.

A mastectomy is unique surgery in many ways. After the skin flaps are dissected, subcutaneous skin fat is stripped away, usually by electrocautery. Fat is the skin's lubricant, and skin slides horizontally over underlying tissue to allow free joint movement. Adhesions form perpendicular to this movement, causing skin to adhere to the chest wall. The treatment of this problem has two aspects: first, the patient learns to stretch her arm in overhead flexion while lying supine with gravity assisting the motion. The stretch can be facilitated by the patient holding a stick in both hands, or grasping her affected wrist with the other hand. The added leverage reduces the discomfort and increases the efficiency of the stretch. Another important stretch position is supine with hands behind the head, pressing the elbows down, which lengthens the pectoralis major muscle.

The second component of treatment of adhered skin is a process called skin mobilization, performed either by the therapist or a family member. The patient herself can learn this technique, sitting in front of a mirror. She places the flat surface of three fingers just above the incision, applies firm pressure and makes slow circular motions to loosen the skin. The circular motions are repeated clockwise and counterclockwise all along the incision. This technique is particularly important for women who are contemplating reconstructive breast surgery, as the looser the skin, the more easily prosthetic implants can be used.

Surgical scarring or radiation fibrosis anywhere in the body may need to be manually stretched. Other effective treatments are connective tissue frictional massage and ultrasound. The use of ultrasound can be particularly effective to soften hardened tissue, and is safe as long as there is no metastatic disease, anaesthetized skin or ischaemic tissue in the planned treatment area.

DIFFICULTY IN AMBULATION

The causes of gait disturbances are numerous. Neurological deficits may result directly from brain or spinal cord tumours, both primary and metastatic. Any tumour of the weight-bearing bones, joints or leg muscles will inevitably cause pain and weakness. Joint stiffness may be the result of treatment, as in radiotherapy to the groin for prostate cancer. One of the most common and easily underestimated causes of poor gait is loss of confidence. The use of assistive devices – parallel bars, walking frames and sticks – may be the most efficient way to restore a patient's confidence in walking. Safety and independence are the primary concerns. A patient may view a walker or walking stick as a symbol of dependency but soon discovers he or she can walk alone with the device, as opposed to being dependent on another person. When assistive devices are clearly unsafe, the patient can support himself/herself between two people, pressing down on their forearms to simulate a walker. Occasionally this is the only way some patients can negotiate steps. Wheelchair-bound patients may feel a sense of control by learning to stand up facing the kitchen sink, with the wheelchair directly behind them. Just standing up relieves skin pressure, straightens the lumbar spine and stimulates muscle action and circulation.

Some patients with pathological fractures or unstable joints may be fitted with lightweight appliances to support the weak joint or extremity. Ambulation with such a device may be quite efficient, whereas it could be impossible without a lightweight, rigid support.

LYMPHOEDEMA

The most important aspect of lymphoedema is prevention, and the only person who can achieve this is the patient, providing he or she has adequate information. Lymphoedema is usually precipitated by cancer treatment, specifically axillary or groin node dissection, with or without radiotherapy. Lymph node dissection frequently obliterates a significant percentage of the extremity's lymphatic vessels as they link up with those of the trunk. Post-radiation fibrosis has also been shown to be a significant cause. Normal body fluid backs up in the extremity, causing oedema and hardening of the interstitial tissue. Fluid accumulation may well be avoided or significantly reduced if no infection occurs. The patient's understanding of the connection between infection and lymphoedema is critical to prevention. If the skin is broken, bacteria can enter the system. In response to this more fluid rapidly seeps into the interstitial cells and gets trapped there. Because the venous and lymphatic drainage systems have no pressure behind them, gravity quickly exacerbates the problem.

It is important to teach the patient skin care precautions, for the same reasons as you would teach foot care to a diabetic. Care of the hands and feet must include instruction to avoid breaking the skin; nail care, including the best way to trim nails and the use of cuticle cream; advice to wear protective gloves when working with sharp objects or caustic materials; and good first aid and basic wound care in case an accident does happen. It is essential to avoid cellulitis or widespread infection in an extremity. Unfortunately, the early warning signs are often insidious – usually warmth and redness. The arm or leg feels feverish and heavy, and may be pink or mottled in appearance. When these symptoms exists, the patient needs to be given antibiotic treatment immediately.

Chronic swelling is treatable, particularly if it is caught early. Circumferential enlargement of the limb greater than 13 mm may be considered significant. The texture of tissue more than the size, however, is the important sign. When the arm or leg feels thick and rigid, particularly if pitting occurs, treatment should be instigated. Not only is such a limb uncomfortable but it is also often immobile and useless. The least complicated treatment is for the patient to wear a pre-measured, tailored elastic sleeve or stocking, designed as a pressure gradient to force fluid into the drainage channels. The correct grade of elastic fabric keeps the tissue soft and the fluid moving. Turgid tissue is literally starving itself, as gelled fluid cannot move osmotically and therefore cannot have its usual transportation functions.

More aggressive treatment requires a pneumatic pump and inflatable sleeve or boot. Two types of equipment are available – intermittent or sequential compression. Intermittent compression is most effective when applied at comfortable pressures over longer periods of time. A practical outpatient programme would be one to two hours of compression each day or every other day. Patients can be treated for six to eight hours daily if intensive fluid reduction is indicated. Upper extremities should be treated at 45–60 mm Hg (intermittent) or up to 100 mm Hg (sequential). Lower extremities should be treated at 50–70 mm Hg (intermittent) and up to 150 mm Hg (sequential). Treatment should be performed with the patient supine to facilitate the effects of drainage. Intermittent pressure should be kept below the patient's diastolic blood pressure. Pressure should be lowered if the patient complains of pins and needles, throbbing or pain. The most efficient intermittent cycles are 60–90 seconds on and 30–45 seconds off. Patients who undergo pneumatic compression treatments should maintain the reduced level by wearing elastic supports between treatments and then for a long time after their measurements stabilize. The limb circumference should be measured at two or three sites before and after each treatment to record progress. Contra-indications to the use of compression pumps include an open wound or established cellulitis, ischaemic tissue, systemic vascular disease or arterial insufficiency, deep-vein thrombosis, or congestive cardiac failure.

Convincing a patient to wear an elastic support may be difficult. The patient's prime concern is cosmetic; while that of the health professional is the health of the limb. It is important that it is not just the appearance of the limb that is at stake. Manual centripetal massage by the patient or a family member is a helpful supplement but is usually not sufficient treatment by itself. Other preventative measures to emphasize are weight reduction and frequent elevation of the limb. Some consider advising patients to restrict their salt intake also. This remains controversial, however, and needs to be balanced with the need for a palatable diet. It is also essential to tell patients that active exercise may make the problem worse, as muscle activity demands fuel, which increases circulation into the limb, and exacerbates the fluid back-up. Instead, encourage the patient to lie supine, elevate the arm to a position perpendicular to the body and then to intermittently squeeze a small rubber ball in the hand. This will help to stimulate venous return.

PAIN

Clearly, pain is one of the most difficult symptoms to assess in cancer patients as it has so many causes. First, one must eliminate the obvious – that for which the tumour itself, or the treatment for it, is directly responsible. The next problem to be addressed is whether or not the pain can be treated by physical measures, by chemical control or by nerve blocks. If possible, it should be determined whether the patient's pain is associated with position or movement. If the patient can intensify or diminish the pain by movement, it may be treatable with physical means. Muscle spasm is usually the cause in this case. Bone pain is more persistent being dull or intense and worse at night or during inactivity. Nerve pain radiates along a predictable dermatome pattern and is the only kind of pain that actually moves around. When the source has been determined and physical measures prove ineffective, use of transcutaneous electrical nerve stimulation (TENS) may provide relief either alone or in conjunction with medication. Before blocking pain, it is important to determine whether the patient needs that pain as a warning mechanism. For example, the amount of weight borne on a painful extremity may need to be controlled by the patient's sensory feedback from the limb. The type of pain to block is pain that is continuous and worse when the person is inactive. More detail on pain control is given in Chapter 13.

LOSS OF SELF-ESTEEM

The final category for referral to rehabilitation services may not be a physical symptom, but may be one of the most important aspects of the impact of cancer that can be treated. In a complex, technological age, the cancer patient quickly feels victimized by the diagnostic process. If the person was symptom free before diagnosis and then undergoes a major surgical procedure, he or she may suddenly find himself/herself disabled in a matter of days. Shock gives way to depression. Feelings of self-confidence and control over one's life may be replaced by fear, resentment and withdrawal. Being subjected to a battery of complex machines, strange faces, a foreign language of medical terminology and physical and emotional pain, is overwhelming at best. Cancer patients may feel as though they have cascaded over the edge of a waterfall. In times past, rehabilitation services were only considered after the crash on the rocks below. Now they can be used to ease the descent and cushion the fall.

Early initiation of physiotherapy can restore independent ambulation before the patient is bed or wheelchair bound. The timely use of occupational therapy helps put patients back in charge of their own self-care and basic functional needs. Following consultation with the patient, referral to a social worker, counsellor or psychologist may also be appropriate in assisting the patient to cope with the disease and its effects. A person who continues to feel capable and physically independent is much less likely to feel hopelessly isolated.

Mobilizing Patients' Resources

Putting cancer patients back in control of their own recovery requires the use of some special skills. Many therapists feel overwhelmed when asked to work with cancer patients. Health care professionals are not immune to cultural attitudes about life-threatening illness and can easily feel inadequate to deal with the complexity of problems. The solution is to stay focused on the patient's functional needs – regardless of their cause. The first step is the process of setting goals. Patients may have to be invited or even persuaded to participate in this process, as they may expect someone else to do it for them; they may therefore need assistance in structuring a realistic timetable for these goals. Regaining range of function in a joint immobilized by surgery and radiation may take longer than patients imagine they can wait. Patients can also discover, however, that it is possible to use that joint effectively before maximum potential is restored.

The next step is to educate those supporting the patient. In their eagerness to help, many loving and distraught family members or friends may inadvertently encourage physical dependence on the part of the patient. If they are too quick to perform basic tasks for the patient, rather than let the patient attempt these himself/herself, a pattern of dependency is easily established. Unfortunately, one's culture tends to encourage one to identify with either the helper or the helpless role. Therapists and nurses are in an excellent position to break these patterns and offer alternative roles and methods. Many patients will surprise themselves when they are left alone and discover that they can perform a simple task such as buttoning a shirt with one hand or getting up from a low chair by shifting their weight forward onto their feet.

Another important resource to conserve is energy. Cancer treatments can drain patients of energy so that they often feel weak and fatigued. They need help to understand that fatigue is the body's way of conserving energy. Many people are angry and resentful when they feel debilitated. They often blame themselves and feel very frustrated. They need to understand that these feelings are appropriate and they need to give themselves permission to be tired, to rest appropriately and to plan activities based on what they know they can cope with. The care-givers must also learn when to encourage the patient to work harder and when to rest. Activity levels must be increased gradually, such as doubling the distance walked every day. Patients may also be taught deep-breathing, and visualization skills. These relaxation exercises can be valuable tools for controlling energy-wasting tension and anxiety.

When patients' own resources are mobilized and operating on a daily basis, they may be able to restore their sense of well-being. To do this entails creating the best possible balance between external and internal disease interventions. Well-ness is promoted by physical movement, participation, communication, touch, independence and self-esteem. Health care professionals need to promote and model well-ness in their language, attitudes and behaviour.

Those patients who recover from their experience with cancer and return to the work force may well benefit from the services of a more specialist rehabilitation service where future employment prospects can be explored and – where necessary – new training given. In the United States, for example, the Rehabilitation Act of 1973 provides cancer patients with this legal right. In the United Kingdom, the local disablement resettlement officer can assist. Whether the patient returns to the same employment, or seeks a new job location or career, timely referral to a vocational counsellor with a background in rehabilitation can eliminate many of the barriers created by apprehension and lack of information on the part of both the employee and the employer. An additional knowledge of, or interest in, cancer in particular can be an invaluable asset to such a counsellor.

An entirely different set of needs is experienced by patients whose disease progresses to death. Patients and families who seek a hospice environment can still benefit from physical therapy. If the patient is mobile, safe ambulation with assistive devices can be taught by the physical therapists to the support personnel at home or in a hospice setting. Bed mobility skills can be reinforced to maintain good skin care and some degree of independence. Simple techniques, such as transferring the patient from bed to wheelchair, may be overwhelming for family members if they have not had proper instruction and demonstration.

The therapist or oncology nurse can also assist the family in setting up a care centre in the home. For many people the bedroom is not the best place to be. Cancer patients can feel very isolated and avoided in a bedroom. The dining room or family room can be turned into the patient's care centre. In the centre of the house, family members cannot avoid contact with the patient, and he or she feels more a part of everyone's activities.

Confronting Attitudes

Rehabilitation must be a positive, self-affirming process. In the face of a life-threatening disease, this attitude requires special effort on the part of patients and the health care delivery teams. When attitudes are destructive or self-defeating, they need to be confronted.

The concept of an integrated and comprehensive rehabilitation service for cancer patients is still not universally provided or even accepted as a necessity. For this reason, all those involved may need to promote actively the available services and convince others of their value. Referrals may not initally come from the medical teams until they are convinced of the value and credibility of therapists and practitioners in this field.

Because of these evolving services, nurses and therapists may well struggle with their own feelings of inadequacy. This is particularly true for those professionals who have not had a great deal of experience in caring for cancer patients. Bringing the disease down to size means assessing functional needs. Look at the patient in terms of what he or she cannot do and what he or she needs to learn to do. With the patient as partner, set goals, establish priorities and agree on a particular timescale. Ongoing treatments may require constant readjustments of goals and priorities. This is when patients need to hear the word 'we'. Help them to remember that they are not alone but that they have support.

Members of the patient's support system, whether they are family or friends, may fall victim to the defeating attitude of over-protection. Pointing this out to them usually frees them of the burden of self-imposed responsibility. It is important for family members to be present during physical therapy treatment sessions so that they can see what is the patient's true level of independence. Spouses, parents and children of cancer patients often struggle with feelings of helplessness, guilt and resentment. These are perfectly normal emotions and it is important that they express these feelings and receive acknowledgement of them. When emotions are denied and suppressed they fester and erupt, causing unnecessary hurt.

Patients themselves may be immobilized in a state of anxiety, anger, denial, hopelessness or withdrawal. Therapists may only need to acknowledge what they observe to the patient. A gentle, direct, well-timed confrontation may be very freeing and may lift a heavy weight off the patient's mind. The patient may subconsciously be begging for someone to do this.

Sometimes patients subconsciously resent the health care professionals who are trying to assist them, simply because they are healthy and in control of their lives. They represent everything the patient wants to be, but cannot be. The therapist needs to be aware of this situation and sensitive to its implications.

Conclusion

A search of current literature on the subject of physical rehabilitation of cancer patients indicates little is being written by the rehabilitation specialists themselves. Much of the literature is about diagnostic and treatment procedures, research and the psychological impact of the disease.

The ultimate goal of rehabilitation of cancer patients is for those patients to be in control of their lives, and to be functioning at their maximum potential. When members of the rehabilitation team encourage patient involvement, that potential is most achievable. When they perform their care-giving roles with attitudes of honesty, support and involvement, they create an atmosphere in which patients can take responsibility for their own well-ness.

Further Reading

Dietz, J. (ed) (1981) *Rehabilitation Oncology*, John Wiley & Sons, New York.

Duncan, M.A., Lotze, M.T., Gerber, L.H, and Rosenberg, S.A (1983) Incidence, recovery and management of serratus anterior muscle palsy after axillary node dissection, *Physical Therapy*, Vol. 63, no. 8, pp. 1243–7.

Flomenhoft, D. (1984) Understanding and helping people who have cancer, *Physical Therapy*, Vol. 64, no. 8. pp. 1232–4.

Gunn, A.E. (ed.) (1984) *Cancer Rehabilitation*, Raven Press, New York.

Molinaro, J., Kleinfeld, A. and Lebed, S. (1986) Physical therapy and dance in the surgical management of breast cancer, *Physical Therapy*, Vol. 66, no. 6, pp. 967–9.

Priest-Naeve, P. and Carter, S.K. (1982) Principles of cancer rehabilitation, in S. Carter, E. Glatstein, and R. Livingstone (eds.) *Principles of Cancer Treatment*, McGraw Hill, New York.

Richmond, D.M. *et al.* (1985) Sequential pneumatic compression for lymphoedema: a controlled trial, *Archives of Surgery*, Vol. 120, pp. 1116–9.

Stumm, D. (1982a) Considering the whole woman: rehabilitation of the breast cancer patient, *Clinical Management in Physical Therapy*, Vol. 2, no. 1, pp. 20–2.

Stumm, D. (1982b) Critical timing: physical therapy in rehabilitation of the cancer patient, *Western States Conference on Cancer Rehabilitation, Conference Proceedings,* Bull Publishing Co., Palo Alto, California.

Taylor, C.M. (1984) The rehabilitation of persons with cancer: is this the best we can do? *Journal of Rehabilitation*, Vol. 50, no. 17, pp. 60–2, 71.

Toot, J. (1984) Physical therapy and hospice, concept and practice, *Physical Therapy*, Vol. 64, no. 5, pp. 665–71.

United States Department of Health and Human Services (1980) *Coping with Cancer: A Resource for the Health Professional*, Publication no. 80-2080, Public Health Service, National Institutes of Health, Bethesda, Maryland.

Wingate, L. (1985) Efficacy of physical therapy for patients who have undergone mastectomies, *Physical Therapy*, Vol. 65, no. 6, pp. 896–900.

Chapter 12

The Cancer Patient in the Community

ELIZABETH A HOULTON BNurs, RGN, NDNCert,
HVCert, ObstCert, OncCert
Senior Nurse
Community Liaison/Self-Care Unit, The Royal Marsden Hospital,
London and Surrey

The Impact of Cancer on the Patient, the Family and the Community

Cancer is often regarded, by both the general public and health professionals, as an acute illness. For some patients, it is. It may have a short history and an even shorter prognosis. However, for the majority of cancer patients and their families, the experience of cancer is that of a chronic illness, with the usual acute exacerbations associated with chronicity. Kaplan (1982) has argued that cancer is perceived to be the most threatening illness that it is possible to suffer; the illness career of a cancer patient has been helpfully described by Sque (1985).

The initial pattern of diagnosis, treatment and its evaluation that characterizes most illnesses is potentially extended for the cancer patient into a lifetime of medical care. Even when initial treatment for acute cancer is successful, cancer patients face regular surveillance of their health. They will always be cancer patients and although learning to cope with the potential threat to their lives, they suffer constant reminders of their illness by undergoing frequent, regular check-ups, in the outpatient clinic. If the initial treatment is not successful, the cancer patient will enter the diagnosis, treatment and evaluation cycle again, perhaps many times. Cancer, like many other chronic illnesses, is punctuated by stages of relapse and remission, each having the potential to compromise the patient's quality of life, and increase the risk of residual damage and disability.

This chapter examines the impact of cancer on patients and their families. The significance of diagnosis and treatment is discussed, and a framework of health care to support the patient through these stages examined. The relationship between the acute treatment centre and the community-based health care services is explored, and examples are given of the formal and informal support services that are available in the community setting in the United Kingdom.

THE IMPACT OF CANCER ON PATIENTS AND THEIR FAMILIES

Edstrom and Miller (1981) state that chronic illnesses present the biggest health problem in our society. As one such illness, cancer demands of the individual patient and his or her family continuous adjustment to the stresses of the disease and its treatment. Wright and Dyck (1984) identify that the diagnostic phase of cancer is emotionally and physically significant for the patient. They also point out that treatment of the disease and its recurrence are psychologically more disruptive and damaging than for other chronic diseases. Holland *et al.* (1977) define a crucial stage in the cancer patient's experience. They call it the 'mid-stage' of cancer – the period between initial treatment and the terminal stage of life. This period is characterized by uncertain treatment outcomes, recurrence, remission and repeated periods of hospitalization. They see it as a time when cancer patients and their families move from one crisis to another with little time for psychological adjustment.

Patients with cancer are now living longer. For example, in the 1930s fewer than one in five patients survived five years following a diagnosis of cancer. In the 1980s, one in three patients can expect to survive more than five years (American Cancer Society, 1981). Because people are living longer the *mid-stage* of the disease will be the longest period in the cancer experience for patients and their families. The responsibility for the day-to-day care of cancer patients rests with the family. Although health care professionals may have that responsibility delegated to them on the patient's admission to hospital, patients and their families are ultimately responsible for care during most of the illness. This can be an enormous burden for them.

Olsen (1970) states that the family is a highly organized system with homeostatic mechanisms for maintaining stability, while at the same time being able to meet the physical and emotional needs of its members. A serious illness, such as cancer, can threaten the whole balance of the family unit, causing disequilibrium and disrupting normal behaviour. Such a threat is defined by family stress theory as a crisis event (Burr, 1973).

The stress caused by a family member having cancer can prevent individuals from successfully fulfilling their normal roles. The patient is often deprived of his or her role within the family and forced to adopt the role of 'person with a serious illness'. Family members may also find their roles compromised because they may have to become a 'carer', or fulfil the role recently vacated by the sick person. If a family member has cancer, the stress caused by the cancer itself, and by the treatment for it, can cause an entire family to experience a crisis situation as described by Burr (1973). This may prevent family members fulfilling their usual role of supporting each other. Many families cannot cope with either the diagnosis of cancer or its threat to the stability of the family as a whole. Wright and Dyck (1984) have identified considerable evidence that families are disrupted by the effects of the treatment on offer for cancer, as well as by the experience of the disease itself.

THE IMPACT OF CANCER ON THE COMMUNITY

The community is also required to absorb the impact of cancer. Anecdotal evidence suggests that much of the cancer patient's time will be spent in the home and therefore the responsibility to support patients and their families will fall to the community to which they belong. The community, however, is not a nebulous collection of professional and lay organizations that will come to the rescue of individuals during a significant crisis in their lives. The community consists of individuals and their families, who will most probably all have had some kind of experience of cancer in their lives. The nature of this experience and the effect that it has had on each individual will determine the corporate response to the disease. Myth, hearsay and unpleasant encounters with cancer and its treatment will produce a more profound corporate response than that of each individual. Health professionals working with cancer patients in hospital have a responsibility to mobilize health care resources when the patient leaves hospital.

A chronic disease like cancer has considerable impact on the use of resources in the community. The current trend for community health services in the United Kingdom is to concentrate efforts and resources towards the care of the chronic sick. For example, in the past five years, the care of mentally handicapped and psychiatric patients has been devolved into the community. In the West, demographic changes in the population over the past 20 years resulting in a larger proportion of old people, have placed further demands on resources. The old, the mentally handicapped and the mentally ill compete for available resources, with patients suffering from chronic illnesses. The total demands placed on the health care system are therefore considerable (Houlton, 1987).

Coping with Cancer – Patients and their Families

Burr (1973) defines a stress event for the family as anything that produces a change in the boundaries, structure, goals, purposes, roles or values of the family system. Any of these changes can precipitate a crisis, particulary if the stress event and the family's perception of it overwhelm the family's resources to deal with it.

The capacity of individuals and families to respond to crises varies considerably. It is dependent on their prior experience of cancer, their ability to adapt to change and their integration with each other and the outside world. Other influencing factors are the family's socioeconomic status, the nature of the extended family and community support. Health professionals must be aware that, for the patient and his or her family, the uncertain nature of many types of cancer means that there may well be many periods of crisis throughout the course of the disease. As the responsibility for caring for cancer patients falls mainly on their families, extra resources to support them should be available.

Bloch (1984) has identified several factors which can seriously affect the competence of the family unit to provide health care. These include the ability of individuals to alter their role within the family in response to a need. They must be able to make sense of the psychologically painful threats to their personal and corporate identity as family members. They should be able to communicate effectively with health care workers to ensure that they receive the help that they need. They may also need to develop skills to monitor the progress of the disease. Learning new skills at the same time as mourning the potential and actual loss of a loved one is demanding for any family member.

If family members feel that they do not have the necessary skills or resources to cope with cancer and its effects, then a crisis will occur, and they too will be at risk from deteriorating physical and mental health (Kaplan, 1982).

The patient and his or her family are the health professional's prime resource in coping with the effects of cancer and its treatment. By promoting the concept of self-care, that is allowing patients to set their own health goals, identify their own needs and be instrumental in meeting them, the health professional maximizes the greatest strength in helping patients to cope with their disease. Self-care activities may include self-medication, oral hygiene or stoma management. Planning teaching in hospital will increase patients' capabilities to care for themselves on returning home and will encourage them to achieve their optimal quality of life. It is also possible to involve patients and their families in activities of health care that are traditionally thought of as the domain of health professionals. Examples of such activities are coping with indwelling urinary catheters, managing skin-tunnelled intravenous catheters or changing dressings. Adopting and promoting a self-care model with the cancer patient prior to discharge allows the patient to develop autonomy, self-reliance and decision-making skills which will be essential on returning home.

Care of the cancer patient at home is primarily about motivating individuals and their families to look after themselves, and then giving them the support to do so. Anecdotal evidence suggests that cancer patients are more likely to be at home than in hospital, so there is little point in promoting the patient's adjustment and coping within an institutionalized setting such as a hospital ward, if it is unlike the home. Although a very important part of the illness experience, cancer care in hospital should be geared towards making the most of patients' potential in their own environment – the community.

Promoting Cancer Care in the Community

Promotion of the relationship between health workers in the hospital and those in the community is essential if continuity of care for cancer patients and their families is to be achieved and maintained. Many patients are diagnosed at one centre, and then find that the treatment recommended is only available at a different one. The potential for frequent, acute exacerbations of cancer, coupled with the often multi-centred approach to treatment, can leave patients and their families bereft of the appropriate support that they need at home. Planning nursing care before the patient's discharge home should be an integral part of the nursing care planning in hospital. It is possible to assess from the outset, some of the significant features of a patient's disease and treatment that will affect coping strategies in the home. A multidisciplinary approach to discharge planning involves nurses, doctors, physiotherapists, occupational therapists, dietitians and, of course, the patients themselves and their families.

It is important to involve community health professionals in planning and implementing care and support with patients and their families as soon as possible. Cancer patients and their families benefit from the continued support and encouragement of community nurses and doctors, even if they themselves are providing most of their own health care needs. The role of the professional is to guide them in identifying potential problems and to assist in the planning of appropriate care. Because of the chronic nature of the illness and its impact on the family unit, considerable adjustment is required so that patients can achieve the best possible life during this experience. Community nurses in particular are in an ideal position to help them to do this.

Many patients and families are unable or unwilling to take responsibility for many of their health care activities when they return home. The responsibility may then return to health professionals. Wherever possible, community doctors and nurses should have the opportunity to consult with hospital staff and patients about their needs before they go home. Cancer treatment protocols, surgical techniques and radiotherapy regimens are often highly specialized and tailored to individual patients' needs. Community nurses and doctors need up-to-date information so that they can provide continuity of care and keep abreast of the changes in treatment as they occur.

Nurses are now familiar with problem-orientated care planning, or the nursing process. Both in hospital and in the community many nurses are using problem-orientated care plans as a means of record-keeping, and sharing nursing care information with other staff members. Care plans are also the most effective way of transferring information from the hospital to the community, and back again. It is important that written information about planned patient care and the potential needs of the patient is communicated as soon as possible between hospital and community in both directions. An example of such a liaison sheet is shown in Figure 12.1. It includes information about the patient's knowledge and understanding of the illness, medications, an assessment of current health status, and suggestions for meeting the patient's needs in the home setting.

Relevant, effective communication between hospital and community nurses is the only efficient way to ensure continuity of care for patients and their families. Many hospitals have appointed a liaison nurse, whose role is to facilitate the smooth transition of patient care from hospital to home. Community liaison nurses can advise hospital staff on the constraints of nursing cancer patients at home and advise community staff on the most appropriate way to deal with

COMMUNITY CARE REFERRAL

Hospital No. _____

NAME_____Date of Birth_____ Religion _____

Address_____Phone No. _____

Address discharged to _____

Next of Kin _____ Relationship _____ Phone No. _____

General Practitioner_____

Date of admission/attendance _____Discharge date_____Ward_____

Consultant_____Next OPD appt. _____Transport_____

Diagnosis_____Allergies _____

Summary of Treatment (past and present)_____

_____

_____

_____

_____

_____

_____

_____

_____

_____

Patient's understanding of Illness _____

_____

_____

Family's understanding of Illness_____

_____

_____

Family/Social support at home _____

Fig 12.1   The Royal Marsden Hospital community care referral form – front cover.

ASSESSMENT FACTORS	
PSYCHOLOGICAL	RESPIRATION
	SIGHT AND HEARING
	COMMUNICATION
NUTRITION	MOBILITY/STAIRS
	ABILITY TO WASH/DRESS
ELIMINATION	ABILITY TO MANAGE TOILET
	PRESSURE AREAS
PAIN	APPLIANCES (e.g. STOMA BAGS)

DRUG REGIME	DOSE	ROUTE	FREQUENCY	HOSPITAL SERVICES INVOLVED
				COMMUNITY SERVICES INVOLVED

Figure 12.1 (continued.) The Royal Marsden Hospital community care referral form – inside front cover.

PROBLEM/NEED	SUGGESTED NURSING ACTION

SIGNED: _____ DESIGNATION: _____ DATE: _____

FOR FURTHER INFORMATION CONTACT:

Figure 12.1   (continued.) The Royal Marsden community care referral form – inside back cover.

the consequences of particular treatments. However, the work of the community liaison nurse is supplementary to the rapport and relationship established between the patient, the hospital, and the community team, and is no substitute for everyone working together on discharge planning.

On returning home after treatment, the cancer patient's family is likely to be the major provider of care (Giacquinta, 1977), even with the appropriate support of a community health service. Edstrom and Miller (1981) identified five areas of concern to family members trying to care for a cancer patient at home:

1. how to prevent skin breakdown;
2. how to supervise medications;
3. how to manage pain and discomfort;
4. how to encourage activity and how to deal with activity limitations;
5. how to deal with family changes or problems arising when living with a family member suffering from a chronic illness.

Hinds (1985) identified physical, financial, affective and psychological needs in families of patients with cancer. These needs were not being met by any health professionals. The persistent presence of these concerns prevented family members from successfully fulfilling their role as carer. This resulted in the development of guilt and anxiety as carers felt they were failing to do their best for their sick relative.

Community nurses can teach family members the necessary skills to overcome these concerns and support them in their efforts to meet patients' needs. The presence of the right nursing aid or appliance in a home can do much to alleviate anxiety among relatives, and prevent undue physical strain on the patient.

Many countries have organizations and charities that will provide information, support and encouragement for cancer patients, their families and the professionals caring for them. Some of these give financial assistance to relieve the burden of cancer on the family. In the United Kingdom, a cancer charity called Cancer Relief has such a financial support system and provides considerable assistance to patients and families. It has also been instrumental in funding and supporting nurses in the community who specialize in palliative care. A separate cancer charity, The Marie Curie Memorial Foundation, provides nursing homes, which give convalescent, respite and continuing care for cancer patients. In conjunction with local health authorities they also run a visiting nurse scheme which supplements the district nursing service by providing nurses at night for families with patients in the late stages of their disease. Details of some of these voluntary organizations are given at the end of this chapter.

Each locality keeps its own information on the provision available for practical help and support for cancer patients, in addition to that provided by statutory services. Cancer information services, such as BACUP (British Association for Cancer United Patients) or CancerLink, keep a current register of local facilities that are available to patients and their families in the United Kingdom. Elsewhere, national cancer charities provide a similar service.

Cancer patients benefit from community support during all phases of their illness. It is traditional to think of the community nurses' involvement with these families as being in the later, terminal stages of the disease. However, this is changing as current treatments for cancer are often given intermittently and patients do not stay in hospital for long periods. Adjusting to the diagnosis, and coming to terms with having the disease, take a considerable amount of time. Patients and families need professional support to cope with the side-effects and sequelae of treatment. Living with cancer, even during long periods of remission, requires psychological adjustment and a re-examination of life goals and values (Kaplan, 1982). Patients and families benefit from informed, professional support (Edstrom and Miller, 1981). If a relationship has been established with community health professionals at the beginning of the illness, a patient will be able to identify when professional help is needed, and can contact the nurse or doctor accordingly. By establishing a trusting relationship with patients and their families, the community nurse is in a better position to help identify potential problems and to respond quickly.

However, it is unrealistic to expect health carers in the community to be able to respond appropriately to all of the cancer patient's needs. Looking after the cancer patient in the increasingly complex context of medical treatments demands that nurses and others who do not specialize in oncology nursing have access to up-to-date information. For nurses, one way this may be achieved is by making contact with an oncology nurse or nurse specialist in the locality. Hospital and community nurses need to communicate freely about their patients' needs. Sensitive, problem-orientated discharge planning will go a long way towards minimizing communication difficulties between hospital and community professionals. However, many of the cancer patient's problems in the community will relate to coping with cancer at home.

These problems may not necessarily be within the range of expertise of hospital nurses.

Developments in the role of clinical nurse specialists, who practise across the hospital–community boundary, have done much to begin to tackle this problem. Clinical nurse specialists should act as mentors for their colleagues when caring for patients with cancer. Their role is to improve the care that the patient receives through practice, teaching, research and management. In the United Kingdom several health authorities have appointed specialist community nurses to care for cancer patients at home. They act as a resource for their colleagues, as well as having a patient case-load. When dealing with a chronic illness like cancer, it seems appropriate to encourage as much of an exchange of information and skills as possible between all health professionals. This ensures continuity of access to specialist expertise for patients and their families and was one recommendation in a recent report on the future of community nursing (Cumberlege, 1986).

The central, constant resource in the care of a cancer patient at home is the family. Family members, too, have to cope with the impact of the disease, its demands in terms of their role change, and their own needs and feelings with reference to the care that they give, and their relationship with the patient. Many close relatives of cancer patients find that their capacity to cope decreases as the patient's needs increase.

Schubin (1978) found that the widows of cancer patients were more vulnerable to anxiety and stress-related health problems than the widows of men who had died of heart disease. This was because they felt increasing helplessness throughout the illness. They felt abandoned by doctors and nurses as the patient's illness progressed, and suffered increased stress as the stigma of the disease grew with time. It is well documented by both Zastrow (1984) and Yasko (1983) that health professionals will withdraw their support from cancer patients and their families when they feel powerless to alleviate distress or manage symptoms.

As the majority of the care of the cancer patient falls on the family members, professionals should focus support on the carers from the time of diagnosis of the disease onwards. Society must accept that living with cancer, for most patients and families, is just as important as coping with treatment. Patients live with their disease at home and need to adapt their lifestyle to cope with it.

Some Voluntary Cancer Help Agencies in the United Kingdom

BACUP (British Association of Cancer United Patients)
121/123 Charterhouse Street,
London, EC1M 6AA.
Tel. 01-608 1661

CancerLink
17 Britannia Street,
London, WC1X 9JN.
Tel. 01-833 2451

The Marie Curie Memorial Foundation
28 Belgrave Square,
London, SW1X 8QG.
Tel. 01-235 3325

Cancer Relief Macmillan Fund
Anchor House,
15–19 Britten Street,
London, SW3 3TZ.
Tel. 01-351 7811

References

American Cancer Society (1981) *Cancer Facts and Figures,* American Cancer Society, New York.

Bloch, D.A. (1984) The family therapist as health care consultant, *Family Systems Medicare,* Vol. 2; pp. 161–9.

Burr, W. (1973) *Theory Construction and the Sociology of the Family*, John Wiley & Sons, New York, pp. 199–217.

Cumberlege, J. (1986) *Neighbourhood Nursing — A focus for care*, Report of the Community Nursing Review, HMSO, London.

Edstrom, S. and Miller, M.W. (1981) Preparing the family to care for the cancer patient at home: a home care course, *Cancer Nursing*, Vol. 4, no. 1, pp. 49–52.

Giacquinta, B. (1977) Helping families face the crisis of cancer. *American Journal of Nursing*, Vol. 77, no. 10, pp. 1585–8.

Hinds, C. (1985) The needs of families who care for patients with cancer at home: are we meeting them? *Journal of Advanced Nursing,* Vol. 10, pp. 575–81.

Holland, J. *et al.* (1977) Psychological aspects of anorexia in cancer patients, *Cancer Research* Vol. 37, pp. 2425–8.

Houlton, E.A. (1987) Cancer — the challenge to primary health care, *Journal of Royal Society of Health*, Vol. 4, pp. 151–4.

Kaplan, D.M. (1982) Intervention strategies for families, in J. Cohen, J.W. Cullen and L.R. Martin (eds.) *Psychological Aspects of Cancer,* Raven Press, New York.

Olsen, E. (1970) The impact of serious illness on the family system, *Postgraduate Medicine,* Vol. 74, pp. 169–74.

Schubin, S. (1978) Cancer widows, *Nursing,* Vol. 8, pp. 56–60.

Sque, M. (1985) What's in a name? *Nursing Mirror,* Vol. 160, pp. 28–30.

Wright, K. and Dyck, S. (1984) Expressed concerns of adult cancer patients' family members, *Cancer Nursing,* Vol. 7, pp. 371–4.

Yasko, J.M. (1983) Variables which predict burnout experienced by oncology clinical nurse specialists, *Cancer Nursing,* Vol. 6, no. 2, pp. 109–16.

Zastrow, C. (1984) Understanding and preventing burnout, *British Journal of Social Work,* Vol. 14, pp. 141–55.

Chapter 13

Symptom Control

PETER J. HOSKIN BSc, MBBS, MRCP, FRCR
Cancer Research Campaign Research Fellow and Honorary Senior Registrar
The Royal Marsden Hospital, London and Surrey

and

BARBARA DICKS BA, RGN, RM, OncCert, FETC
Nurse Adviser to Caner Relief Macmillan Funds, and Course Tutor
The Royal Marsden Hospital, London and Surrey

Introduction

The main characteristic of cancer is that of uncontrolled growth and spread to sites distant from its origin. The common patterns of spread by direct invasion, lymphatic and blood-borne dissemination result in frequent involvement of bone, liver, lungs and brain with metastatic tumour. It is, therefore, not surprising that the patient with advanced cancer may present a complex array of interrelated symptoms which, if left untended, will result in misery and disability before death intervenes. Of the many symptoms which can arise in this situation, pain is the most prominent and often the most feared by the patient, occurring in some 60 per cent of patients managed in a general oncology unit and in up to 85 per cent of patients referred for hospice care (Twycross and Lack, 1983). In addition, around two-thirds of patients will complain of anorexia, one-half will have symptomatic dry mouth and constipation and one-third nausea, vomiting, insomnia, dyspnoea, cough or oedema (Hanks, 1983). Other symptoms which, although less frequent, cause considerable distress include confusion and drowsiness, diplopia, urinary frequency and incontinence and itching.

It will be clear from these statistics that most patients will have more than one symptom which requires active attention. The basis of management in these patients is a careful detailed assessment of their presenting problems with attention to identifying each individual symptom and, of equal importance for effective treatment, identifying the underlying cause for each symptom. Having identified the underlying cause for each symptom, some of which may be closely interrelated, rational treatment kept as simple as possible and individualized for each patient can then be instituted. Inevitably, however, not all symptoms will be identified accurately or their underlying pathology clearly defined. For this reason, having implemented an initial treatment regimen, it is vital to follow this with regular and frequent review and appropriate modifications to treatment. Furthermore, patients with advanced cancer are in a dynamic state as a result of which their symptoms profile will change from week to week and even from day to day. This means that regular monitoring must continue beyond the initial control of symptoms in order that the best treatment can be maintained.

Management of Chronic Cancer Pain

Four basic steps in the approach to pain control may be defined.

1. PAIN ASSESSMENT

The pain associated with progressive cancer is different from the acute pain such as that due to trauma, headache or toothache, with which most people are familiar. A simple model divides pain into two components: the physical stimulus (the cognitive component) and the related emotional response (the affective component). As the affective component is particularly important and may predominate in cancer pain, particular attention must be paid to factors that modulate pain sensitivity such as anger, depression, anxiety and fear. Furthermore, it has been shown that fewer than 20 per cent of patients will have a single site of pain and that around one-half of patients will have three or more individual sites of pain (Twycross and Fairfield, 1982).

The clinical picture which the patient presents reflects a summation of these physical stimuli and the associated emotional reaction. Careful analysis of individual pains and their specific underlying cause, without which rational treatment cannot be proposed, is, therefore, fundamental. This involves a detailed history from the patient and, where appropriate, selected investigations such as X-rays, ultrasound and computerized tomography (CT) scans to define the underlying pathology. Body charts in which sites and severity of individual pains are marked on a body diagram are a useful means of analysing individual pains. More complex pain assessments using visual analogue and ratings scales have the added advantage of including patient assessment of pain and provide a valuable tool not only in initial assessment, but also in subsequent monitoring of response to treatment (Jones *et al.*, 1987).

2. GOAL DEFINITION

Since an important component of patients' subjective sensation of pain is their emotional response to it, careful explanation of its causes and treatment options at the outset is essential. The knowledge that the pain can be explained by specific mechanisms and that similar situations have been met before and controlled can allay a considerable amount of fear and anxiety in the patient. The setting of realistic goals in patient management reinforces a positive approach to pain control. For most patients, three stages of pain control may be recognized:

a. pain free at night;
b. pain free at rest during the day;
c. pain free on movement.

These provide easily defined landmarks on which to build the patient's confidence.

3. TREATMENT

Having carefully defined the underlying pathological processes resulting in pain, suitable therapeutic modalities can then be applied to modify the nociceptive (painful) stimulus. While the mainstay of treatment is based on specific analgesic and co-analgesic drugs it is important at this early stage to identify those patients who will benefit from specific palliative tumoricidal treatment where this remains appropriate. Advanced symptomatic metastatic disease is not in itself a contra-indication for appropriate chemotherapy or radiotherapy in the hands of experienced teams who can evaluate not only the likelihood of benefit but also the associated toxicity. Consideration of other modalities such as specific nerve blocks, massage, relaxation therapy or acupuncture, is also valuable at this stage. In this way, the best treatment can be achieved for all patients with individualization and simplicity as the main aims.

4. REASSESSMENT

While many patients will achieve some degree of pain relief with the initial therapeutic manoeuvre, for most, modifications to their treatment regimen will be required with titration of analgesic doses to their pain. Constant reappraisal of the underlying pathology is necessary to identify developments which may require alterations in treatment strategy.

DRUG TREATMENT OF CHRONIC CANCER PAIN – CHOICE OF DRUG

Appropriate analgesic medication will form the framework of effective pain control. In pain due to progressive malignant disease, analgesics should always be given regularly and continued even though the patient may be pain free. There is no value in witholding analgesia only for the pain to return. Analgesics of appropriate strength and in adequate doses should be employed. The use of a simple three-stage analgesic ladder is recommended, in which patients start on a mild simple analgesic and progress to a moderate analgesic (weak opioid) and thence a strong opioid analgesic whose dose will be escalated as necessary to achieve pain control (Figure 13.1). Within each class of analgesic a single drug should be chosen with an alternative for use where idiosyncratic intolerance is encountered. There is no value in changing from one drug which is ineffective to another of similar analgesic strength, for example from coproxamol to dihydrocodeine,

			Severe pain
		Moderate pain	Morphine or diamorphine (oxycodone suppositories) Phenazocine
	Mild pain	Coproxamol (dihydrocodeine)	
Drug of choice (alternative drug)	Paracetamol (aspirin)		
Drugs to avoid	Compound preparations	Pentazocine Nalbuphine Meptazinol	Dextromoramide 'Diconal' Pethidine Buprenorphine

Figure 13.1 Analgesic ladder.

and no merit in attempting to withhold strong opioids, that is morphine or diamorphine, until the patient is moribund (Hanks and Hoskin, 1986).

Morphine

Most patients will eventually find moderate analgesics such as coproxamol ineffective and require regular medication with a strong opioid analgesic. Morphine remains the drug of choice for oral use. Many fear the introduction of morphine, which may be seen as a drug given only to dying patients, and it is important to discuss these fears openly with the patient. Patients should know that they are receiving morphine and that it is the most appropriate agent for symptom control in this situation.

Side-effects should be anticipated and prevented. All patients requiring opioid analgesics will become constipated and should receive a regular laxative, again titrating the dose until the desired effect is achieved. Nausea and, less frequently, vomiting may occur but can be controlled with regular anti-emetics such as haloperidol 1.5-3 mg nocte. Sedation may occur particularly when initiating treatment or escalating doses but this usually resolves spontaneously, particularly if anticipated with careful explanation and reassurance.

Reluctance to use adequate doses of morphine remains and is often based on fears of either respiratory depression or addiction developing. Respiratory depression does not occur when the morphine dose is carefully titrated to control pain. This has been demonstrated using objective measures of respiratory function in patients being treated for chronic cancer pain (Twycross and Lack, 1983). Similarly, addiction is not seen in this setting, since psychological dependence does not develop although some degree of physical dependence and tolerance will inevitably occur. This means that over a period of time some increase in dosage may be required (tolerance) and that if suddenly stopped, a physical withdrawal will be seen (physical dependence). Other features of addiction do not occur. Where definitive treatment for the pain is possible, such as radiotherapy for bone pain or a nerve block, morphine can be reduced or withdrawn (Twycross and Lack, 1983).

Route of Administration

The use of subcutaneous infusions of strong opioid drugs, of which diamorphine is the drug of choice due to its greater solubility, has gained in popularity. It is important, however, to emphasize that parenteral opioids are not intrinsically more active than the same drug when given orally and are, therefore, only indicated where the oral or rectal route of administration is impracticable such as in severe nausea, vomiting or dysphagia. Similarly the use of slow-release oral preparations (MST-Continus) is simply a more convenient means of administering morphine using a twice daily tablet rather than using a four-hourly elixir. Conversely, unless morphine requirements are defined and stable, such slow-release preparations are disadvantageous since their delayed absorption characteristics make dose adjustment and titration difficult.

Dose Equivalents

As a patient's clinical condition varies it is likely that changes will be made in the strong opioid preparation of choice, using oral morphine elixir initially, converting to MST tablets once stable and changing back to morphine elixir if pain recurs or converting to parenteral diamorphine when oral medication is no longer possible. In making these changes, it is important to consider the equivalent dose for each preparation and route of administration. Morphine elixir and controlled-release morphine sulphate tablets are dose equivalent so that in changing from 4-hourly morphine elixir, the requirements over 12 hours, that is three doses, are calculated and given as the 12-hourly MST dose. When given orally there is little difference between the potency of morphine or diamorphine although it has been suggested in the past that diamorphine may be up to one and a half times more potent than morphine (Hanks and Hoskin, 1987). The major difference, however, arises when oral medication is converted to parenteral medication. This is because when given orally, these drugs pass directly through the liver where they are metabolized before reaching the systemic circulation where they have their effect. In contrast, when given parenterally they enter the systemic circulation directly, which means that both morphine and diamorphine are far more potent when given parenterally than orally. When changing from oral morphine to parenteral diamorphine, therefore, the dose must be reduced to produce an equivalent effect. The factor for this dose reduction is a source of some debate but a reduction to one-third of the oral dose works well in clinical practice (Hanks and Hoskin, 1987). An example of these dose adjustments is shown in Figure 13.2.

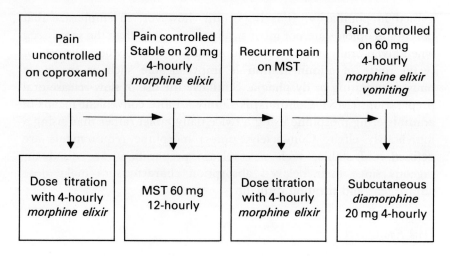

Figure 13.2   Dose equivalents in the use of morphine and diamorphine.

Co-analgesics

In addition to drugs with recognized analgesic properties, a number of other drugs are used in the control of cancer pain; while these may not be true analgesics, they do contribute considerably to pain control. Drugs in this group are called co-analgesics (Twycross and Hanks, 1984). Their use depends on careful assessment and diagnosis since their efficacy is based on specific properties of the drug (Table 13.1).

OTHER TREATMENTS FOR PAIN RELIEF

While the mainstay of treatment is the use of appropriate analgesic and co-analgesic drugs, other methods of pain control should also be considered for individual patients.

Radiotherapy

Radiotherapy remains the treatment of choice for localized bone pain due to metastatic infiltration and, for pain relief, a single fraction is as effective as a prolonged course of treatment (Hoskin, 1988).

Nerve Blocks

Nerve blocks may be considered where localized pain is attributed to a specific nerve distribution which is accessible to the anaesthetist or

Table 13.1   *Co-analgesics*

Drug	Indication
Non-steroidal anti-inflammatory drug (NSAID), e.g. aspirin, ibuprofen, flurbiprofen	Bone pain Soft tissue infiltration
Steroids: dexamethasone or prednisolone	Nerve compression, Raised intracranial pressure Soft tissue infiltration Hepatomegaly
Antidepressants, e.g. dothiepin, mianserin	Depression Nerve root pain
Anxiolytics, e.g. diazepam, lorazepam	Anxiety
Muscle relaxants, e.g. baclofen	Muscle spasm
Anticonvulsants, e.g. sodium valproate	Paraesthesia or dysaesthesia
Diuretics	Oedema
Antibiotics	Infected ulcers or fungating tumour

neurosurgeon (Churcher, 1983; Clarke, 1984). Sympathectomy may also be advocated in some situations (Boas, 1983).

Surgical Fixation

Surgical fixation of pathological fractures should always be considered for the patient who may be returned to a pain-free, ambulant lifestyle. Control of the pain due to an unstable fracture is otherwise often difficult to achieve (Philips, 1984).

Transcutaneous Electrical Nerve Stimulation (TENS)

This is a simple technique which many patients find helpful, particularly for paraesthetic or dysaesthetic pains (Lundeberg, 1984).

Neurosurgical Techniques

Techniques such as cordotomy, rhizotomy or thalotomy may rarely be considered. Pituitary ablation by either surgery or irradiation may produce dramatic pain relief in advanced cancer in selected patients (Lipton, 1984).

Relaxation Therapy

Relaxation therapy can be of value where anxiety is a major component in the patient's symptomatology (Copley Cobb, 1984).

Acupuncture

This is undoubtedly effective in selected situations that are unresponsive to drug therapy (Richardson and Vincent, 1986).

Management of Other Symptoms

The considerable array of symptoms which the patient with advanced cancer presents may appear daunting when first encountered. The same principles of management can, however, be applied to these symptoms as to pain, with careful assessment and diagnosis of the underlying cause being the most important steps towards achieving symptom control. Once the underlying cause or causes for a particular symptom have been identified, rational treatment can be instigated.

ANOREXIA

Anorexia is perhaps the commonest symptom encountered in patients with advanced cancer, often compounded by emotional tension as close relatives become intent on feeding patients to get them well again. It is important to dispel this myth so that the patient does not feel guilty at declining well-meant, but inappropriate offerings. Frequently, a specific physical cause can be identified, such as a sore mouth, oropharyngeal candidiasis, uraemia, hypercalcaemia or hepatic metastases. Anorexia may also be secondary to other symptoms, such as persistent pain, nausea or vomiting, constipation, dyspnoea or insomnia. The effects of treatment by chemotherapy or radiotherapy are often cited as further causes of anorexia but often these effects can be overemphasized. Ulcerated lesions, in particular fungating breast cancer or node metastases in the neck, will have adverse effects on appetite, especially if they are infected and offensive.

Treatment of anorexia involves both attention to the underlying cause and general measures, such as providing small appetizing meals, and avoiding rigid adherence to meal times. Alcohol is a useful appetite stimulant and both patients and relatives should be reassured that this will do no harm since many misconceptions persist, particularly where other drugs are being taken or there is known liver involvement. Steroids are frequently prescribed for their non-specific appetite stimulant action which can be achieved with relatively low doses, such as dexamethasone 2–4 mg daily or prednisolone 20 ml daily (Hanks, 1983). Progestogens, such as medroxyprogesterone, may also have a similar effect. It is important to ensure that appetite stimulation is appropriate since increasing appetite in the patient with a sore mouth, dysphagia or vomiting may only exacerbate these underlying problems, emphasizing again the importance of careful assessment before instituting treatment.

CONSTIPATION

Constipation will inevitably occur in patients who are increasingly weak, immobile and anorectic. All patients taking opioid drugs, whether weak opioids such as coproxamol or dihydrocodeine, or strong opioids such as morphine, will become constipated and several other common drugs including phenothiazines, antihistamines and antidepressants have anticholinergic activity which also reduces bowel motility. In patients with advanced cancer, more specific causes may include hypercalcaemia, hypokalaemia, dehydration and intestinal obstruction due to intra-abdominal or pelvic tumour masses.

For drug-induced constipation, anticipation and prophylactic treatment are preferable, which means the patient should take a regular laxative. More specific causes should, where appropriate, be reversed and adequate fluid intake encouraged. Equally important is for the patient to be able to have a bowel motion without embarrassment, receiving assistance to reach the toilet or providing a commode without delay and trying to avoid the use of a bedpan which many patients find inhibiting.

Many laxative drugs are available and these may be classified into four main groups: bulking agents, osmotic agents, bowel stimulants and softening agents. While undoubtedly having a sound physiological basis the use of bulking agents, such as methyl cellulose or bran, is rarely welcomed by the patient who has a poor diet, dry mouth or nausea and, unless an established part of their usual diet, such unpalatable measures may be best avoided. Since the basis of opioid-induced constipation is reduced colonic motility probably due to a direct action on peripheral opioid receptors, a bowel stimulant, such as bisacodyl or senna, is the most appropriate drug to prevent constipation in this situation. The addition of a faecal softening agent, such as dioctyl, is also often of value. Where constipation is resistant to the combination of a bowel stimulant and faecal softener, then addition of an osmotic agent to draw fluid into the bowel acting as a small bowel flusher may be successful. Lactulose is effective in this way and tends to have a less dramatic effect than magnesium salts, which may also be used.

In established constipation, local measures either by suppository or enema may be necessary but it is important to complement this with regular oral treatment. The presence of a colostomy does not prevent constipation and equal attention is required to bowel function. Where necessary, suppositories or enemas can be given through the colostomy although poor retention may make colonic irrigation preferable.

NAUSEA AND VOMITING

Nausea and vomiting are distressing features of advanced cancer when they tend to be a persistent and recurrent problem distinct from acute, self-limiting episodes such as those associated with gastrointestinal infection or chemotherapy. There may be many causes of nausea or vomiting in this situation, often several interacting to produce the clinical picture. These may be classified as mechanical, such as gastric stasis, reflux or intestinal obstruction; chemical, such as drug induced, uraemia, hypercalcaemia or hepatic failure; and miscellaneous causes, including persistent nausea due to chronic anxiety, fear or depression.

As with other symptoms it is important to consider the individual cause because not only will correction of this help to achieve control but also vomiting may be stimulated through one of two specific areas in the brain – the emetic centre or the chemoreceptor trigger zone (CTZ) for which anti-emetics have selected activity (Figure 13.3).

Metoclopramide has a dual action both on the CTZ and directly on the upper gastrointestinal tract where it promotes gastric emptying and is, therefore, the drug of choice for reflux and stasis. Domperidone also acts in the same way as metoclopramide. These drugs are, however, best avoided in established intestinal obstruction where their

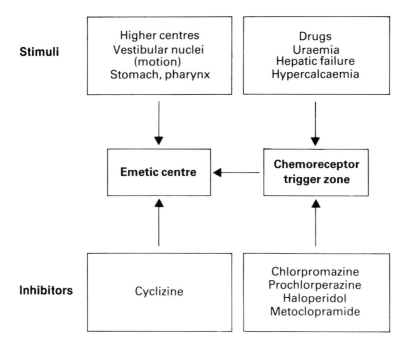

Figure 13.3 Vomiting mechanisms and drug action.

effects may exacerbate symptoms. In this situation and others where a direct effect on the emetic centre is required, cyclizine is of value. Steroids, such as dexamethasone, also have anti-emetic properties and may be effective where other measures fail.

SORE OR DRY MOUTH

Sore or dry mouth may be a prominent symptom and contributes to reduced food and fluid intake and anorexia. Possible causes and appropriate treatment are shown in Table 13.2.

COUGH AND DYSPNOEA

Cough and dyspnoea are common problems since both primary lung cancer and pulmonary metastases are common in patients with advanced cancer. They are usually due to the effects of tumour in the lungs or pleural involvement resulting in an enlarging effusion. It is however, important to consider the many other benign causes of cough or dyspnoea. Pulmonary embolus, cardiac failure and chronic

Table 13.2   *Management of sore or dry mouth in advanced cancer*

Cause	Treatment
Oral candidiasis	Nystatin suspension Miconazole gel if resistant

Drugs,
  e.g. morphine, antidepressants,
  phenothiazines
	Avoid or choose drugs with least
	  anticholinergic activity, e.g.
	  dothiepin instead of
	  amitriptyline, haloperidol
	  instead of chlorpromazine

Dehydration	Fluids

Irreversible causes,
  e.g. drugs, local radiotherapy,
  mouth breathing
	Mouth care: antiseptic
	  mouthwashes, frequent small
	  drinks, crushed ice, carbonated
	  drinks, effervescent ascorbic
	  acid, etc.

obstructive airways disease are common in any population of debilitated middle-aged and elderly patients. In general, cardiac failure and acute exacerbations of bronchitis should continue to be treated actively while they are symptomatic, but careful selection is required of those patients likely to benefit from anticoagulation after pulmonary embolus. Patients who have been troubled by asthma or any of the rarer lung diseases before presenting with cancer will continue to have these problems, which will require active treatment as before.

Where respiratory symptoms are attributable to tumour within the chest, then specific treatment offers the best chance of palliation. Thus local radiotherapy to a tumour occluding a main bronchus may allow shrinkage and re-expansion of distal collapse, and aspiration of pleural effusions will allow re-expansion of the lung and improved respiratory capacity. For intrinsic tumour or lymphangitis carcinomatosa, however, drug treatment aimed at reducing subjective respiratory distress and cough is usually most appropriate. An opioid drug, such as morphine elixir given in low doses of 10–20 ml four-hourly, is useful and a benzodiazepine with anxiolytic properties, such as diazepam or lorazepam, is of value. Steroids may improve respiratory symptoms due to lung infiltration or lymphangitis. Bronchodilators, such as salbutamol, are only of value where there is clear evidence of wheeze and bronchoconstriction, although undoubtedly some patients benefit from the placebo effect of an inhalation or nebulizer. Mucolytic agents are, in general, disappointing but where sticky foul sputum is the prominent problem, carbocisteine may help together with antibiotic treatment of symptomatic infection.

For cough suppression morphine elixir is an effective agent. Since it is the opioid action which accounts for its efficacy, there is no value in using codeine linctus, weak opioid, or methadone linctus for cough in a patient already taking morphine elixir. Simple linctus has a useful placebo and local soothing action in these patients.

Clinical Conditions

The wide range of symptoms which may be encountered in the patient with advanced cancer has already been discussed with emphasis being placed on the need for careful assessment and diagnosis of the underlying cause before instituting treatment. This is important not only for devising rational therapeutic regimens but also because several symptoms may be closely interrelated with a single unifying cause.

HYPERCALCAEMIA

Hypercalcaemia is a common complication, seen particularly in carcinoma of the lung, breast and prostate and myeloma. It usually occurs as a result of multiple bone metastases causing release of calcium from bone, but is also due to humoral factors related to parathyroid hormone or prostaglandins being released by the tumour (Mundy and Martin, 1982). Hypercalcaemia is, therefore, often associated with bone pain but may also present with confusion, anorexia, nausea, vomiting, polyuria, polydipsia, dehydration and constipation. The diagnosis of hypercalcaemia is an important one to consider where these symptoms occur and can be made simply from an estimation of the calcium and albumin in the blood.

The initial treatment will usually be based on diuresis, aided by frusemide which has calciuric properties, aiming at an input and output of at least 4 litres per day. However, care needs to be taken not to increase the existing problems of profound dehydration and the timing of diuretic administration is important (see Chapter 6 of Volume 1). A moderate dose of steroids, such as dexamethasone 4 mg twice a day, is also usually given. In resistant cases or where the blood level is very high and rapid reduction is thought desirable, mithramycin 1 mg/m^2 given intravenously is usually effective. Calcitonin is also useful where simple measures are ineffective but has the disadvantage of requiring regular injections. Since both these drugs cause nausea or vomiting, an anti-emetic should be given with them. Diphosphonates, in particular aminohydroxypropylidene diphosphonate (APD), given intravenously are effective and a single infusion may be sufficient for long-term control (Cantwell and Harris, 1987). Oral phosphates reduce calcium absorption in the bowel but may cause troublesome diarrhoea and, if absorbed, can result in hyperphosphataemia or precipitation of calcium phosphate.

RENAL FAILURE

Renal failure in advanced cancer is usually due to obstruction of the urinary tract by tumour within the pelvis or retro-peritoneal tissues. The progressive uraemia which results may present with a variety of symptoms including anorexia, sore mouth, nausea, vomiting, diarrhoea, confusion, drowsiness, tremor, fits, itching, hiccups, dyspnoea, cough, polyuria and oliguria, together with loin pain or discomfort where there is significant hydronephrosis. Again the diagnosis can usually be confirmed by simple blood biochemistry in which elevated urea and creatinine are found with hyperkalaemia and acidosis developing in more advanced cases.

Active treatment of renal failure in this situation is often inappropriate although in selected patients with localized pelvic disease urinary diversion or ureteric stents to relieve the obstruction may be considered. Usually, where the underlying cancer is advanced, simple treatment of the individual symptoms and attention to fluid balance to avoid overloading patients with fluid they cannot excrete provide the most suitable management.

HEPATIC METASTASES

Hepatic metastases occur in most common cancers, in particular those arising in the lung, breast and intra-abdominal organs. The liver has a large reserve capacity and large amounts of tumour may develop within the liver before a significant degree of hepatic failure develops. However, before evidence of hepatic failure is found, several symptoms attributable to non-specific effects of liver metastases may present, in particular anorexia and nausea together with discomfort and pain as the liver enlarges stretching its capsule. At a more advanced stage jaundice, itching, confusion and ascites may develop.

In the treatment of symptoms due to hepatic metastases steroids in moderate doses, such as dexamethasone 4 mg twice a day, are often useful. Cholestyramine or antihistamines will help itching due to obstructive jaundice and chlorpromazine will suppress troublesome hiccups. In the management of patients with advanced metastatic liver disease (as opposed to patients with advanced benign liver disease, such as cirrhosis) there is no evidence to suggest that opioid drugs or phenothiazines should be withheld, although drug metabolism may result in increased sensitivity and lower dose requirements (Bennett, 1981).

DRUG-INDUCED SYMPTOMS

It is regrettably true that, in many instances, the symptoms of which patients complain may be related to their medication. Common situations in which this occurs have already been mentioned and careful attention to minimizing drug-related side-effects is particularly important in this situation.

When Death is Imminent

Despite the presence of advanced cancer and limited life expectancy, active diagnosis and management of symptoms should continue throughout. There will, however, come a time when death is inevitable within a short period and the emphasis in management will shift towards reducing the traumas of these final hours for both the patient and relatives.

In most cases the patient will have impaired consciousness and be unable to take oral medication. Oral morphine should be changed to rectal morphine or subcutaneous diamorphine either as an intermittent injection or, where the patient may remain alive for some time, a subcutaneous infusion, remembering to make the appropriate dose reduction in converting from oral to parenteral medication. Where an anti-emetic is still required chlorpromazine, prochlorperazine or cyclizine suppositories are useful.

Additional symptoms which may arise at this time are agitation and restlessness, for which diazepam administered rectally in a dose of 5-10 mg is usually effective, and pooling of secretions in the throat causing discomfort and a characteristic noisy rattle which can be suppressed using an anticholinergic agent to dry up the secretions. Hyoscine is preferable to atropine in this situation, being relatively sedative, and is given subcutaneously in a dose of 0.2-0.4 mg.

Less frequently an acute event may precipitate death in a patient with advanced cancer either by massive pulmonary embolus, myocardial infarction or haemorrhage from the lung, gastrointestinal tract or a major vessel eroded by tumour. In these situations sedation, using diamorphine given parenterally for rapid action and diazepam given rectally, is the only active treatment required. Of equal importance, however, is to deal with the problem calmly and efficiently, providing reassurance for both patient and relatives in what is a very frightening and distressing event for them.

Summary

The principles of symptom management in the patient with advanced cancer should not differ from those in other branches of medicine. Careful assessment and identification of individual problems are followed by a diagnosis of their causes using both clinical information and appropriate investigations, on the basis of which the best treatment, individualized for each patient, can be instituted. Continuous monitoring of response to treatment with appropriate modifications is then essential to ensure continuing symptom control and to reduce treatment toxicity. While the emphasis of treatment may change as the patient nears death, the need for active treatment of specific symptoms using the above principles will remain.

References

Bennett, P.N. (1981) The influence of cancer on drug metabolism, in H.F. Woods (ed.) *Topics in Therapeutics 6,* Pitman Medical, Tunbridge Wells, pp. 103-10.

Boas, R.A. (1983) The sympathetic nervous system and pain relief, in M. Swerdlow (ed.) *Relief of Intractable Pain,* Elsevier, Amsterdam, pp. 215-36.

Cantwell, B. and Harris, A. (1987) Effect of single high dose infusions of amino-hydroxypropylidene diphosphonate on hypercalcaemia caused by cancer, *British Medical Journal,* Vol. 294, pp. 467-9.

Churcher, M. (1983) Peripheral nerve blocks in relief of intractable pain, in M. Swerdlow (ed.) *Relief of Intractable Pain,* Elsevier, Amsterdam, pp. 147-74.

Clarke, I.M.C. (1984) Nerve blocks, *Clinics in Oncology,* Vol. 3, pp. 181–93.

Copley Cobb, S. (1984) Teaching relaxation therapy to cancer patients, *Cancer Nursing,* Vol. 7, pp. 157–61.

Hanks, G.W. (1983) Management of symptoms in advanced cancer, *Cancer Update,* Vol. 27, pp. 1691–702.

Hanks, G.W. and Hoskin, P.J. (1986) Pain control in advanced cancer: pharmacological methods, *Journal of the Royal College of Physicians (London),* Vol. 20, pp. 276–81.

Hanks, G.W. and Hoskin, P.J. (1987) Opioid analgesics, *Palliative Medicine,* Vol. 1, pp. 1–25.

Hoskin, P.J. (1988) Scientific and clinical aspects of radiotherapy in-the relief of bone pain, *Cancer Surveys,* Vol. 7, no. 1, pp. 69–86.

Jones, V.A. *et al.* (1987) Pain assessment charts in chronic cancer pain management, *Palliative Medicine,* Vol. 1, pp. 111–16.

Lipton, S. (1984) Cordotomy and hypophysectomy, *Clinics in Oncology,* Vol. 3, pp. 195–208.

Lundeberg, T. (1984) Electrical stimulation for the relief of pain, *Physiotherapy,* Vol. 70, pp. 98–101.

Mundy, G.R. and Martin, T.J. (1982) The hypercalcaemia of malignancy: pathogenesis and management, *Metabolism,* Vol. 31, pp. 1247–77.

Philips, H. (1984) Orthopaedic surgery, *Clinics in Oncology,* Vol. 3, pp. 75–87.

Richardson, P.H. and Vincent, C.A. (1986) Acupuncture for the treatment of pain: a review of evaluative research, *Pain,* Vol. 24, pp. 15–40.

Twycross, R.G. and Fairfield, S. (1982) Pain in far advanced cancer, *Pain,* Vol. 14, pp. 303–10.

Twycross, R.G. and Lack, S.A. (1983) *Symptom Control in Advanced Cancer: Pain Relief,* Pitman, London.

Twycross, R.G. and Hanks G.W. (1984) Co-analgesia, *Clinics in Oncology,* Vol. 13, pp. 153–64.

Chapter 14

Death, Dying, Bereavement and Loss

MARILYN MARKS BA(Hons), RGN, DipN(London),
RCNT, OncCert
Senior Nurse/Clinical Nurse Specialist
Continuing Care Unit, The Royal Marsden Hospital, London and Surrey

Death

A HISTORICAL PERSPECTIVE

> Death closes all; but something near the end
> Some work of noble note, may yet be done
>
> (Alfred Tennyson, 'Ulysses')

Dying remains one of the few certainties in life today. However, in recent years attitudes to death have changed substantially. In ancient civilization death was acknowledged as one of the major *rites de passage* with great ceremony and many rituals. Until the Middle Ages dying was a public event and death took place in the presence of family, friends, neighbours and children. The progression from life to death was expected and death was not seen as the failure of life.

A slow transformation from the theological to the scientific view of life began in mediaeval times when sickness and death were seen as punishment for wrong doing. Death became the shadowy grey figure stalking about – the final enemy. Despite this fear of death there was a certain familiarity about it. The Great Plague (1665) and The Great War (1914–18) rendered to death an accepted inevitability. 'All those with whom I had really been intimate were gone: not one remained to share with me the heights and depths of my memories' (Brittain, 1933).

In the twentieth century, due to a major shift in patterns of disease, chronic illness has become one of the leading causes of death. Treatments for more acute illnesses are effective, technology can eradicate many diseases and public health measures have shifted the trends in mortality. Death has become taboo in the twentieth century, and replaces sex as a forbidden subject (Gorer, 1967). As Victorian constraints on morality changed, attitudes to 'the pornography of death' also changed.

Caring for the dying has always been the responsibility of nurses. From the battlefields of Europe and the New World to the many infants and families who died from the major epidemics of diphtheria, typhoid and smallpox, nurses have been present to ease the mental and physical discomfort of death.

DEATH FROM CANCER

Medical technology has advanced considerably and the expectation of the public (and indeed of some professionals) is that disease can be eradicated. Now, aggressive treatment often continues until the moment of death. In cancer, where a fatal outcome is by no means certain, the curative approach is the one to which most nurses are exposed. Perception of success in a multidisciplinary team may vary from a partial regression of the disease process to a peaceful and comfort-orientated death.

These changing facets of treatment have led to alterations in a patient's place of death. Earlier in this century two-thirds of the people who died were under the age of 50 years, and the majority of these died at home. In 1966, 54 per cent of deaths in the United Kingdom occurred in hospital, rising to 68 per cent in 1983–84 (Office of Population Censuses and Statistics, 1984). It can be argued that many people feel ill-equipped to cope with the basic care of the dying patient at home since all their life they have been sheltered from exposure to death.

Approaches to Care: Hospice, Home and Hospital

Hospital deaths are often impersonal and technologically orientated. People dying at home may be isolated and may have inadequate symptom control. The hospice movement, which has evolved during this century, has attempted to combine the best of home and hospital care. Corr and Corr (1983) describe the hospice as a philosophy rather than a facility. The *Shorter Oxford Dictionary* defines 'hospice' as a house of rest and entertainment for pilgrims, travellers or strangers. It is seen as a place where those travelling on to an after-life may rest, be refreshed, find relief from their symptoms and attain peace before their death. In practical terms the hospice movement was developed by the Irish Sisters of Charity who established hospices at the turn of the century. The modern initiative was begun by Dame Cicely Saunders when she established St Christopher's Hospice in Sydenham, England, in 1967.

The past 10 years have witnessed the worldwide development of a movement based on the philosophy of the hospice, which endeavours to bring expertise in symptom control and relief of all suffering, whether mental, physical, emotional or spiritual. Now many hospices provide home care and day care in addition to inpatient units. In hospitals, continuing care units have developed, providing those same principles with continuity of care and a multidisciplinary-based team approach.

Home care for the dying has been revolutionized by the advent of home care teams attached to inpatient units and by the work of Cancer Relief Macmillan Fund, a cancer charity which has steadfastly pioneered the concept of Macmillan nursing. These specialist nurses funded by Cancer Relief Macmillan Fund are skilled practitioners and expert advisers on all aspects of symptom control. They also offer emotional support to patients and their families at home. Working in conjuction with the community health care services they assist community nurses and general practitioners and are able to provide additional psychological support to those families who wish the patient to remain at home.

In hospitals the concept of the hospital support team has been developed for the terminally ill. In the United Kingdom the first team was started at St Thomas' Hospital, London and has formed a prototype for many other hospital developments. A specialist nurse works within a multidisciplinary framework, providing advice on symptom control and support while the patient is within the hospital. On discharge, the home care nurses attached to the hospital support team take on a similar responsibility to Macmillan nurses. Thus patients do not move their treatment base from the hospital in which they have previously been treated but rather have continuity of care.

This approach may avoid an issue ably expressed by Krakoff (1979): 'In seeking death with dignity we may overlook treatable disease and provide patients with the indignity of a premature death... It is important both to differentiate and understand what is truly terminal and what is reversible.'

It is vital that hospices and continuing care units maintain an approach to treatment which explores every avenue of palliation of the disease, balancing this against the issues surrounding quality of life. The difficulties involved in the question of euthanasia have been best described by Jackson (1958): 'Would this procedure give him a *reasonable* chance of an *appreciable* duration of *desirable* life at an *acceptable* cost of suffering?'

When considering treatment and what Vere (1971) would describe as a 'trial of therapy' all those adjectives of quality need careful deliberation. Other ethical issues concerning nutrition, hydration and the use of opioids are discussed in Chapter 13.

Reaction to Death

Two major studies (Craven and Wald, 1975; Davidson, 1979) have revealed that there are certain primary concerns of the dying patient:

1. the fear that the patient and his or her family will be abandoned;
2. the loss of self-management and independence;
3. the fear of intractable pain and distressing symptoms.

These concerns may be greatly eased by an understanding of some of the problems of communication and emotional reactions experienced by patients and their families as death approaches.

COMMUNICATION

In establishing communication with the dying person, good rapport and respect for the individual are essential. No meaningful conversation can take place, however, unless the symptoms of advanced cancer are first alleviated. People will cope with impending death often in the same way they cope with other crises in their life. They may use a variety of coping mechanisms, such as denial, displacement and dependency. Glaser and Strauss (1964), in their books on the awareness of communication between dying patients, family and staff, describe four awareness contexts:

1. closed awareness;
2. suspicion awareness;
3. mutual pretence;
4. open awareness.

In the first context, patients are not aware of their impending death and staff members collaborate or collude with them by encouraging patients to make plans which do not acknowledge the possibility of death. In the suspicion awareness context, patients have some idea of the seriousness of their condition but staff do not confirm this and do not confront the question. In the mutual pretence context both staff and patient are aware of the patient's terminal condition but do not discuss it either implicitly or explicitly. The open awareness context allows more free discussion and planning for short-term goals in the future. The patient has control of his or her life and there is sharing of feelings among family and staff. Open awareness is encouraged in continuing care settings as patients who discuss their concerns are less likely to experience anxiety, depression or anger (Hinton, 1979).

No chapter on death and dying would be complete without mentioning Elizabeth Kubler-Ross who, in 1969, described for the first time the stages through which a person may pass as he or she faces death. Modern medicine and nursing owe much to Dr Kubler-Ross for highlighting the various emotions which can arise in attaining the acceptance of one's own mortality. Though her work has given us much, there is an inherent danger in her five stages becoming prescriptive. Caution must be exercised to allow patients and their families to be and feel as they are at that moment in time without any expectation of which stage they might be reaching. It is also spurious to suggest that all patients should aim to reach a passive and peaceful acceptance of their condition. Patients will die as they have lived.

DENIAL

This commonest of defence mechanisms is also the first reaction of many patients to the realization of the seriousness of their disease. Pattison (1977) has contributed substantially to our understanding of the denial mechanism by differentiating between three forms:

1. *Existential denial*, which is the capacity held by all human beings to believe that one's mortality is not threatened by impending danger in everyday life.
2. *Psychological denial*, which is the defence against the anxiety which is produced by the threat of danger. Patients who persistently 'forget' that they have been given answers to their questions or constantly search for reassurance, are operating this defence mechanism. It is a recognized and acceptable form of coping behaviour.
3. *Non-attention denial* is partly conscious and occurs when patients

have accepted their prognosis, made plans accordingly, and then live day to day as though they have a full and normal lifespan in front of them. Many patients operate at this level as it enables them to live well without the pain of continuously acknowledging their mortality. Few patients can maintain total denial in the face of a deteriorating body. Therefore non-attention denial provides many advantages to patients as a way of coping.

ANGER

Anger may often appear as a general reaction against the unfairness of the situation. Often the question 'Why me?' is asked and frequently the patient, and indeed often the relatives too, will look for someone or something to blame for the disease. Those who believe in God may blame him. Alternatively, the medical staff may be berated for their inability to cure the cancer. Extremely angry patients will direct their anger at anyone prepared to listen and this may be one of the most difficult responses for the multidisciplinary team to handle. A recipient of a patient's anger needs to be sensitively helped to bear with the anger and should be supported in recognizing that it is seldom a personal indictment.

BARGAINING

Often patients will negotiate with God, with the medical staff and with themselves, to bargain for some extra time. This is usually a private negotiation and may serve as an incentive and motivating factor in the patient's life.

DEPRESSION

There are often many losses which patients will have sustained during the course of their illness. They will have natural and understandable sorrow at the loss of their health, their security and possibly their role within the family, work and social life. As an attitude to death, sadness is an appropriate reaction and needs to be distinguished from a clinical and therefore treatable depression.

ANTICIPATORY GRIEF

This is more commonly seen in modern times as the dramatic advances in medicine have significantly changed the nature of terminal illness. It is now quite common for patients and their families to face an extended period anticipating death. During this time, emotional, spiritual, financial and physical concerns attack those who are struggling to cope with an altered lifestyle. As a result of achieving a high level of symptom control, Stedeford (1985) describes patients who are now free to contemplate what they are losing. The expectations of nursing staff are always that symptoms are there to be relieved and it may help to realize that some of this emotional suffering is inevitable. Well-intentioned staff should try to accept that this variety of painful exploration of the soul is normal and expectations of total relief are sometimes inappropriate.

ACCEPTANCE

A stage of peaceful expectation and quiet acceptance may appear to be the ultimate aim for some patients. However, in many cases a resignation and a wish to die with dignity are more prominent. Escaping the weariness and exhaustion which accompanies terminal illness may well be a more realistic assessment of the emotional state in which many people die. Several factors may affect the ease with which acceptance can be reached, and for many patients it may be inappropriate to expect it at all. Sometimes an old person will accept death with more equanimity. Those with a firm belief in the after-life may gain comfort from the knowledge that they will meet loved ones after death. A patient's personality and previous coping mechanisms will influence the resilience with which he or she accepts death.

The manner in which a person's prognosis is imparted will lead to trust and confidence in the team caring for him or her and an openness in discussion will help towards acceptance.

Lastly, a supportive family whose difficulties have been resolved and who are united in their sadness but strengthened with hope on a daily basis generally will ease someone towards acceptance.

HOPE

It is often argued that truth may destroy hope and consequently the truth should be withheld from patients. As previously seen (non-attention denial) it is possible for a patient to hold two incompatible ideas at the same time. Without hope life is meaningless. Short-term goals, aiming for small accomplishments and attainable ideals, encourage hope. When patients are looking for information to complete and fulfil their lives, the sensitive imparting of knowledge is mandatory (see Chapter 7).

The Impact of Death on Family and Friends

Do not go gentle into that good night,
Old age should burn and rage at close of day;
Rage, rage against dying of the light
                    (Dylan Thomas, 'Do not go gentle')

It is sometimes difficult to combine the two facts – that a patient is alive and that he or she is soon going to die – into an easily maintainable pattern of care. Often the living find relating to dying hard and will isolate the patient, sometimes because they are afraid of what is happening, and sometimes because they believe that it is genuinely the best thing not to bother that person. The dying person may have relinquished hope of recovery and hope of the maintenance of a good quality of life. The patient's role may have changed substantially from that of head of the household, money-earner and active member of the community, holding down a responsible job. In a position of weakness, having to accept help from others the sick person fights to retain as much independence as is possible.

Relatives and family must invest emotional capital in caring for someone whose situation can only lead to their own distress. Often members of the family will have feelings of guilt. They may have delayed the initial consultation with the doctor, they may indeed feel angry with the individual for becoming ill in the first place. They may be frightened and withdraw prematurely from the patient's side. Often they will find difficulty in expressing emotions or in maintaining a normal relaxed conversation and lifestyle. Through all of this the family needs intense support, understanding and patience. Where members are angry and distressed by a patient's impending death, often they will encourage the patient, wearied and ready to die, to hang on to life and to fight at all costs, because they themselves wish to fight the prognosis.

Nursing and the Issues of Dying

Our ability to care is in direct proportion to our vulnerability.

                                        (Prophit, 1984)

In a major study on stress in home care and hospital support nurses, Yardley and Hunt (1987) found that a patient's death alone is not a major cause of stress. Stress did, however, arise when the patient was moved to a different institution. Wilkinson (1987) found that job satisfaction was high in terminal care nursing, where patients were allowed to die a peaceful and pain-free death and were permitted free and open discussion about their situation. This is in direct contrast to the research findings of Stoddard (1979) who showed that nurses take, on average, twice as long to respond to the bell of a dying person as they do to those who are apparently recovering. In a review of nursing literature on terminal care, Conboy-Hill (1986) found many studies where nurses described feelings of helplessness, inadequacy and depression associated with terminal care (Benoliel, 1972; Friel and Tehan, 1980; Wilson, 1985). Many other studies would seem to validate the findings of Hinton (1979) that increased distress is noted when 'closed awareness' is routine. When patients are allowed to discuss openly the truth of which they are aware, staff stress levels drop dramatically. Vachon (1978) lists five ways of improving coping skills for staff working with the dying:

1. encouragement of personal insight to understand and acknowledge one's own limits;
2. healthy balance between work and outside life;
3. the promotion of a team approach to care;
4. an ongoing support system within work and outside work;
5. for those working in isolation, continuing guidance and support, from peers and superiors.

NURSING EDUCATION

The last and possibly most important addition to the field of stress reduction is education. In the United States of America, death education, commencing at high school, is now common. Before entering nursing in the United Kingdom most young people have been relatively protected from seeing and talking with a dying person and have had no education about death. The need for skilled nursing care and a quick adaptation to the problems surrounding death are an essential part of general nurse training. In post-registration training, education should provide nurses with the ability to assess a symptom, suggest interventions, set realistic objectives with and for the patient and evaluate the outcome.

In addition to a fundamental pharmacological knowledge for symptom control, there are other factors to be considered in preparing nurses for the care of the dying patient, to assist nurses to function at a level where their colleagues recognize and respect their expertise. 'If nurses are to take charge of terminal care they will need to demonstrate special skills in the communication of painful information and in dealing with its effects on the individual' (Conboy-Hill, 1986). These skills are not just acquired. Many need to be taught with adequate support and constant appraisal. These special skills of communication need sensitive management. It cannot just be assumed that nurses automatically develop these particular attributes.

Nurses must develop reasearch-based education methods in both basic and post-basic education. Until recently, research-based training has existed only in general nursing education but has now been employed in continuing care. The lack of standardization among continuing care educational programmes is of concern as there are no national standards of assessment in this area. All continuing care units and hospices have a high teaching commitment and responsibility. Only 36 per cent of the units in the United Kingdom are currently running courses to equip specialist nurses for this work. The two recognized English National Board short courses (ENB 931 and 285) in the care of dying patients and their families are currently examining some of these issues. The need for further education into aspects of terminal care has been addressed by the Department of Health and Social Security and the National Association of Health Authorities in their guidelines, which have made very specific recommendations for the future. A totally multidisciplinary approach is necessary to set the standards and allow for development and improvement in the care of the dying.

EVALUATION OF CARE OF THE DYING PATIENT

With any area of care it is vital that there is constant evaluation and revision of practices. To assess suffering and relief of suffering is a complex problem. Many quality-of-life studies have been undertaken recently (MacAdam and Smith, 1987; Twycross, 1987) and there are numerous dimensions to be considered. Some studies are based purely on clinical observations, others on interview, others on self-report by patients. A common theme in quality-of-life studies shows the patient's rating of their life quality is higher than that of an observer. For a patient and relative to evaluate the care is a purely subjective phenomenon but may nevertheless give valuable indications of areas where improvements can be made. For nursing care, an evaluation package such as MONITOR (Goldstone *et al.*, 1983) can be valuable in identifying areas of nursing practice which fall below a required and preset standard. Developments in the future will lead to a form of nursing audit system specific to care of the dying. Currently those questionnaires designed for the evaluation of cancer nursing and geriatric nursing contain many questions pertinent to terminal care but the future lies with recognized standards of care and agreed practice. Then those various institutions and units responsible for care of the dying can evaluate their performance, both locally and nationally, with regard to the care to which everyone is entitled at the end of their lives.

At the Time of Death

During the final hours of life nursing care becomes intensified. It is helpful when both doctors and nurses jointly accept that the patient's death is imminent, preparing the family, allowing the relatives to participate in care when they wish, permitting close relatives to stay near to the patient and gently easing them into the knowledge that death is approaching. For the patient, care should be totally comfort orientated. He or she may be very weak, even unconscious, but at no point should the patient's physical, emotional or spiritual needs be neglected. The unit should have sufficient staff to allow a nurse to be present with someone during their dying moments and, if it is the patient's or family's wish, a minister of the appropriate religion should be called. Sacrament of the sick or the equivalent in other religions is often a great comfort to the patient and to the family. Aiming for as peaceful and gentle a death as possible, the nurse must remain sensitive to the wishes of the family who may be frightened and appreciate the presence of a professional. Some may find it an intensely personal moment when they would rather be alone with the dying person.

Bereavement

But in my spirit when I dwell,
And dream my dream, and hold it true;
For though my lips may breathe adieu,
I cannot think the thing farewell.

(Alfred Tennyson, 'In memoriam')

Cancer, more than many of the other potentially fatal illnesses, carries with it a certain symbolic power. The popular image of cancer is of a relentless destruction and a death which cannot be averted. Because of this, anticipatory grief is often experienced by both patient and relatives and this may ease the bereavement process as it acts as forewarning of the loss to come. It allows time for goodbyes, for preparation and for practical arrangements.

Bereavement is a reaction to the loss of a close relationship. In bereavement, certain psychological processes assist the bereaved person to lessen gradually the psychological ties which bound him or her to the deceased. These bonds, which have been demonstrated in Bowlby's (1980) attachment theory, are those which have added security and safety to the fabric of human existence. In the animal kingdom, many species show signs of grief and mourning behaviour, and for human beings grief in bereavement is a partly instinctive and biological reaction (Parkes, 1972). Grief can be both physiologically and emotionally traumatic but mourning plays an essential part in the return to a healthy and functional lifestyle. The adaptation to the loss of a loved one is, therefore, a normal and essential process which can be greatly helped if health care professionals understand the processes and emotions involved. Although no two losses are the same, it is recognized that there are certain tasks of mourning (Worden, 1983) which must be accomplished before a relative or friend can adjust to a bereavement:

1. to accept the reality of the loss;
2. to experience the pain of grief;
3. to adjust to an environment in which the deceased is missing;
4. to withdraw emotional energy and reinvest it in another relationship.

TO ACCEPT THE REALITY OF THE LOSS

The initial responses of relatives or friends to the death of someone they love is usually extreme shock and numbness, however well prepared they have been. Here the professional team may encourage acceptance by allowing relatives to spend time with the deceased and by allowing those who have not been present to view the body while still on the ward. Allowing relatives to return to view or to visit the undertaker to see the person who has died, again has an important function in bringing them gently to reality. Formalities of death have functions in reinforcing the facts of loss and often the preparations for the funeral, the registering of the death and the gathering of the family and friends can assist in this process.

Mourning rituals have changed substantially from the 'wake' which was common at the turn of the century but this ritual had benefits in offering an acceptable arena for the release of emotions and for allowing natural 'goodbyes' to be said. The intense searching behaviour described by Parkes (1972) is part of this process of acceptance. While accepting the facts of the loss, some people may deny the meaning of the loss and may find it difficult to move to the second task.

TO EXPERIENCE THE PAIN OF GRIEF

The pain of intense grief is that described as separation pain when intense yearning, pining and longing for the loved one may totally disrupt the physical and psychological parameters of life. The physical manifestations are those of an acute stress reaction. People may experience a feeling of hollowness in the stomach, tightness in the chest and throat, breathlessness, weakness of muscles, lack of energy, sweating, diarrhoea, dizziness, irritability and sensitivity to noise, loss of appetite and concentration, insomnia and a sense of depersonalization. Grief is sometimes experienced as total pain and the restlessness and agitation while pining for the dead person may sometimes be an extremely frightening reaction. Psychological mourning processes often lead to a certain disorganization. Frequently the dead person is idealized and sometimes there is an overlay of guilt that the relationship may not have been perfect. Some people find they stay orientated to the rituals of their previous life with no real changes and then experience acute grief when they realize that life will not be as it was before.

TO ADJUST TO AN ENVIRONMENT IN WHICH THE DECEASED IS MISSING

This task may take a long time to accomplish. Changes in practical matters and lifestyle may be not only difficult but unwelcome. Often people must find new skills and adopt new roles. Parkes (1972) states that in any bereavement it is seldom clear exactly what is lost. This is a time of great adjustment and the gradual undoing of the bonds which have tied people for many years. The symbolic development of 'shrines' (for example untouched bedrooms) may hamper this process and birthdays and anniversaries will often make people experience again an upsurge of grief, which may lead them to feel this task is not accomplished. The bereaved may suffer from hallucinations of their loved ones and continue with routines of their past existence. However, in wanting recovery, which may take several years, this task is usually completed.

TO WITHDRAW EMOTIONAL ENERGY AND REINVEST IT IN ANOTHER RELATIONSHIP

Some people may view new relationships as being disloyal to the memory of the deceased person and for many this is the hardest task to accomplish. Although it may appear unbelieveable that life can ever be good again, for many a new relationship can signify that all the tasks of mourning have been completed.

Abnormal Grief Reactions

For most people, grieving following a major bereavement is a long, difficult and lonely process. The majority of people will survive. Some will grow through their bereavement, others will need help and for some their grief may become pathological or abnormal.

DETERMINANTS OF THE OUTCOME OF BEREAVEMENT

In some establishments where death is a frequent occurrence 'at risk' assessments are performed to ascertain which relatives and friends might be vulnerable to pathological grief. People who score highly on these assessments may be channelled to a support network or counselling programme such as those run by many of the hospices or by local trained volunteers in organizations such as CRUSE. CRUSE is an organization for widows, widowers and their children, founded in 1959 in the United Kingdom, to offer help regardless of age, nationality or belief.

Parkes (1972) lists the determinants of bereavement outcome as:

1. *Antecedent*: those factors existing prior to the death including previous experience and life crises, relationship with the deceased and mode of death.

2. *Concurrent*: those factors determining a person's existence – sex, age, personality, social, religious and cultural characteristics.
3. *Subsequent*: social support, additional stresses and life opportunities.

Worden (1983) has listed more simply the six categories which he feels encompass the determinants of grief:

1. who the person was;
2. the nature of the attachment;
3. the mode of death;
4. the historical background;
5. personality variables;
6. social variables.

Help for the Bereaved

It must never be forgotten that the staff, both professional and ancillary, are also bereaved at the time of death when a patient has been known to them for a long period of time. Often staff need support themselves to be able to help the relatives and friends. Bereavement counselling is becoming an increasingly familiar phenomenon. In the United Kingdom, as elsewhere, there are now courses run by bereavement organizations or by independent counsellors to prepare people for this difficult and sensitive task.

Several factors are important in the provision of guidance and support for the bereaved during the process of mourning:

1. to be there and available;
2. to help the bereaved to recognize the loss;
3. to assist in the practicalities of survival;
4. to assist with the expression of emotions;
5. to recognize the warning signs of abnormal grief;
6. to be able to emphasize and yet not become overwhelmed by the intensity of an individual's grief;
7. to recognize the patterns of normal grief and the strength of the attendant feelings;
8. to be able to recognize when other skilled help is necessary;
9. to not become disheartened by the length of the bereavement process;
10. to believe that life can be good again;

11. to be able to let go at the end of the supportive relationship;
12. to have adequate personal support.

Death is one of the few certainties of this life. It is feared by many, misunderstood by some and, when caused by cancer, is often untimely. For the professional whose tasks are to ease the physical, emotional and spiritual suffering of the patient at the end of his or her life, the future must lie in adequate education for the necessary knowledge and skills and continuous support to enable them to be exercised.

References and Further Reading

Benoliel, J. (1972) Nursing care for the terminal patient; a psychological approach, in I. Schoenberg *et al.* (eds.) *Psychosocial Aspects of Terminal Care*, Columbia University Press, New York, p. 145.

Bowlby, J.C. (1980) *Attachment and Loss*, Vol. 3: *Loss, Sadness and Depression*, Hogarth Press, London, p. 582.

Brittain, V. (1933) *Testament of Youth*, Victor Gollancz, London.

Cancer Relief Macmillan Fund, Anchor House, 15/19 Britten Street, London, SW3 3TY.

Conboy-Hill, S. (1986) Terminal care: Their death in your hands, *The Professional Nurse*, Vol. 2, no. 2, pp. 51–3.

Corr, C. and Corr, D. (eds.) (1983) *Hospice Care: Principles and Practice*, Faber & Faber, London.

Craven, J. and Wald, F. (1975) Hospice care for dying patients, *American Journal of Nursing*, Vol. 75, pp. 1816.

CRUSE, Cruse House, 126 Sheen Road, Richmond, Surrey, TW9 1UR.

Daland, E.M. (1948) Palliative treatment of patients with advanced cancer, *Journal of the American Medical Association*, Vol. 136, pp. 391–6.

Davidson, G. (1979) Hospice care for the dying, in H. Wass (ed.) *Dying; Facing Facts*, McGraw Hill/Hemisphere, New York.

Engel, G. (1964) Grief and giving, *American Journal of Nursing*, Vol. 64, no. 9, pp. 93–8.

English National Board for Nursing, Midwifery and Health Visiting, 170 Tottenham Court Road, London, W1P 0HA.

Freud, S. (1917) Mourning and melancholia, in *Sigmund Freud: Collected Papers, Vol. 4*, Basic Books, New York.

Friel, M. and Tehan, C. (1980) Counteracting burnout for the hospice caregiver, *Cancer Nursing*, Vol. 3, no. 4, p. 285.

Friel, P. (1982) Death and Dying, *Annals of Internal Medicine*, Vol. 987, pp. 767–71.

General Register Office (1967) *The Registrar-General's Statistical Review of England and Wales for the Year 1966*, Part 1, Tables Medical, HMSO, London.

Glaser, B. and Strauss, A. (1964) Awareness contexts and social interaction, *American Sociological Review*, Vol. 29, pp. 669–79.

Glaser, B. and Strauss, A. (1966) *Awareness of Dying*, Aldine, Chicago.

Goldstone, W., Ball, J. and Collier, H. (1983) *MONITOR – An Index of the Quality of Nursing Care for Acute Medical and Surgical Wards*, Newcastle upon Tyne Polytechnic.

Gorer, G. (1976) *Death, Grief and Mourning,* Anchor Books/Doubleday & Co., New York.

Hinton, J. (1979) Comparison of places and policies for terminal care, *Lancet*, Vol. i, pp. 29–32.

Holing, E. (1986) The primary caregiver's perception of the dying trajectory, *Cancer Nursing*, Vol. 9, no. 1, pp. 29–37.

Jackson, D. (1958) *Human Life and Worth*, Christian Medical Fellowship, London.

King Edward's Hospital Fund for London/National Association of Health Authorities (1987) *Care of the Dying: A Guide for Health Authorities*, KEFH/NAHA, London.

Kitson, C. (1986) The practical reality, *Nursing Times*, 19 March, pp. 33–4.

Krakoff, I. (1979) The case for active treatment in patients with advanced cancer: not everyone needs a hospice, *CA – A Cancer Journal for Clinicians*, Vol. 29, no. 2, pp. 108–11.

Kubler-Ross, E. (1969) *On Death and Dying*, Macmillan, New York.

MacAdam, D.B. and Smith, M. (1987) An initial assessment of suffering in terminal illness, *Palliative Medicine*, Vol. 1, pp. 37–47.

Office of Population Censuses and Statistics (1984) *Theories*, DH1, Table 14, HMSO, London.

Olivant, P. (1986) Last offices, *Nursing Times*, 19 March, p. 32.

Parkes, C.M. (1972) *Bereavement: Studies of Grief in Adult Life*, Tavistock, London.

Pattison, E. (1977) *The Experience of Dying*, Prentice Hall, London.

Pincus, L. (1974) *Death and the Family*, Faber & Faber, London.

Prophit, P. (1984) The place of prayer in nursing care. Paper presented at RCN Oncology Nursing Society Conference, September.

Rando, T. (1986) *Loss and Anticipatory Grief*, Lexington Books, Lexington, USA.

Raphael, B. (1984) *The Anatomy of Bereavement*, Hutchinson, London.

Richardson, J. (1979) *A Death in the Family*, Lion Publishing, Tring, Hertfordshire.

Robbins, J. (ed.) (1983) *Caring for the Dying Patient and the Family*, Harper & Row, London.

Stedeford, A. (1985) *Facing Death*, William Heinemann, London.

Stedeford, A. (1987) Hospice: a safe place to suffer, *Palliative Medicine*, Vol. 1, no. 1, p. 73.

Stoddard, S. (1979) *The Hospice Movement*, Jonathan Cape, London.

Tennyson, A. 'In memoriam', in H. Gardner (ed.) (1972) *New Oxford Book of English Verse*, Oxford University Press.

Tennyson, A. 'Ulysses', in H. Gardner (ed.) (1972) *New Oxford Book of English Verse*, Oxford University Press.

Thomas, D. 'Do not go gentle', in H. Gardner (ed.) (1972) *New Oxford Book of English Verse*, Oxford University Press.

Twycross, R. (1987) Quality before quantity — a note of caution, *Palliative Medicine*, Vol. 1, no. 1, pp. 65–72.

Vachon, M. (1978) Motivation and stress experienced by staff working with the terminally ill, *Death Education*, Vol. 2, pp. 113–22.

Vere, D. (1971) Lecture to Christian Medical Fellowship, 4 November.

Wilkinson, S. (1987) The reality of nursing cancer patients, *Lampada*, no. 12, pp. 12–19.

Wilson, C. (1985) Stress in hospice nursing, *Newsletter of the British Psychological Society*, no. 48, p. 5.

Worden, J.W. (1983) *Grief Counselling and Grief Therapy*, Tavistock Publications, London.

Yardley, J. and Hunt, J. (1988) Stress in home care and hospital support nurses for the terminally ill, in M. Watson, S. Greer and C. Thomas (eds.) *Psychosocial Oncology*, Pergamon Press, London.

Chapter 15

The Impact of Cancer on Specific Groups

Children with Cancer

BETH SEPION RSCN, RGN, RM, OncCert, FETC
Senior Nurse, Paediatric Unit, The Royal Marsden Hospital
London and Surrey

Introduction

In the past 20 years there have been major breakthroughs in the treatment of childhood cancer. Of the 1,200 children diagnosed as having cancer each year, over half of them are expected to survive. Cancer is no longer viewed as a rapidly progressive fatal disease, but as a chronic illness requiring intensive treatment. The aim now is to ensure that the child and his or her family survive emotionally and psychologically as well as physically. This requires paediatric oncology nurses to shed their traditional role as primary care-giver and adopt a new one of educator and supporter to parents as they continue *their* role as the primary care-givers. Although the title of this chapter refers only to the child with cancer, it is particularly relevant that the family is included in all issues discussed.

Research (Spinetta and Deasy-Spinetta, 1981; Fotchman and Foley, 1982) has shown that the whole family will be affected when a child is diagnosed as having cancer, and the best way to help them to cope is by involving and supporting the whole family. The goal of family-centred care is to educate the family about the disease, the treatment, the side-effects and the prognosis, where this is possible. Giving them a realistic picture will help to relieve their anxieties, their confusion and their feelings of hopelessness. Primary nursing is a system designed to provide individualized family-centred care. It is based on the foundation that a nurse with the appropriate qualifications and skills will accept the responsibility of assessing, planning, implementing and evaluating the care of the child and his or her family.

The introduction of a primary nurse, at this time, can facilitate the establishment of a relationship with the family and decrease the number of hospital personnel involved in the care of the child.

Investigation and Diagnosis

Parents require a great deal of support during the child's investigation period. They may be already aware of the potential diagnosis but need to continue to hope that it is not true or that mistakes have been made. Procedures carried out to aid or confirm diagnosis are often numerous, uncomfortable and can be painful for a child. They occur soon after admission when relationships are newly formed and trust may not yet be fully established. The parents and the child may require frequent explanation in preparation for these investigations. Children can be brave for one procedure, but at an early stage it is necessary to gain their trust if they are going to co-operate and cope not only with the investigations, but with their treatment as well.

The use of general anaesthesia has reduced the traumatic effect of invasive procedures. Routine investigations including bone marrow aspirates, lumbar punctures, computerized tomography (CT) scans, blood tests and insertion of cannulae, can be performed with the same general anaesthetic with the minimal amount of physical and psychological pain to the child.

As soon as the diagnosis is confirmed parents need to be told about it as the agony of waiting is protracted enough without delaying further. The way that the information is given to the parents is important. It is better if both parents are present, for this gives them the opportunity of checking with each other afterwards their own interpretation of the information. Telling only one parent imposes a tremendous strain and responsibility on that parent to be able to absorb the information and relay it back to his or her partner. Telling parents individually may lead to feelings of mistrust with the medical and nursing staff, because parents may have interpreted the news in different ways and consider that they have been given entirely different information.

In the early stages, parents require the confirmation of diagnosis, an outline of the suggested treatment, the side-effects of that treatment and the likely prognosis. Once the words 'tumour', 'cancer' or 'leukaemia' are used the parents may not hear or understand anything else that is said. One must, therefore, be aware of the necessity to repeat the same information over and over again. If the primary nurse is present with the parents at this interview, the information the doctor has given can be reinforced or clarified afterwards. The primary nurse can also ensure that the other members of the health care team are aware of the discussion and decisions made. Written confirmation of these first communications can be recorded on a communication sheet and kept in the child's care plan.

All members of the specific health care team can then have access to the information that the parents were given, to enable them to care intelligently for the child and family. The parents themselves also have access to these records and find it helpful to see the facts in writing. Often at this stage the parents' main worries are that it was something they could have prevented, something they had or had not done or something they should have detected earlier. They need a great deal of reassurance that they are not to blame for the occurrence of cancer.

When the parents have discussed the confirmed diagnosis, it is important that the child is told. The parents may be reluctant to do this at first, thinking that they can protect their child by not telling him or her, but there are several reasons why a child needs to be told the truth.

Truth-Telling

From the moment cancer has been suspected children will have picked up the anxieties of their parents and others surrounding them; they may interpret these as being very serious and will, therefore, be very frightened. Like adults, children in hospital often compare their own signs and symptoms with another patient in the bed next to them. This may cause confusion and may also lead the child to consider an even more serious or frightening diagnosis. Children may perceive the treatment as some kind of punishment. Also, if they feel that the medical and nursing staff are not telling them the truth at the beginning they are unlikely to trust them.

Subsequently, children need information about their illness, including its name, what it is, that it is treatable, what this treatment involves and the side-effects. This should be given at the child's level of understanding and therefore requires the skill of someone specializing in paediatric care. The effect that this will have on the child depends on age and previous experiences. Children under the age of five years are more concerned about separation and abandonment from parents than about dying. Children of five or six years of age, however, do appear to be able to grasp the seriousness of their illness and what it may mean, but may not be able to verbalize their fears. This will lead to intensification of those fears and the child may feel isolated if he or she continues to be treated with secrecy and avoidance of the truth. If children need to talk about their disease or its treatment but recognize that their parents do not or cannot, they may try to protect or please the parents by talking about it themselves. This may add to the child's own feelings of sadness, fear and guilt. If the primary nurse has formed a good relationship with the child she may well be able to detect this and facilitate communication between the child and the parents.

Siblings

The next hurdle for the parents to face is how to tell the other children in the family. Obviously it is important that this is done at a level of their individual development and understanding. The siblings need the same information as the patient but, in addition, they need reassurance that it is not contagious and it is not something that they have caused. Rivalry for parental attention is apparent in every family and if the well siblings do not have an understanding of why the sick child's demands are so great they may make excessive demands themselves. The siblings should be encouraged to visit the ward and be involved as much as possible. Primary nurses should get to know them by name and help them to recognize that they have an important role to play.

At this stage the parents may channel all their love, energy and care to the sick child and not recognize that the well children will be experiencing their own feelings of fear, guilt and grief. If help is not given to the parents to recognize this, the psychological well-being of the siblings could be affected long after the patient dies or is cured. Several studies (Koocher and O'Malley, 1981) have shown that there is no compelling evidence that when cancer is diagnosed in a child it increases the likelihood of divorce. There is, however, evidence that the diagnosis of cancer in the family does threaten the psychosocial development of the siblings (Lansky *et al.*, 1978).

Treatment

Paediatric tumours are treated with surgery, chemotherapy or radiotherapy or a combination of two or of all three. Paediatric tumours can develop and spread quite rapidly, therefore creating an urgency to start treatment before the family has had time to come to terms with the disease. One of our first priorities is to make the treatment acceptable. This again emphasizes the importance of an open, honest relationship. The parents have a wealth of information about their child, the primary nurse has knowledge about the treatment and by working together they can formulate a plan of care that is realistic and acceptable to the child and the family.

Major advances have been made in the treatment of childhood cancer. As with everything else, each child should be treated as an individual when assessing his or her capability for coping with the proposed management. Many children have commented that they feel well until the treatment starts. For this reason they need to maintain a degree of control. This can be encouraged by giving them the choice of which bed they have, what time they have their treatment and making other decisions for themselves, for example choosing their own food from the menu.

Children with cancer have identified that the treatment is worse for them than the disease itself (Fotchman and Foley, 1982). As previously stated most children can be brave for one unpleasant procedure, but most will have treatments lasting weeks or months and therefore it is important to establish a relationship of trust and co-operation. The parents may also experience feelings of helplessness and loss of control in giving over the care of their child to others. The primary nurse again plays an important role by educating the parents in their new role of primary care-giver to a sick child. Parents will require a great deal of support and reassurance from the health professionals, but many of them will be able to take on the day-to-day care of their child. Some parents may take on more responsibilities than others, keeping records of their child's fluid intake and output and temperature. However, it must be recognized that not all parents can cope with this and they will need reassurance that the role they do adopt is acceptable.

CHEMOTHERAPY

The use of skin-tunnelled catheters or other central lines facilitates the administration of chemotherapy, anti-emetics, analgesia and blood products and allows painless access for blood samples, without creating a needle phobia or placing too much restriction on the child's mobility.

Chemotherapy regimens are frequently complex due to the use of a combination of different cytotoxic agents. This requires nurses to have a wide understanding of their administration and side-effects. The rationale for combination therapy is to maximize the treatment effect on the tumour, with minimal toxicity to the patient, by using drugs that act on cells in different stages of the cell cycle. Common side-effects of chemotherapy agents in paediatrics are nausea and vomiting, alopecia, myelosuppression, mucositis and anorexia. Parental and child education of these potential side-effects prepares them to take an active role in the prevention and early detection of any problems.

The primary nurse can advise the child on the variety of anti-emetics available and can find the one that is most suitable for the individual child. Establishing an effective oral hygiene routine that children will perform themselves is more beneficial than having regimens that are rigid and do not allow for individual preferences and capabilities. Encouraging the parents to cook for their child on the ward enables them to maintain control over their child's nutritional needs. Children will often eat more because it is their mother's cooking and they can eat it when they feel like it rather than at set meal times.

RADIOTHERAPY

The restrictions that radiotherapy place on patients in requiring them to lie still in a room on their own with a large piece of equipment are often too much for a child to cope with. Sedation or general anaesthesia can be used in such cases. A major problem identified when using medication strong enough to sedate the child is that it takes a long time for it to wear off. This interferes with meal times and normal sleep patterns and can cause major disruption in family life if it continues. There should be no age restrictions as to who qualifies for a general anaesthetic but criteria should be based on the needs of the individual child. Observing another child having treatment, playing with the equipment and meeting the staff who will be responsible for the child during the procedure, all help the child and the parents to decide what he or she can or cannot cope with. Again there must be flexibility within the department in case the child has a change of mind.

Children receiving a daily general anaesthetic for radiotherapy can still be treated as outpatients with the parents taking the responsibility to administer the premedication when appropriate. Side-effects of radiotherapy are related to the area being treated. The parents and patient will require advice on the short- and long-term side-effects. Skin care with specific advice on the use of soap and water and creams again needs to be assessed on an individual basis. Parents will also require warning of the somnolent period that children experience about six weeks after completing cranial irradiation. It is important to give reassurance that it is normal for them to experience intermittent low-grade pyrexias and general lethargy for up to a week and that this should only require hospital admission on the rare occasion that there is inadequate oral intake. Long-term side-effects such as growth retardation due to irradiation of the spine, or to the growth rate of long bones may cause psychological problems which may require skilled help in the future. Children usually cope very well with their radiotherapy. If they remain in hospital to have it, boredom is their worst enemy.

SURGERY

Surgery may be performed as a means of obtaining a diagnosis, assessing the extent of the spread of the disease, or for removal of the tumour. The child requires both physical and emotional preparation. Visits to the anaesthetic and recovery area may be appropriate. The parents will also require explanation and reassurance at this time. The opportunity of escorting their child to and from the operating theatre is usually appreciated by both the child and the parents.

Play

The child's environment during this treatment is important. Children will continue to grow and develop during their illness and therefore an environment must be provided that is conducive to their physical and emotional growth.

Play is an important part of the child's development. It therefore needs to be continued and encouraged in hospital. It may be diversional or therapeutic. The availability of syringes, bandages, stethoscopes, blood pressure cuffs and intravenous equipment may help children to identify, verbalize and act out their fears. The parents, play therapist or primary nurse can help the child to find an acceptable way to come to terms with the different instruments and procedures. Play can also be used to introduce the next stage of treatment.

Remission and Relapse

When the first treatment is given in hospital the parents may experience problems on returning home for the first time and coping on their own. They need reassurance that they can cope, information about potential side-effects they may encounter and guidelines on any restrictions or limitations there may be. They also need a telephone number for them to contact someone whom they know and who knows them and their child. Statistically, general practitioners will probably only see one case of childhood cancer during their entire practice and will, therefore, need adequate communication from the hospital if they are to continue the support in the community.

Each stage of the disease and treatment will bring new stresses to the family. When the child's disease is in remission the side-effects of the treatment are easier to cope with and the family can begin to take on more than a day-to-day existence, but the fear of relapse is always in their mind (Lansky *et al.*, 1979).

For the sake of the children, normal life needs to be re-established as soon as possible. The parents need support and guidance to discipline the child as they would have done before the illness was diagnosed. The parents need help to recognize that the child needs the security of being treated the same as his or her siblings. It is unfair to cure children of their disease and then cause them to be in social exile with their peers because they are over-protected.

If the disease recurs, the whole family will enter a crisis situation again. They understand the implications of relapse and may experience the more severe feelings of shock, anger, grief and fear than at the time of diagnosis. The recommencement of treatment may cause more psychological problems for the patient than the initial treatment.

Terminal Care

When the stage is reached where active treatment is no longer appropriate to achieve cure or remission, alternative ways must be identified to continue the care and support of the child and the family.

The parents may have already prepared for this stage. Futterman and Hoffman (1973) defined this anticipatory mourning as 'a set of processes that are directly related to the awareness of the impeding loss, to its emotional impact and to the adaptive mechanisms whereby emotional attachment to the child is relinquished over time'.

The issue of discussing death is difficult. Elizabeth Kubler-Ross (1974) states:

> No patient should be told that he is dying. I do not encourage people to force patients to face their own death when they are not ready for it. Patients should be told that they are seriously ill. When they are ready to bring up the issue of death and dying, we should answer them, we should listen to them, we should hear their questions, but you do not go around telling patients they are dying and deprive them of a glimpse of hope that they may need in order to live until they die.

Children may well adopt a similar coping strategy as at the time of diagnosis, namely protecting their parents by not discussing things that they feel may distress them. The primary nurse may well be the person with whom the child chooses in this instance to share his or her fears and anxieties. Decisions on where the child dies should be made by the child, the parents and the members of the multidisciplinary team. The parents will require information about the support available in the community, to help make this decision. The primary nurse can introduce the support of the community liaison sister or support team, where available.

Parents who have developed the skills of administering medication via their child's central venous line may well wish to administer intravenous analgesia, anti-emetics and hypnotics at home. Guidelines may need to be drawn up for this within individual health authorities.

In the terminal stages of the disease, the paediatric oncology nurses are required to develop skills in recognizing different coping mechanisms and helping the family to realize that their feelings of anger, hope, despair, sadness and depression are normal and need to be expressed.

Pain is a major concern of both the child and the parents. Analgesia needs to be given in doses that control the pain but leave children alert and able to do the things that are important to them. The fear that the children may become addicted to drugs is not an issue in this case and there should be no limits on the doses prescribed to control the pain.

The use of blood products and antibiotics has a place in symptom control if used to improve the quality of life not the quantity.

Support links and bereavement follow-up need to be established before the child dies. Families need to know in advance that their acute feelings of grief and mourning may last several months and that anniversaries of birthdays and Christmas may act as painful reminders of the child. It is important that the parents feel that they can come back to the ward either to visit or to discuss any issues that are worrying them.

Staff Support

Nurses working in paediatric oncology must learn to recognize their own coping mechanisms and also those of their colleagues. Support should be available in the form that is most acceptable to the individual members of the health care team and at the most appropriate time.

Paediatric oncology nursing is demanding both physically and emotionally. Nurses must not develop emotional immunity to the death of a child but must learn to recognize the positive skills they have to offer to the whole family to help them all live with the cancer.

References

Fotchman, D. and Foley, G. (1982) *Nursing Care of a Child with Cancer*, Little Brown & Co., Boston, USA.

Futterman, E. and Hoffman, I. (1973) *Crisis and Adaptation in the Families of the Fatally Ill Children*, John Wiley & Sons, New York.

Koocher, G.P. and O' Malley, J.E. (1981) *The Damocles Syndrome*, McGraw-Hill, New York.

Kubler-Ross, E. (1974) *Questions and Answers on Death and Dying*, Macmillan & Co., New York.

Lansky, S.B. *et al.* (1978) Childhood cancer: parental discord and divorce, *Paediatrics*, Vol. 62, no. 2, pp. 184–8.

Lansky, S.B. *et al.* (1979) *The Family Of the Child with Cancer*. American Cancer Society.

Spinetta, J. and Deasy-Spinetta, P. (1981) *Living with Childhood Cancer*, C.V. Mosby, St Louis.

Adolescents with Cancer

JENNY THOMPSON RGN RSCN, OncCert, FETC

Director of Nursing Services

The Royal Marsden Hospital, London and Surrey

Introduction

Before the significant advances in the diagnosis and treatment of cancer many young people died quickly of the disease. Now, cancer in the adolescent age-group is considered a chronic disease. Chronicity has considerable implications for the care and support of this particular age-group. As with younger children, cancer in the adolescent years is rare, yet accounts for significant morbidity and mortality (Klopouvich and Cohen, 1984).

For the adolescent with cancer, developmental concerns of maturity, independence and a sexual identity are of no less importance than those of their well peers. Health care professionals must recognize that adolescents with cancer need to master these developmental tasks together with the additional stress of the diagnosis of a life-threatening illness. The types of cancer most commonly found in the adolescent population are listed in Table 15.1.

Table 15.1 *Most common types of cancer in adolescents*

---

(1) Acute leukaemia
    (a) lymphocytic
    (b) non-lymphocytic

(2) Central nervous system tumours

(3) Lymphomas
    (a) Hodgkin's disease
    (b) non-Hodgkin's lymphomas

(4) Bone tumours
    (a) osteogenic sarcomas
    (b) Ewing's sarcomas

Adolescent Growth and Development

The word 'adolescence' is derived from the Latin verb *adolescere* – 'to grow up'. The length of time generally recognized as a transition from childhood to adulthood varies in different cultures. However, in all cultures this transitional period encompasses not only the physical changes of puberty but also the emotional, physiological and social differences between adults and children.

During the present century many theories have been put forward concerning adolescence. Hall (1962) regarded adolescence as a period of 'storm and stress'. He emphasized the importance of the developmental process but tended to underplay the effect of environmental influences on the developing individual. Brook (1985) states that the age-range for the start of adolescent growth may be between 9 and 13 years in girls and 10 and 15 years in boys.

Differences in the speed of growth and development, especially in adolescence, make it difficult to give an exact chronological age-range to define adolescence. In modern, Western societies most people would support the suggestion that adolescence includes the years approximately from the ages of 12 to 19 years. Crow and Crow (1965) state that no two individuals are alike and at no age are these differences more apparent than during adolescent years.

Kuykendall (1985) describes the period of adolescence as being complex. He emphasizes that during different stages and at differing times there are specific tasks that the adolescent addresses. He describes stages of early, middle and late adolescence. In early adolescence he states that the development of peer-groups, primarily of the same sex, is important, whereas in middle and late adolescence peer-groups remain important but tend to be of mixed sexes.

Adolescence can therefore be described as a time of tremendous change characterized by high and low mood swings as individuals seek to find their own identity. Acceptance by peer groups is important for a sense of self-confidence and self-worth. The diagnosis of cancer may threaten and interrupt the adolescent who is striving for independence and an adult future.

Cancer and its Impact on Adolescent Development

Cancer – its image and treatment – is likely to threaten the adolescent's sense of worth and competence. Probably the most devastating effect the adolescent will experience is losing control of his or her life and body at a time when self-image, self-esteem and independence are crucial to that individual.

Moore *et al.* (1969), discussing the management of cancer in the adolescent, state that the treatment given for the cancer may result in undesirable changes in body image that cause further stress. Alopecia is one such change. To the female, it may signify the loss of femininity and to the male, loss of virility. This effect on sexuality at such a vulnerable time may cause a profound loss of self-esteem.

Other outcomes of treatment may interfere with body image, independence and sexuality. Scarring following surgery and changes in skin colour and texture as the result of drug therapy or radiotherapy may result in the adolescent not wanting to reveal parts of his or her body. Reacting in this way will limit the choice of clothing at a time when fashion and copying others' dress are all-important.

The adolescent who is not acceptable as he or she wishes to appear before friends and family may use a visible change in body image as an excuse: one such patient said, 'I'm not popular because I have lost my hair due to treatment'. They may also engage in attention-seeking behaviour just to be noticed. Hammer and Eddy (1968) state that rebellion in the adolescent with chronic illness is not unusual; it is often an exaggeration of normal adolescent rebellion, but because the consequences of such behaviour in the chronically ill youngster may be more serious it becomes extremely threatening to those entrusted with that person's care. Hammer and Eddy (1968) also describe the behaviour of the adolescent who appears to overcompensate for his or her feelings and concerns about self and about the illness. Describing the dedicated athlete with an amputation or the determined scholar with a chronic disease, they support the fact that the fantastic amounts of energy and perseverance to succeed should not be discouraged, but should be encouraged. Given time and freedom to try, the handicapped adolescent will generally adjust to the situation and set his or her own realistic goals.

Gabriel and Hoffman (1983) have divided the tasks of adolescence into three main groups: independence, identity and a functional role. Independence is described as mastering control over self, the environment and gaining a sense of autonomy. Identity makes reference to the acquisition of a positive body image. A functional role is described as that which results from the completion of education and training, the plans for future employment and the prospect of marriage. The impact of cancer on these three groups is described in Table 15.2.

Table 15.2   *The effect of cancer on adolescent development*

Developmental task	Effects caused by cancer
Independence	Increased dependence on parents and family members for care and financial support. Dependence on health care professionals. Dependence on significant others. Limited autonomy
Identity	Decreased peer contact due to periods of hospitalization; impaired body image due to effects of treatment, for example hair loss, weight loss or gain, scarring. Decreased self-esteem and sexual identity.
Functional Role	Limited or changed lifestyle. Interrupted education and training. Compromised future goals. Question of marriage prospects. Question of gaining employment, life insurance and mortgage.

Until recently the unique difficulties experienced by the adolescent cancer patient have received little attention. Two studies carried out by Koocher and O'Malley (1981) and Spinetta and Deasy-Spinetta (1981) look at the psychosocial consequences of living with and surviving childhood cancer. Both studies examine the special needs of the adolescent patient. One unresolved problem that they highlighted was the number of surviving cancer patients who had difficulty obtaining or retaining employment due in part to the persistent negative attitude of employers towards cancer. Plumb and Holland (1974) investigated the reaction of adolescents to the side-effects of cancer treatment. They report that for the adolescent, side-effects such as impaired athletic ability and the loss of physical attractiveness may be much more alarming than the threat of death.

Care and Support – for the Patient

Since more sophisticated treatment has resulted in some cures and better control of cancer, the adolescent patient's focus will be on living and coping with cancer. The patient and his or her family will live with a great deal of uncertainty during this time.

The special problems of caring for and supporting the adolescent are not always recognized and understood by health care professionals. Brook (1985) states that in medical terms adolescents are badly catered for. He says that their problems fall between the spheres of the expertise of paediatricians and the various specialties of adult medicine. Burman (1982) stated that there is a lack of awareness among the medical profession as to the problems of the adolescent as there was with children 30 years ago.

The way that adolescents are treated by their family, friends, health care professionals and others is crucial in giving them encouragement to face a diagnosis of cancer. Previous experience of hospitalization and how adolescents view health care professionals, helps to determine how they perceive themselves and their ability to cope with the diagnosis. Donovan and Pierce (1976) state that the initial reaction of others immediately after the threat to oneself is realized, seems to be more important than the visible effects or the severity of the diagnosis.

With an understanding of adolescent growth and development care must be directed towards helping patients in this age-group to find appropriate methods of coping and adapting to a changed lifestyle. Trust is only established when the adolescent receives honest and accurate information. Knowledge of the disease and treatment can strengthen the adolescent's sense of worth. Fochtman (1979) states that the strengths of the adolescent must be fostered by the staff throughout the course of the illness. The staff can help patients to identify their feelings by discussing some of the reactions expressed by other patients. Using this approach may help adolescents to recognize their own feelings and also to realize that if others experience similar anxieties, their reactions are not peculiar or unusual. Morrow (1978) suggests that care must therefore be directed towards supporting the adolescent from diagnosis through treatment in an atmosphere conducive to his or her developmental progress and a full life.

Care and Support – for Parents

The family usually needs the same kind of help as the adolescent patient. They too are trying to cope with the effect of cancer on the patient. When a family tries to accept a diagnosis it should be recognized that feelings of anger and resentment may be displaced onto health care professionals. Such anger need not be taken personally and staff should not become involved in defending themselves or colleagues. Accepting the reasons for resentment, they must strive to give the best comprehensive care. Listening and accepting feelings of the adolescent and family are often all that are required. Giving inappropriate advice or being defensive will only create more problems. In their study Koocher and O'Malley (1981) considered family relationships. Most parents described the importance of feeling able or permitted to express their own emotions. The tone set by health care professionals in both inpatient and outpatient settings was of major importance. How procedures were carried out and the way in which news was communicated seemed far more important than the specifics of actual treatment. The study showed that, contrary to popular myth, marital stability seemed unaffected by the cancer experience. Many parents described the experience as having a positive effect on their marriage. They tended to draw closer and become more sensitive to each other's needs. Whether or not the findings would be similar if the child or adolescent had died requires further investigation.

Care and Support – for Siblings

One of the most stressful consequences faced by the healthy siblings is frequent separation from their sick brother or sister caused by repeated hospitalization and visits to outpatient clinics. Sourkes (1981) noted that siblings expressed concern about the cause of the illness, the visibility of the illness and the effects of treatment. Fears were also expressed that cancer may be contagious. Koocher and O'Malley (1981) asked 101 siblings to describe their feelings and experiences about the diagnosis of cancer in a brother or sister. They described feelings of resentment and jealousy but also reported feeling ashamed of such negative thoughts.

Clearly, healthy siblings have a unique set of problems with which they must cope. Kramer and Moore (1983) describe a programme that was developed to facilitate healthy siblings' adjustment to the experience of cancer in a brother or sister. The purpose of the programme was to provide siblings with an opportunity to discuss their feelings and concerns. Following evaluation, the benefits of the programme were encouraging. They reflected increased sibling adjustment. Health care professionals therefore need not only to be aware of the needs of siblings themselves but also must remind families of those needs.

Conclusion

With knowledge of adolescent growth and development, health care professionals and others will have a better understanding of the impact of a diagnosis of cancer on this vulnerable group. Brook (1985) suggests that it often appears that the health professional's own inability to deal with the adolescent is because adolescent development is not part of the curriculum of most training courses, medical or otherwise.

However, with honesty and support from care-givers who understand them, many adolescents will survive a serious illness with minimal psychological scarring.

References

Brook, C.D.G. (1985) *All About Adolescence*, John Wiley, Chichester.

Burman, D. (1982) *Adolescents in Hospital*, edited papers from Adolescents in Hospital Conference, The National Association for the Welfare of Children in Hospital (NAWCH), London.

Crow, L. and Crow, A. (1965) *Adolescent Development and Adjustment* (2nd edn), McGraw-Hill, New York.

Donovan, M. and Pierce, S. (1976) *Identity and Body Image*, Appleton Crofts, New York.

Fochtman, D. (1979) How adolescents live with leukaemia, *Cancer Nursing*, Vol. 2, no. 1, pp. 27–31.

Gabriel, H. and Hoffman, A. (1983) Managing chronic illness, in A. Hoffman (ed.) *Adolescent Medicine*, Adison-Wesley, Menlo Park, California, p. 351.

Hall, G. (1962) in R.E. Muuss (ed.) *Theories of Adolescence*, Random House Inc., New York.

Hammer, S. and Eddy, J. (1968) *Nursing Care of Adolescent*, William Heinemann Medical Books, London, pp. 73–74.

Klopouvich, P. and Cohen, D. (1984) An overview of paediatric oncology nursing for the adult oncology nurse. *Oncology Nursing Forum*, Vol. 11, pp. 56–63.

Koocher, G. and O'Malley, J. (1981) *The Damocles Syndrome*, McGraw-Hill, New York/London.

Kramer, R. and Moore, I. (1983) Childhood cancer. Meeting the special needs of healthy siblings. *Cancer Nursing*, Vol. 6, no. 3, pp. 213–17.

Kuykendall, J. (1985) *Adolescents in Hospital*, edited papers from Adolescents in Hospital Conference, The National Association for the Welfare of Children in Hospital (NAWCH), London.

Moore, D. *et al.* (1969) Psychological problems in the management of adolescents with cancer, *Clinical Paediatrics*, Vol. 8, pp. 464–73.

Morrow, M. (1978) The effect of cancer chemotherapy on psychosocial development, in M. Klopouvich and B.J. Clancy, Sexuality and the adolescent with cancer, *Seminars in Oncology Nursing*, Vol. 1, no. 1, pp. 42–8.

Plumb, M. and Holland, J. (1974) Cancers in adolescents. The symptom is the thing, in B. Schoenberg *et al.* (eds.) *Anticipating Grief*, Columbia University Press, New York.

Sourkes, B. (1981) Siblings of the paediatric cancer patient, in J. Spinetta and P. Deasy-Spinetta (eds.) *Living with Childhood Cancer*, C.V. Mosby, London/St Louis/Toronto.

Spinetta, J. and Deasy-Spinetta, P. (1981) *Living with Childhood Cancer*, C.V. Mosby London/St Louis/Toronto.

The Elderly with Cancer

DEBORAH WELCH-McCAFFREY RN, MSN
Oncology Clinical Nurse Specialist
Good Samaritan Medical Center, Phoenix, Arizona

Introduction

The single greatest risk factor for the development of cancer is growing old. With every five years of life, the risk of developing cancer doubles. In a 25-year-old person, this risk is 1 in 600; by the age of 70, the risk is increased to 1 in 10. So, the longer you live, the more likely you are to develop cancer.

As a whole, the elderly represent a small proportion of the total population – 11 per cent in the United States of America and 8 per cent in the United Kingdom. Yet the elderly account for a disproportionate number of cancer cases given that more than half of all cancers are diagnosed in those over 65 years of age. This problem will also become accentuated during the next 20 years as a result of an exponential growth in the total number of those individuals surviving beyond 65 years of age (Baranovsky and Myers, 1986; Crawford and Cohen, 1987).

Unlike other oncology specialties, such as paediatrics, geriatric oncology has received comparatively little attention. In the light of the statistical evidence now available the time has come to focus attention on that subset of cancer patients which represents a significant proportion of the total population of cancer patients. The unique needs of the older cancer patient have not been uniformly addressed nor systematically researched. A blending of knowledge between oncology and geriatric nurses is desperately needed if a sound practice base is to be formulated so that elderly patients receive expert care.

This section identifies critical themes to assist health care professionals in expanding their knowledge base related to geriatric oncology nursing. It reviews the problem of cancer in the elderly; discusses dilemmas encountered in treating elderly cancer patients with antineoplastic therapies; and highlights issues in nursing care that require ongoing assessment and intervention.

Cancer in the Elderly – the Problem

Ongoing research addresses the relationship of ageing to cancer without coming to any finite conclusion. Two main schools of thought may be identified. One feels that cancer is not a consequence of ageing while the other argues that ageing does facilitate tumour development (Butler and Gastel, 1979; Goodell, 1985; Lipschitz *et al.*, 1985; Ponten, 1985).

The normal process of ageing is postulated to predispose the older person to cancer (Table 15.3). As DNA becomes progressively

Table 15.3   *The relationship of cancer to ageing*

Process of general ageing
DNA instability
Loss of genetic information required for the control of cell division

NORMAL PROCESS:	ABNORMAL PROCESS:
Cellular ageing	Cancer

unstable as a correlate of normal ageing, genetic information necessary to control cell division is lost. Two distinct end-products may result.

First, there is the normal process of cellular ageing evidenced by changes in the elasticity of the skin, functional neurosensory impairment in vision, hearing and touch and modifications in gastrointestinal function which effect secretion, digestion, absorption and motility. A reduction in vital organ mass also occurs with normal ageing which results in compromised cerebral, renal and cardiac circulation.

Second, the end-product of DNA instability in relation to ageing may be malignancy. As the genetic information required for normal cell reproduction becomes lost or miscoded, an abnormal growth of cells may be promoted and cancer develops. Concurrent factors within the host may also foster the growth of cancer (Table 15.4).

Table 15.4   *Theories of cancer causation in the elderly*

(1)	Accumulation of somatic mutation
(2)	Increased sensitivity to oncogenic viruses
(3)	Increased sensitivity to external carcinogens
(4)	Decreased immunological resistance to neoplastic cells
(5)	Increased tendency for hormone imbalance

In particular, the relationship of ageing with compromised immune system functioning is critically important to the study of prevalence of cancer in the elderly. Alterations in cell-mediated immunity and a reduction of the functional reserve capacity of the bone marrow with age are thought to affect the older person's ability to both recognize and eradicate evidence of early proliferation of cancer. This reduced immunological functioning also influences the older patient's ability to tolerate antineoplastic therapies.

Prominent cancers in the elderly population are identified in Table 15.5. These cancers represent 70 per cent of all cancer diagnoses in the elderly. Non-melanomatous skin cancer is also a frequent malignancy

Table 15.5   *Prominent cancers in the elderly*

Male	Female	Combined
Prostate	Breast	Colo-rectal
Bladder	Uterus	Lung
Stomach	Ovary	Pancreas

in the elderly population. Other cancers with less frequent incidence, but of significance in that they occur almost exclusively in the older person, include cancer of the gallbladder, multiple myeloma and some forms of chronic leukaemia affecting both males and females.

Prostate cancer in the elderly male represents a significant health care problem. Currently in the United States, between 3 and 4 million men are thought to have prostate cancer yet fewer than 2 per cent of these men are diagnosed each year (Cape, 1983; Ahmann, 1985). It is still not understood why prostate cancer becomes clinically apparent in only a small percentage of men who have the disease. Prostate cancer will present an immense health care problem in the future as the number of elderly men surviving increases dramatically.

Breast cancer in elderly women is the most common malignancy found in those over 65 years of age. Additionally, elderly females have twice the incidence rates of breast cancer compared with women between the ages of 45 and 64 years. A change in the nature of breast cancer relative to age, however, appears to make this malignancy less aggressive.

Elderly women with breast cancer, having a greater incidence of oestrogen receptor-positive tumours, have added treatment options open to them in the form of hormonal therapy. The tumour itself may also be a biologically less aggressive variant, due to fewer numbers of cells in the S (synthesis) and G2 (where the cell prepares for mitosis) phases of cell reproduction, than that found in younger patients with breast cancer.

An important determinant to any patient's prognosis is the stage of disease at initial diagnosis. Special consideration must be addressed to this issue in geriatric oncology as it has a bearing on the efficacy of treatment, ultimate prognosis and, importantly, screening programmes for the elderly.

The primary question confronting all practitioners and researchers in geriatric oncology concerns the relationship between the stage of cancer and host resistance. Are the differences in survival attributable to the reduced physical capacity of older people to survive even early cancer or to the point at which older people enter the medical system and receive a primary diagnosis and initial therapy? The tendency to be diagnosed at a more advanced stage of cancer may reduce the chances for survival in the elderly. The fault would appear to lie with both the patient and the health care system. In general, the elderly appear less compliant with routine health screening than are their younger counterparts. Ongoing monthly breast self-examination and annual cervical smears, for example, are not always undertaken as a necessary cancer screening practice. Reasons for this are plentiful. Access to screening or transport problems may interfere with the screening process. The elderly often resist costly screening (where cost is a factor) especially if they are asymptomatic. Emotional reactions may also play an important part in avoiding cancer screening options. A fatalistic attitude – 'It's too late' – or an overwhelming fear that cancer will indeed be detected, are often responsible for the elderly avoiding cancer screening programmes.

Health professionals may also be eager to assume that a particular cluster of signs and symptoms, attributable to normal ageing or another chronic disease, is indicative of cancer. Bone pain, for example, may easily be related to a history of arthritis rather than to a new presenting symptom of bone metastases associated with oat cell lung cancer or multiple myeloma. Rectal bleeding may be correlated with old haemorrhoids rather than a potential colo-rectal tumour. The differential diagnosis of cancer in the elderly is frequently difficult as the cancer-related symptoms often arise among multiple disease processes. Successful treatment of one cancer should not negate the possibility of new symptoms of a second cancer, the incidence of second and third primaries being higher in the elderly population.

Antineoplastic Therapies in the Elderly

Problems are many when treatment modalities in the elderly are evaluated. Often, decisions on treating elderly cancer patients are based on anecdotal observations rather than on the results of validated research findings.

Few well-controlled clinical trials have compared the elderly with their younger counterparts in terms of the intensity of treatment, the response to it, and toxicity incidence. The existence of an arbitrary cut-off age (65 years) for dose reduction in many treatment protocols has compromised the development of appropriate treatment regimens for the elderly cancer patient. By excluding *all* elderly patients from the treatment protocols on the basis of age alone, the decision to treat or not to treat or to what extent to treat, is founded on speculation. It has recently been stated, however, that chronological age should never be the sole criterion on which treatment decisions are made (Serpick, 1978). Because the elderly are a heterogeneous group, consideration must be given to physiological as well as chronological age. To date, all people over 65 years of age are categorized as similar, little attention being given to the fact that an 80-year old may have a distinctly different state of health from a 70-year-old and that within each group there are variations of a health status based on individual norms.

Automatic reduction or omission of treatment in the elderly has been based on information describing normal ageing. Acknowledging functional decreases in size of vital organs due to age, concern about toxicity tolerance in elderly cancer patients has been the impetus for excluding the elderly from many treatment protocols. Table 15.6 outlines these changes and identifies cancer-related implications.

Table 15.6   *Normal physiological changes of ageing and their implications for cancer treatment*

Functional decrease in size	Result	Concurrent cancer-related concern
Skeletal muscle: 40%	Anorexia/cachexia syndrome pronounced; cardiac index decreased	Nutritional compromise from multimodality therapy; reversal of catabolism; cardiotoxicity
Liver: 18%	Drug metabolism decreased	Drugs given in usual concentration range may result in exaggerated responses
Bone: 15%	Marrow reserve decreased; circulating granulocytes decreased	Bone marrow depression
Kidney: 10%	Renal plasma flow decreased	Nephrotoxicity
Lung: 10%	Decrease in vital capacity	Pulmonary toxicity

Elderly patients with lymphoreticular tumours may be particularly vulnerable to the side-effects of chemotherapy and radiation therapy. Older patients with acute leukaemia, in particular, may not be able to withstand the rigours of intensive chemotherapy. Concern is also expressed that the coronary circulation and myocardium in the elderly cannot withstand the stress of haemorrhage, anaemia, infection and the cardiotoxic effects of the anthracyclines. This, coupled with the decreased regenerative capacity of the ageing bone marrow, may influence treatment-related morbidity in the elderly cancer patient. Elderly patients must be assessed individually, however, for their overall pre-treatment health status as chronological and physiological age may be dissimilar.

The problem of the elderly and surgical procedures is yet another example of the need to view the elderly not as a homogeneous but as a heterogeneous group. It is thought that it is the presence of other medical complications, not age alone, that is the primary variable influencing surgical mortality in cancer-related procedures. Thus, it is the general effect of age in reducing the competence of the body that is often responsible for perioperative complications in the older person with cancer.

The fact that many elderly people have not received the most therapeutically effective doses when treated may also account for poor response to treatment rather than the variable of age alone. Hodgkin's disease presents another example where chronological age has determined treatment decisions (Austin-Seymour *et al.*, 1984). The fact that aggressive investigation is rarely used for initial staging of elderly patients with Hodgkin's disease may mean that less accurate treatment is given, leading to an overall poorer response.

Nursing Implications in Geriatric Oncology

In the United States the Oncology Nursing Society (1979) has developed and published *Outcome Standards for Cancer Nursing Practice*, which define the high-incidence problem areas for cancer patients and cite expectations of oncology nurses in intervening in these areas. Four major categories within these standards are listed below with reference to nursing actions associated with the care of elderly cancer patients.

PREVENTION AND EARLY DETECTION

It is paramount that the elderly and their families possess adequate information about prevention and detection of cancer. The assumption that it is too late to stop smoking, change dietary habits, have routine cervical smears or practice breast self-examination must be addressed. Whether in a public forum or on an individual basis, nurses are effective teachers if they are perceived as credible sources by their elderly clients. Nurses can assist older people to recognize factors that place them at risk, acknowledging warning signs of cancer and encouraging them to respond promptly to suspicious signs and symptoms (Stromborg, 1982).

Programmes specifically oriented to self-detection measures must be tailored to the needs of the elderly. In teaching about prevention and early detection the use of large, bold print in a non-cluttered design in printed materials helps to compensate for sensory impairment. Taking programmes to the elderly may overcome the transport problems often associated with such screening events. Addressing the problem of avoidance of screening opportunities by the elderly also requires deliberate work. Nurses are becoming increasingly involved in cancer prevention and early detection activities. This focus will become more prominent in the years to come.

INFORMATION

Working with elderly cancer patients to gain knowledge about their cancer and its treatment is often fraught with multiple barriers (Welch-McCaffrey, 1986). Prior to instituting teaching, a specific assessment must be undertaken to identify barriers to learning. Some of these barriers include disinterest in the therapy, misconceptions, non-compliance, neurosensory impairment and anxiety. With no prior knowledge of deterrents to learning, time invested in patient/family education will be time lost. This assessment helps with mutual goal-setting and the identification of what indeed the patient needs to know. The assessment will also assist in determining the rate and level of information-giving appropriate for each patient/family unit.

With reference to the education of the older cancer patient, some general trends have evolved which warrant mention. Although these are not listed to promote stereotyping the elderly's needs, they are identified to help anticipate some common themes in geriatric oncology patient education. They include patients' difficulty in using the word 'cancer'; feeling uncomfortable airing their views in a group setting; difficulty in expressing their feelings when the diagnosis of cancer has been made; and uneasiness in seeking further information. Since securing information has a direct effect on how the individual copes with cancer, both information and coping should be addressed together.

COPING

The stress of coping with a diagnosis of cancer is moderated by various factors. Two important ones are the experience of dealing with crises and the number of role responsibilities a person may have.

Because the elderly have had, theoretically, a greater opportunity to be exposed to life's crises and have fewer role responsibilities than their younger counterparts, the degree of stress produced by the diagnosis of cancer may be less. Also, there may even be an *expectation* of a chronic disease like cancer affecting them. They may witness friends and family developing cancer and, if diagnosed themselves, exhibit little surprise that they too have contracted the illness.

On the other hand, the death of relatives and friends due to multiple losses to cancer may confuse the elderly individual's coping mechanisms. It may be hard to muster hope and keep an open mind about one's own cancer when vivid recollections of those close to the patient surface and complicate emotional reactions. It is at this point that cancer phobias may develop with elderly patients left feeling that everyone around them has cancer.

Confusion in the elderly cancer patient, ranging from memory loss to disorientation, is one symptom often attributed to ageing (Welch-McCaffrey and Dodge, 1988). However, confusion has many cancer-related aetiologies that are both acute and reversible. Drug-related causes often stem from the use of multiple drugs with central anticholinergic properties such as antipsychotics, antihistamines and antispasmodics. Infection, dehydration, ischaemia and metabolic imbalances, such as hypercalcaemia, may also cause varying degrees of confusion. To determine the cause of confusion, it is important to ask the family if this is a new symptom or a gradual worsening of an insidious problem. Interventions to correct confusion will then be based on deliberative assessment.

Another emotional reaction commonly attributed to ageing in the elderly cancer patient is depression. It would, however, appear that the best indicator of a depressive response in elderly cancer patients is a pre-morbid history of depression rather than old age alone.

In helping elderly patients to cope with cancer it is important that we honour their usual style in coping with crises. Patients who for 40 years have never expressed their feelings openly, may find it hard to do so within the context of the cancer experience. Although probably well meaning, putting pressure on such patients to talk about their feelings may increase rather than decrease stress. Thus, early in the relationship the nurse must ask the patient how he or she deals with crises. The individual answers to these questions help to predict coping style in the present and offer guidance as to how best to support the patient throughout the illness.

COMFORT

Multiple factors influence comfort in the geriatric oncology experience. Interventions which promote psychobiological comfort must be planned in an ongoing fashion throughout the patient's illness (Dellefield, 1986). Cancer-related sources of discomfort such as pain, oesophagitis and vomiting, must be considered as possible aetiologies along with non-malignant sources. Often, it is the non-cancerous chronic illness that is distressing the patient more than the cancer. This is an important consideration as most elderly cancer patients may be coping with several chronic illnesses simultaneously.

Sleep disturbance may be a particularly troublesome deterrent to comfort. In general, the elderly are characterized by more frequent awakenings during the night, an increase in the total time spent awake, longer time in bed before the onset of sleep, subjective expression of poor sleep and early morning awakening. The presence of pain and anxiety associated with cancer experience, as well as changes in orientation associated with being in hospital, may exaggerate these symptoms of sleep disturbance. Subjective feelings of overall comfort are then often influenced by sleep alterations in a negative way.

The effective pharmacological management of symptom distress in the elderly cancer patient is hampered by inadequate information about dose requirements for common drugs used. The use of narcotics, anti-emetics and anti-anxiety agents in treating symptom distress in the elderly is similar to the treatment in all age-groups. There are general dose modifications for children but few exist for the elderly. Hence, the prescription of medications to promote comfort is often characterized by the need to titrate the drug longer to reach effective therapeutic and non-toxic levels.

In working with elderly cancer patients and their families to promote comfort, defined goals must include those that encourage the patient and family to report alterations in comfort level and identify measures which enhance comfort. The nurse's documentation of efficacious regimens to promote comfort is essential if effective protocols in symptom management are to be identified. The promotion of comfort with elderly cancer patients represents a major area of nursing intervention. Success in this area also correlates with the elderly patient's ability to remain at home rather than in institutionalized care (Berkman *et al.*, 1983). For many, living at home is, in itself, a major contributor to the feeling of overall comfort.

Conclusion

Currently, and increasingly in the future, the prominence of cancer in the elderly will demand significant increases in the allocation of supportive services and general attention to the unique needs of geriatric oncology patients and their families. Challenges for cancer health care professionals will include the creation of innovative cancer screening programmes targeted at the needs of the elderly; making best use of patient and family education approaches; providing ongoing, individualized emotional support; and reducing physical distress associated with cancer and its treatment.

There are still many unanswered questions in geriatric oncology. Extensive research is needed to describe the experience of cancer in the elderly and to evaluate the effectiveness of interventions in meeting patients' needs. This sub-specialty offers fertile ground for those innovative cancer health professionals eager to address the needs of geriatric cancer patients.

References

Ahmann, F. R. (1985) Dilemmas in managing prostate carcinoma, Part I: localized disease. *Geriatrics*, Vol. 40, no. 7, pp. 34–42.

Austin-Seymour, M.M. *et al.* (1984) Hodgkin's disease in patients over sixty years old, *Annals of Internal Medicine*, Vol. 100, no. 1, pp. 13–18.

Baranovsky, A. and Myers, M.H. (1986) Cancer incidence and survival in patients 65 years of age and older, *CA — A Cancer Journal for Clinicians*, Vol. 36, no. 1, pp. 22–37.

Berkman, B., Stolberg, C., Calhoun, J., Parker, E. and Stearns, N. (1983) Elderly cancer patients: factors predictive of risk for institutionalization, *Journal of Psychosocial Oncology*, Vol. 1, no. 1, pp. 85–100.

Butler, R.N. and Gastel, B. (1979) Ageing and cancer management. Part II: research perspectives. *CA — A Cancer Journal for Clinicians*, Vol. 102, no. 6, pp. 333–9.

Cape, R.T. (1983) Geriatric perspectives in prostate cancer, in R. Yancik *et al.* (eds.) *Perspectives in Prevention and Treatment of Cancer in the Elderly*, Raven Press, New York, pp. 171–9.

Crawford, J. and Cohen, H.J. (1987) Relationship of cancer and ageing, *Clinics in Geriatric Medicine*, Vol. 3, no. 3, pp. 419–32.

Dellefield, M.E. (1986) Caring for the elderly patient with cancer, *Oncology Nursing Forum*, Vol. 13, no. 3, pp. 19–27.

Goodell, B.W. (1985) Neoplasia, in R. Andres, E.L. Bierman and W.R. Hazzard (eds.) *Principles of Geriatric Medicine*, McGraw-Hill, New York, pp. 461–76.

Lipschitz, D.A. *et al.* (1985) Cancer in the elderly: basic science and clinical aspects, *Annals of Internal Medicine*, Vol. 102, no. 2, pp. 218–28.

Oncology Nursing Society and the American Nurses' Association (1979) *Outcome Standards of Cancer Nursing Practice*, Pittsburgh, Pennsylvania, USA.

Ponten, J. (1985) Abnormal cell growth (neoplasia) and ageing, in C.E. Finch and L. Hayflick (eds.) *Handbook of the Biology of Ageing* (2nd edn), New York, Van Nostrand & Reinhold, pp. 536–60.

Serpick, A.A. (1978) Cancer in the elderly, *Hospital Practice*, Vol. 2, no. 2, pp. 101–12.

Stromborg, M. (1982) Early detection of cancer in the elderly: problems and solutions, *International Journal of Nursing Studies*, Vol. 19, no. 3, pp. 139–56.

Welch-McCaffrey, D. (1986) To teach or not to teach? Overcoming barriers to patient education in geriatric oncology, *Oncology Nursing Forum*, Vol. 13, no. 4, pp. 25–31.

Welch-McCaffrey, D. and Dodge, J. (1988) Acute confusion in elderly cancer patients: a nursing framework for assessment and intervention, *Seminars in Oncology Nursing* (in press).

Men with Cancer

STEVE GENTZLER RN, BSN
Head Nurse, Outpatient Department, Ellis Fischel State Cancer Center
Columbia, Missouri

Introduction

Worldwide more men die of cancer than do women (Silverberg and Lubera, 1987). In Western countries cancer is the second most common cause of death in men. It is surpassed only by heart disease (Muir and Nectoux, 1982; Page and Asire, 1985). To provide holistic care to men with cancer, oncology nurses need to understand their psychosocial and psychosexual behaviour. This is important in primary and secondary prevention, early detection, treatment and in the terminal stages of illness.

Understanding the male sex role is important not only in providing nursing care to men with cancer, but also in understanding why men are at risk from cancer. In the following pages certain male psychosocial and psychosexual characteristics and their relation to cancer are explored as is the general impact of cancer on men. The major cancers associated with men are also discussed.

Gender and Gender Role

Humans are complex beings, ever-changing products of ongoing biological and sociocultural factors (Tiedt, 1975; Krumm, 1982; Fisher, 1983). An initial definition of 'man' is based on certain biological sex indicators associated with males. Franklin (1984) identifies these as consisting of the penis, testicles, seminal vesicals, prostate gland, male and female hormones and XY chromosomes. Secondary sex characteristics, such as hair distribution, muscle–fat ratios and voice pitch, are also included in the biological definition.

Gender and gender role identity complete a description of the concept of male identity. Gender includes social attitudes, behaviours, values; it involves the expectations a society has for individual socialization to the role of a culturally acceptable male or female (Allen and Whatley, 1956; Pleck, 1981; Franklin, 1984). The degree to which an individual fulfils society's expectations by demonstrating appropriate gender characteristics determines his 'masculinity' or her 'femininity'.

Pleck (1981) states that the sex, or gender, role includes culturally typical and normal behaviours and characteristics. An individual's perception of his or her relation to the masculine or feminine role determines the gender role identity. The traditional stereotype male of the Western world is described as assertive, aggressive, independent, autonomous, competent, self-confident, dominant, powerful, strong, capable of endurance, hardy, courageous, logical, ambitious, productive and lacking emotional expression (Allen and Whatley, 1956; Pleck, 1981; Shipes and Lehr, 1982; Vetterling-Braggin, 1982; Franklin, 1984). Shifts are occuring in the male sex role, although it is difficult to determine how rapid and encompassing they are. Doyle (1983) provides us with some of the characteristics of the 'modern male' in contemporary Western middle-class society: the male is emotionally expressive with women, but not men; anger and hostility are contained; the male should satisfy female sexual needs, a role which is validated through power over others; a male should also achieve economic success. To understand how men regard health and interact with health care systems, nurses must understand and recognize these male gender traits.

The Susceptibility of Men to Illness

Men, by their very nature, are at greater risk from health-related problems than are women. In fact, men in Western society have a substantially lower life expectancy than females. Various explanations for this have been offered and are pertinent to men with cancer and men at risk from cancer. Most conclusions are based on male sex role behaviours. Men are more likely to take risks because they are less willing to acknowledge personal weaknesses. Men consume more tobacco and alcohol than females. Many men work in occupations with high health hazards and are not likely to take preventative action. Finally, men can suffer from stress incurred as a result of the demands of the male sex role (Cowling and Campbell, 1986; Forrester, 1986; Kronenfeld, 1986; Ossler, 1986).

Illness is both biologically and socially undesirable. In trying to maintain the gender role stereotype of the strong, healthy and self-sufficient male, a man may be reluctant to seek health information, to use health care providers or even admit to having an illness (Shipes and Lehr, 1982; Cowling and Campbell, 1986; Forrester, 1986; Kronenfeld, 1986).

Cancer in Men

The diagnosis of cancer and its subsequent treatment can result in a need for dependency in males. Conflict and frustration will occur for men with cancer who perceive a need to maintain society's expectations of autonomy, capability and power when forced to relinquish control of their body, time and money (Goldberg and Tull, 1983; Hughes, 1986; Priestman, 1986). Feelings of anger, hostility, depression, hopelessness and loneliness in a man expected to have control of his emotions can create additional stressors (Goldberg and Tull, 1983; Priestman, 1986). The stereotypical courageous and logical male may be confronted with fears of disfigurement or pain, and may be preoccupied with this situation. The stalwart male, supposedly able to handle anything that comes his way, may feel just the opposite but believes that any expression of his true feelings would call into question his masculinity. Dealing with a health care system that can at times seem very inefficient and unresponsive can be frustrating for the male socialized to be self-reliant and efficient. The male 'breadwinner' who is separated from his job as a result of cancer may also experience anxiety and distress (Kaplan, 1983). A loss of productivity associated with the more chronic aspects of cancer and its treatment, coupled with potential economic strain, both of which can place stress on a man's family and friends, places additional stress on male self-esteem.

ECONOMIC IMPLICATIONS

The economic impact of cancer on men can be long term and discrimination for re-employment has been noted (Dietz, 1981). The possibility of time-off for treatments and ongoing medical follow-ups, together with the assumption that the man may not live long, can contribute to employment problems. Perceived expectations of friends and community pose additional problems for a man with cancer whose casual appearance denotes wellness but who cannot work because he is easily fatigued (Goldberg and Tull, 1983; Scallion, 1984; Carr and Powers, 1986; Leinster, 1986).

SEXUAL FUNCTION AND DYSFUNCTION

Potential sexual dysfunction poses a direct assault on the man with cancer. For the stereotypical male, sex is the very essence of a man's masculinity (Shipes and Lehr, 1982). Cancer and its treatment and the man's responses to both can all have a bearing on his expectations of himself. Sexual performance can be affected by loss of self-esteem, body image alterations, depression, anatomical alterations, such as head and neck operations, ostomies, pelvic autonomic nerve and vascular damage, and by other symptoms, such as malaise, fatigue, pain, dyspnoea, nausea, vomiting, alopecia and hormonal changes. Alterations in sexual performance may range from transient disinterest or decreased desire to complete dysfunction (Grubb and Blake, 1976; Wabrek, Wabrek and Burchill, 1980; Yeager and van Heerden, 1980; Bracken, 1981; Swanson, 1981; von Eschenbach, 1981; Krumm, 1982; Shipes and Lehr, 1982; Fisher, 1983; Nevidjon, 1984; Andersen, 1985; Spaulding and Spaulding, 1985). The male confronted with such assaults on his masculinity may respond with behaviours intended to re-establish control and autonomy. Such behaviour may not be linked with the fact that his needs have not been acknowledged and may be seen as some new problem. The psychosocial and psychosexual effects of the disease, and/or its treatment, must be individually assessed in order to plan appropriate interventions (Morris, 1985).

Types of Cancer and their Effects

Cancer generally occurs in men over 40 years of age. Cancers of the lung, stomach, colon and rectum, and prostate are the leading causes of male mortality due to cancer. Cancer incidence and mortality, according to site, sex and background, vary along with the cultural and environmental factors of different countries (Muir and Nectoux, 1982; Page and Asire, 1985; Silverberg and Lubera, 1987). Oral, respiratory, colo-rectal and genito-urinary cancers are most significant to the masculine role.

ORAL AND RESPIRATORY CANCERS

The incidence and mortality rates of oral and respiratory cancers for men are double those for women. This group of cancers affects the lip, tongue, mouth, pharynx, larynx and lung. Smoking is the primary risk factor associated with lung and laryngeal cancer and may cause 85 per cent of lung cancer deaths and 75 per cent of laryngeal cancer incidence (Page and Asire, 1985; Greenwald and Weisburger, 1986). For men, occupational exposure is a major risk factor for lung cancer. Of special note are uranium miners exposed to radon gas (Muir and Nectoux 1982). A decline in male smoking, from 52.1 per cent in 1963 to 35.4 per cent in 1985, marks a positive trend in the United States of America. Fewer white-collar workers are smoking than blue-collar workers (Greenwald and Weisburger, 1986). The incidence and death rates for oral cancers in men are double those found in women. Men's use of alcohol and tobacco and their synergistic effects put men in a high-risk category for these cancers (Page and Asire, 1985). Smokeless tobacco use is associated with increased oral cancer occurrence. Advertisements using male sports figures or rugged cowboy types are used to promote smokeless tobacco. The typical male is susceptible to these stereotypes and may use tobacco because of its perceived association with 'real men'.

COLO-RECTAL CANCER

The incidence of colo-rectal cancer in males and females is roughly equal, although mortality is slightly higher in men (Page and Asire, 1985; Silverberg and Lubera, 1987). This site is of particular importance to men because of potential sexual dysfunction. Treatment for colo-rectal cancer frequently involves neurological impairment of erectile and ejaculatory capabilities (Wabrek, Wabrek and Burchill, 1980; Yeager and van Heerden, 1980). Men with colostomies have greater sexual disruption than those having a colon resection and anastomosis. Male rectal cancer patients with stomas reported erectile difficulty, premature or dry ejaculation and less frequent sexual intercourse (Grubb and Blake, 1976; Andersen, 1985). Significant body image alteration and lowered sexual drive may occur with altered elimination routes, such as a colostomy. For men, the genito-urinary cancers (bladder, testicular, penile and prostate) have obvious implications with reference to their masculinity.

BLADDER CANCER

Bladder cancer occurs most frequently in men who are over 65 years old and at a 2:1 male–female ratio. Occupational groups at risk include rubber and leather industry workers; truck drivers; paint, chemical, print and metal workers and machinists. Smoking is the most common risk factor associated with bladder cancer. An estimated 40 per cent of bladder cancers are caused by smoking (Page and Asire, 1985; Silverberg and Lubera, 1987).

Transurethral resection of bladder tumours generally causes no anatomical impairments that could change sexual response but altered response of a psychogenic origin is possible. Radical cystectomy results in erectile dysfunction and the absence of ejaculation in a significant percentage of men. Although the effect of radiation therapy is significantly less than that of surgical intervention, it may damage the nerves necessary for erection, emission and ejaculation (Swanson, 1981; Shipes and Lehr, 1982; Andersen, 1985).

Some types of chemotherapy, such as bladder-instilled thio-TEPA, can cause fatigue and urethritis. The fatigue that accompanies cancer can reduce sexual desire.

PENILE CANCER

Although penile cancer has a very low incidence and mortality rate in the Western world, it does have obvious implications for male sexuality. Following excision of the tumour, erection capabilities will be generally retained for the penile stump. However, body image disturbances may interfere with sexual functioning (Bracken, 1981).

TESTICULAR CANCER

Testicular cancer is a cancer of young men. It occurs most frequently in white males between 15 and 39 years of age. It is one of the most frequently occuring cancers in this age-group although it is rare in those with black skin (Page and Asire, 1985; Pattern and Goedert, 1986). Testicular cancer survival rates are very good if the disease is diagnosed early. Fortunately, this disease is relatively easy to detect and monthly testicular self-examination may help to promote early detection.

A unilateral orchidectomy with chemotherapy is used to treat non-seminoma testicular cancer while radiation is used for seminoma. A unilateral orchidectomy should not result in decreased sex drive or fertility loss. However, psychosexual disruption can occur approximately 20 per cent of the time (Andersen, 1985). A 90 per cent reduction in ejaculate is reported with retroperitoneal node dissection (Bracken, 1981). Infertility can occur from radiation therapy and chemotherapy depending on dosage and duration of treatment. Alkylating antineoplastic drugs have the greatest gonadal effect (Schilsky *et al.*, 1980; Bracken, 1981; Spaulding and Spaulding, 1985).

PROSTATIC CANCER

Prostate cancer is a disease of older men and particular races. For example, in the United States of America it is most frequently found in black males. Worldwide, prostate cancer accounts for approximately 17 per cent of all male cancer deaths (Chisholm, 1986; Silverberg and Lubera, 1987). Dietary fat and occupational exposure to cadmium have been associated with prostate cancer (Page and Asire, 1985). The effects of treatment on sexual function are variable. An absence or reduction of ejaculate due to retrograde ejaculation has occurred in 57 per cent of men having a transurethral resection; erectile dysfunction has also been reported. Radical prostatectomy can result in impaired erectile function in 90 per cent of men having this procedure. Depending on the approach, retropubic or perineal ejaculation difficulties may occur at rates of 78 and 100 per cent respectively. Men having bilateral orchidectomy and oestrogen as treatment will generally all have erectile, ejaculatory and sex drive problems following surgery. For those having only radiation therapy, erectile and ejaculatory problems will be reduced to half those of individuals who have undergone surgery (Swanson, 1981; Andersen, 1985). Gynaecomastia can occur with those men receiving hormonal treatment (oestrogen).

Conclusion

The male sex role has been demonstrated as interfering with men recognizing their needs and seeking help. An understanding that the male sex role and the man cannot be separated has significant implications for nursing care. The nurse must avoid sexual stereotypes and remember that male sex role shifts are occurring. Individualized assessments of sexuality for all cancer patients are essential (Rodriguez, 1981; Krumm, 1982; Morris, 1985).

Cultural assessment of the male population will allow the development of more effective strategies in promoting prevention and early detection activities, such as testicular self-examinations and anti-smoking programmes. Occupational hazards that put men at risk of cancer must also be considered. Initial nursing encounters with men diagnosed as having cancer should include provision for information about personal, family and social concerns within the context of the male sex role (Derdiarian, 1986). Nurses should be aware of the potential communication gap about emotional issues between the male physician and the man with cancer. It is beneficial to allow the venting of feelings in a relaxed, accepting manner. By promoting independent decision-making and autonomy and by involving the male patient in his treatment plan, the nurse can help him to come to terms with any subsequent effect on his masculinity.

References

Allen, D.G. and Whatley, M. (1956) Nursing and men's health: some critical considerations, in F.L. Cohen and J.D. Dunham (eds.) Men's health, *Nursing Clinics of North America*, Vol. 21, no. 1, pp. 3–13.

Andersen,B.L. (1985) Sexual functioning morbidity among cancer survivors, *Cancer*, Vol. 55, no. 8, pp. 1835–42.

Bracken, R.B. (1981) Cancer of the testis, penis and urethra: the impact of therapy on sexual function, in A.C. von Eschenbach and D.B. Rodriguez (eds.) *Sexual Rehabilitation of the Urologic Cancer Patient*, G.K. Hall, Boston.

Carr, J.A. and Powers, M.J. (1986) Stressors associated with coronary bypass surgery, *Nursing Research*, Vol. 35, no. 4, pp. 243–6.

Chisholm, G.D. (1986) Natural history of prostatic cancer, in J.P. Blandy and B. Lytton (eds.) *The Prostate*, Butterworths, London.

Cowling, W.R., III and Campbell, V. (1986) Health concerns of ageing men, *Nursing Clinics of North America*, Vol. 21, no. 1, pp. 75–83.

Derdiarian, A.K. (1986) Informational needs of recently diagnosed cancer patients, *Nursing Research*, Vol. 35, no. 5, pp. 276–81.

Dietz, J.H., Jr (1981) *Rehabilitation Oncology*, John Wiley and Sons, New York.

Doyle, J.A. (1983) *The Male Experience*, William C. Brown, Dubuque.

Fisher, S.G. (1983) The psychosexual effects of cancer and cancer treatment, *Oncology Nursing Forum*, Vol. 10, no. 2, pp. 63–8.

Forrester, D.A. (1986) Myths of masculinity: impact upon men's health, *Nursing Clinics of North America*, Vol. 21, no. 1, pp. 15–23.

Franklin, C.W., II (1984) *The Changing Definition of Masculinity*, Plenum Press, New York.

Goldberg, R.J. and Tull, R.M. (1983) *The Psychosocial Dimensions of Cancer*, The Free Press, New York.

Greenwald, P. and Weisburger, E.K. (eds.) (1986) Cancer control objectives for the nation, *NCI Monographs*, 2.

Grubb, R.D. and Blake, R. (1976) Emotional trauma in ostomy patients, *AORN Journal*, Vol. 23, no. 1, pp. 52-5.

Hughes, J. (1986) Depression in cancer patients, in B.A. Stoll (ed.) *Coping with Cancer Stress*, Martinus Nijhoff, Dordrecht.

Kaplan, M. (1983) Viewpoint: the cancer patient, *Cancer Nursing*, Vol. 6, no. 2, pp. 103-7.

Kronenfeld, J.J. (1986) Health and the health care system in F.A. Bourdreau, R.S. Sennott and M. Wilson (eds.) *Sex Roles and Social Patterns*, Praeger, New York.

Krumm, S. (1982) Psychosocial adaptation of the adult with cancer, *Nursing Clinics of North America*, Vol. 17, no. 4, pp. 729-37.

Leinster, S.J. (1986) Coping with cancer surgery, in B.A. Stoll (ed.) *Coping with Cancer Stress*, Martinus Nijhoff, Dordrecht.

Morris, C.A. (1985) Self-concept as altered by the diagnosis of cancer, *Nursing Clinics of North America*, Vol. 20, no. 4, pp. 611-30.

Muir, C.S. and Nectoux, J. (1982) International patterns of cancer, in D. Schottenfeld and J.F. Fraumeni (eds.) *Cancer Epidemiology and Prevention*, W.B. Saunders, Philadelphia.

Nevidjon, B. (1984) Sexuality, in S.N. McIntire and A.L. Cioppa (eds.) *Cancer Nursing: A Developmental Approach*, John Wiley & Sons, New York.

Ossler, C.C. (1986) Men's work environments and health risks, *Nursing Clinics of North America*, Vol. 21, no. 1, pp. 25-36.

Page, H. and Asire, A. J. (1985) *Cancer Rates and Risks* (3rd edn), publication no. 85-691, National Institute of Health.

Pattern, L.M. and Goedert, J.J. (1986) Epidemiology of testicular cancer, in N. Javadpour (ed.) *Principles and Management of Testicular Cancer*, Thieme Medical, New York.

Pleck, J.H. (1981) *The Myth of Masculinity*, MIT Press, Cambridge, Massachusetts.

Priestman, T. J. (1986) Impact of diagnosis on the patient, in B.A. Stoll (ed.) *Coping with Cancer Stress*, Martinus Nijhoff, Dordrecht.

Rodriguez, D. B. (1981) The problem for the nurse, in A.C. von Eschenbach and D.B. Rodriguez (eds.) *Sexual Rehabilitation of the Urologic Cancer Patient*, G.K. Hall, Boston.

Scallion, L. (1984) Loss, in S.N. McIntire and A.L. Cioppa (eds.) *Cancer Nursing: A Developmental Approach;* John Wiley & Sons, New York.

Schilsky, R.L., Lewis, B.J., Sherins, R.J. and Young, R.C. (1980) Gonadal dysfunction in patients receiving chemotherapy for cancer, *Annals of Internal Medicine*, Vol. 93, no. 1, pp. 109-14.

Shipes, E. and Lehr, S. (1982) Sexuality and the male cancer patient, *Cancer Nursing*, Vol. 5, no. 5, pp. 375-81.

Silverberg, E. and Lubera, J. (1987) Cancer statistics, *Ca—A Cancer Journal for Clinicians*, Vol. 37, no. 1, pp. 2-19.

Snyder, C. (1986) *Introduction to Oncology Nursing*, Little & Brown, Boston.

Spaulding, M. and Spaulding, S. (1985) Chemotherapy and gonadal function, in W.L. McGuire and D.J. Higby (eds.) *The Cancer Patient and Supportive Care*, Martinus Nijhoff, Boston.

Swanson, David A. (1981) Cancer of the bladder and prostate: the impact of therapy on sexual function, in A.C. von Eschenbach and D.B. Rodriguez (eds.) *Sexual Rehabilitation of the Urologic Cancer Patient*, G.K. Hall, Boston.

Tiedt, E. (1975) The psychodynamic process of the oncological experience, *Nursing Forum*, Vol. 14, no. 3, pp. 264–77.

Vetterling-Braggin, M. (ed.) (1982) *'Femininity', 'Masculinity', and 'Androgyny'*, Rowman & Littlefield, Totowa, NJ, USA.

von Eschenbach, A.C. (1981) Sexual dysfunction and rehabilitation: definition of the problem, in A.C. von Eschenbach and D.B. Rodriguez (eds.) *Sexual Rehabilitation of the Urologic Cancer Patient*, G.K. Hall, Boston, p. 322.

Wabrek, A.J., Wabrek, C.J. and Burchill, R.C. (1980) Sexual implications of bowel diversion, *American Journal of Proctology, Gastro-enterology and Colon and Rectal Surgery*, Vol. 31, no. 8, pp. 23–7.

Yeager, E.S. and van Heerden, J.A. (1980) Sexual dysfunction following proctocolectomy and abdominoperineal resection, *Annals of Surgery*, Vol. 191, no. 2, pp. 169–71.

Women with Cancer

RUTH McCORKLE RN, PhD

*Professor, School of Nursing
University of Pennsylvania*

Introduction

This section presents current information about women and cancer. Although it reflects the situation in the Western world, many of the actual examples given and the research quoted are from the United States of America. The cancers associated with the female reproductive system have a unique impact on women, primarily because the incidence of these diseases is so high and because sexuality becomes a central concern (Derogatis, 1986). The specific characteristics of these cancers, their diagnoses and treatments are presented in Volume 1. In addition, an excellent overview of the psychological impact of having cancer and its effects on living is presented in Chapter 2.

Women in the United States and the United Kingdom tend to live longer than men, but they are ill more frequently, have more disability days and use more health services than do men (Verbrugge, 1979). Women generally show a higher incidence of acute illness, minor chronic conditions, short-term restricted activity and more use of medicines. In contrast, men have higher rates of life-threatening chronic conditions, injuries and long-term disability. In short, women are more frequently ill than men, but with relatively minor illnesses. Men are less often ill but when they are, their illnesses and injuries are more serious. These morbidity differences help to explain differences in the sexes in relation to health behaviour. For women, frequency of symptoms leads to more restricted activity, more physician visits and more drug use. For men, the severity of symptoms leads to more permanent limitations, hospitalizations and premature death (Verbrugge, 1982).

Numerous biological and sociocultural factors are thought to contribute to this paradox of greater morbidity and longer life for women. These major social and cultural factors affect both women's health and their access to, and utilization of, health services. Employed mothers, for example, continue to assume almost full responsibility for housework and child care, even while ill.

By the year 1990, many current demographic and social trends will have had a predictable effect on the social status of women in society and consequently on their health status and need for health services. A task force on women's health issues in the United States (Merritt and Kirschstein, 1985) identified the following three important social changes affecting women's health:

1. the increasing number of women living in poverty;
2. the unprecedented entry of women into the labour force, including women with infants and young children;
3. the continuing increase in the longevity of women.

These changes will ultimately affect women's health, the types of illness they develop, and the care they receive.

This section discusses three specific topics related to women and illnesses: health-seeking behaviours, shifts in roles and responsibilities during illness, and care-giving abilities.

Health-Seeking Behaviour of Women

Several authors have reported consistent differences in the ways men and women use health care services. Women use physicians and hospital services more frequently than men (Nathanson, 1977;

Verbrugge, 1979), have higher rates of morbidity than men, and express their distress differently than do men (Nathanson, 1975; Mechanic, 1976). These differences have been a source of considerable debate and empirical investigation over the past 10 years. Some authors maintain that women report their symptoms more often than men because they are more interested in health and are more knowledgeable about health care (Feldman, 1966). Gove (1984) suggests that women are more willing to admit to psychological distress and to seek treatment for it, because they place less stigma on these actions. Another explanation is based on the relative convenience and accessibility of services for men and women. Most women are described as having fewer work and time constraints on their behaviour and greater flexibility in arranging medical appointments. Also, women suffer less cost associated with medical care in relation to time-off from work. This may be due to differences in pay structures and work responsibilities.

Mounting evidence suggests that gender differences in health are largely a consequence of social and psychological factors rather than biological or genetic factors (Nathanson, 1975; Gove and Hughes, 1979). A consensus is emerging that sex differences in morbidity reports and the differences in the uptake of health services in Western industrial societies are due to differences in the way symptoms are perceived, evaluated and acted on (Mechanic, 1976; Hibbard and Pope, 1986).

In view of their higher morbidity and utilization rates, women should be diagnosed and treated early for diseases such as cancer. In fact, delay in seeking treatment for some women has been associated with such diagnoses as early stage breast cancer (Elwood and Moorehead, 1980; Huguley and Brown, 1981). Hackett, Cassem and Raker (1973) found that breast cancer patients overall responded rapidly in seeking health care, with nearly 75 per cent getting care in less than one month. Approximately 20 per cent, however, delayed reporting symptoms for at least one year. Lierman (1987) reported that over 35 per cent of her sample of breast patients delayed seeking treatment for months and in several instances years. All of the women who delayed for over a year had a close relative with cancer. Lierman (1987) defined delay as the amount of time lapse between initial discovery of the symptom and first seeking professional assistance. Based on data from sixteen women whose symptoms were discovered outside the health care system, four behavioural responses were identified:

1. early help seeking (one to four weeks);
2. ignoring symptoms (weeks to months);
3. wait and see (months to years);
4. preparation for death (years).

The majority of Lierman's sample (70 per cent) reported that their initial symptom was a breast lump, the most common presenting symptom for breast cancer. However, the initial symptom in 30 per cent of the women was an inverted nipple, nipple discharge or a burning sensation. Bullough (1980) and Gould-Martin *et al.* (1982) reported similar findings. These findings indicate the importance of describing symptoms other than lumps when teaching breast self-examination.

Magarey, Todd and Blizard (1977) identified five psychological factors associated with an increased length of delay in women with breast cancer. These factors, identified as unconscious mental processes, included marked use of denial and suppression, intellectualization, isolation, anxiety and depression. Similarly, Watson and her asociates (1984) cited avoidance and denial as the most frequent observed coping responses in women with breast cancer. In their study, however, deniers and acceptors did not differ in the length of delay in seeking treatment.

Gould-Martin and associates (1982) noted that women who found breast lumps by breast self-examination (BSE) were actually more likely to delay than women whose lumps were discovered accidentally. Funch (1985) points out conflicting evidence in the literature about the relationship of BSE and delay in seeking treatment. Her study found no significant relationship between frequency of BSE and delay in seeking treatment. Practising BSE women were most likely to delay if they had less education, larger breasts, were older, or had a family member who had died of breast cancer.

Women might also delay in seeking treatment for other types of cancers. Marshall and Funch (1986) have distinguished between patient delay – the time-lapse between the patient's initial recognition of symptoms and first physician contact, and diagnostic delay – the time-lapse between the first physician contact and treatment. Their study of 154 men and 152 women with cancer of the colon or rectum, found that women were more likely than men to delay in seeking treatment (diagnostic delay). Both men and women had similar symptoms, the most common being bleeding, general weakness and abdominal pain. They also reported similar severity of symptoms. However, differences occurred in the way the two groups *responded* to their symptoms. When the findings for both colon and rectal cancers were combined, gender differences in diagnostic delay were not significant, although women tended to delay about 10 per cent longer than men. When the findings for the two types of cancer were separated, distinct differences emerged. Among patients with colon cancer, males tended to delay slightly longer than women. On the other hand, among patients with rectal cancer, women delayed on the average over 100 days. Marshall and Funch (1986) concluded that gender differences in health-seeking behaviours depended heavily on the site of cancer. Yet they acknowledge that, since the symptom patterns for the two gastrointestinal cancers were slightly different, physicians might have responded differently in recommending treatment. The authors added that 'substantial delay among female patients rather than among male patients may indicate that symptoms of these two cancers are overlooked as a function of the sex of the person presenting the symptoms' (Marshall and Funch, 1986).

These findings may suggest that the symptoms of rectal cancer presented by women might not have been taken seriously by physicians, causing a delay in treatment. Women who reported longer physician delays had visited the doctor more times than men before a diagnosis was reached. A separate analysis revealed that the number of physician visits before diagnosis was related to the length of physician delay. When the number of visits before diagnosis was held constant, there were no differences between men and women in delay. This additional finding suggests a substantial proportion of the male–female difference in physician delay was a function of the excessive visits required by women before the physician arrived at a diagnosis. The women identified the following reasons for their delays:

1. scheduling problems (office or laboratory);
2. physician related (e.g. misdiagnosis, 'watching and waiting');
3. patient related (e.g. cancelling follow-up visit).

Differences in the symptomatology of these diseases and their relationship to delay, warrant further investigation.

The primary implication of these findings for nurses is to encourage women to continue to express themselves and their symptoms to a health care provider. Nurses can listen to women's complaints of their symptoms and help them to express their distress. Women need to be encouraged to seek a second opinion if they feel their complaints are being discounted or if no physical basis for their complaint is identified. Nurses can help patients to identify who can best help them and when referral to a specialist consultant may be needed.

Shifts in Roles and Responsibilities During Illness

It has been widely assumed that as women's participation in the labour force increases, the morbidity and mortality patterns in women would show greater similarity to those of men. Morbidity and mortality data have been examined between the sexes and no new differences have emerged but the effect on women's health of actively contributing to the labour force awaits further study. What is clear is that women are taking on new roles outside the home without giving up their old roles.

Living with cancer creates disruptions in family roles and responsibilities (Edstrom and Miller, 1981). Adult females clearly carry a disproportionate percentage of household responsibility prior to illness. What happens to family roles and household responsibilities during illness is less clear.

Green (1986) interviewed nine non-partnered families and eighteen partnered families in which the adult woman had breast cancer, in order to identify the responsibilities of individual family members at the woman's diagnosis of cancer and 6–12 months later. Green found that women carried considerably more responsibility for household duties than did any other single family member, and often more responsibility than all other family members combined. Prior to diagnosis, partnered and non-partnered women were primarily responsible for shopping, meal preparation, kitchen cleaning, housework, clothing upkeep, pet care, child care, co-ordination of children's activities and financial management. Partners often assisted the women with these activities, but assumed primary responsibility for outside upkeep, vehicle maintenance and repair, household repairs and financial input. In non-partnered families, the women assumed primary responsibility for these latter activities. Women in both types of families worked outside the home.

Family responsibilities lessened for women after diagnosis. A portion, but less than all of their workload, was assumed by one or more other people. Friends and relatives, including children, became much more visible, especially in non-partnered families. This redistribution of responsiblity, however, was short lived. By the second interview, all families had returned to their prediagnostic patterns and, in several instances, women had assumed more responsibilities than they had before.

Several interesting findings emerged during the initial treatment phases. Families reported that chemotherapy and radiation therapy constituted new family activities that required additional distribution of responsibility in the weeks and months after diagnosis. Additional treatment meant that someone had to take responsibility for making appointments, arranging for transport, and taking women to treatment if they needed assistance. The families stated that health care professionals assisted with these activities, but the women, their families, friends and relatives had to assume the majority of care. For a small number of families, the patient with cancer needed temporary assistance with activities of daily living after surgery and during recovery. These new responsibilities were shared by the family group, friends and relatives.

During the recovery period, the distribution of responsibility for some activities shifted more dramatically than for others. These 'high-shift' activities were defined as transfer of 15 per cent or more of total responsibility from one member to another. The greatest shifts for partnered families occurred in shopping, housework, co-ordination of children's activities, child care and clothing upkeep. With the exception of co-ordination of children's activities, the same high shift in activities occurred in non-partnered families. In addition, non-partnered women experienced high shifts in five other activities: meal preparation, kitchen cleaning, assisting with activities of daily living, outside upkeep and vehicle maintenance. Overall, a greater percentage of responsibility was shifted in non-partnered families than in partnered families.

Family members and friends who took on new roles and responsibilities reported spending less time in wage-earning activities. For both types of families, the hours spent in financial input (employment responsibilities) decreased by approximately one-third during the weeks after surgery. Time spent in outside upkeep decreased for both groups. In contrast, the time commitment to children and to shopping remained stable.

Although exploratory in nature, Green's (1986) study provides evidence that shifts in roles and responsibilities do occur in illness. The effects of a long-term or progressive illness on the redistribution of roles and responsibilities in families have not yet been determined. Strauss (1975) identified the need for health care providers to assist patients with management of treatment regimens and symptoms, and with reduction of social isolation. These factors clearly affect a woman's ability to perform her own roles or redistribute roles to others in the family unit.

In research with lung cancer patients, individuals reported relinquishing recreational and social roles before their work roles, activities in the home or self-care behaviours (McCorkle and Quint-Benoliel, 1983). Role shifts in families seem less disruptive if the patient is a man rather than a woman. For men, being ill typically translates into staying home from work and retreating into an environment where they can be taken care of. When a woman is ill, she must confront her role as a pivotal adult female in the family. She cannot escape the work within the home, even if she is employed outside the home. She is expected to recuperate in the very arena in which she is seen by herself and others as a responsive and continued worker (Sandelowski, 1981). Nurses are in a unique position to assist women by informing them of the areas where high role shifts can occur and by exploring with them ways to plan the redistribution of responsibilities.

Few women are informed of what to expect once they are discharged. Quint (1963) found that women are poorly prepared to deal with their concerns about the future and the potential for recurrence of disease once they are home. Mechanic (1976) noted that a woman's symptoms may limit her activity and interfere with her role obligations. Nurses need to establish ongoing mechanisms to monitor patients' symptoms and assess patients' perceptions of what they think is interfering with their activities and responsibilities. The nurse is then in a position to help the woman to find the best solution for her situation.

Women's Care-Giving Abilities

Living with cancer often requires continuing care management by a team of specialists. Care is usually provided to women through follow-up visits to ambulatory or outpatients clinics and consulting rooms, rather than through hospitalization. Families are relied on to be the major provider of care outside the health care institution during treatment, as well as during the advanced phases of illness. Currently, little is known about differences in care-giver responsibilities assumed by male and female family members or about differences in the ways men and women react to their care-giver roles.

Horowitz (1985) studies 131 adult children identified as the primary care-giver to an older frail parent. Sons tended to become care-givers only in the absence of an available female sibling and they were more likely to rely on the support of their own spouses. Sons provided less overall assistance to their parents than daughters, especially with regard to 'hands-on' services. Sons also reported less stressful care-giving experiences independent of their degree of involvement.

Stetz (1986) documented the demands reported by sixty-five spouses taking care of a terminally ill spouse with cancer, in the home. The majority of spouses, twelve men (57 per cent) and thirty women (68 per cent), reported that managing the physical care, treatment regimens and imposed changes was the most difficult part of their spouses' illness. Other demands commonly cited were managing the household and finances, standing by, alterations in their own well-being, unmet expectations from the health care system, constant vigilance, anticipating the future, and alterations in their relationship with their spouses. Major differences in the care-giving demands were noted between male and female care-givers. Overall, women reported more demands than men. On average, each woman reported between two or three demands whereas each man reported zero to two. Men may have reported less overall concerns than women because family members may be willing to offer greater assistance and support to male care-givers than to female care-givers.

Women rated 'standing by' as more difficult than 'managing the household and finances', while men reported the reverse ratings for these demands. Approximately one-third of the women (n = 13) experienced alterations in their own pattern of living and health as a direct result of the care-giving experience. As part of their research on morbidity and mortality of cancer widows, Vachon and her colleagues (1977) noted that these widows, unlike women whose husbands died of other causes, felt worse after the death than they had at the time of death. In addition, significantly more women whose husbands had died of cancer felt they were in poor health during the illness as compared with other widows. Thus, individuals who experience alterations in their own health during the care-giving experience could be at greater risk for illness in the ensuing months. Germino (1984) found that adult children were more concerned about the father's health when the mother was the patient, than vice versa.

Ekberg, Griffith and Foxall (1986) in a study of thirty married couples, found that chronic illness in one partner can result in increased responsibilities for the spouse and eventually lead to spouse burnout. The authors concluded that nurses have a responsibility to care for spouse care-givers as well as for the patient. Nurses need to be knowledgeable about common physical and emotional symptoms of burnout. With that knowledge, nurses are better prepared to assist the spouse in early recognition of problems and to plan interventions accordingly.

One such intervention is to arrange respite care. Respite care is designed to provide relief to family care-givers for limited time periods when long-term home health care is a non-institutional alternative and where the nursing therapeutic regimen is brought into the patient's own home (Miller, 1985). Investing in care-givers' physical, financial and emotional well-being may be more effective than providing the care required when care-givers become 'patients' (Bader, 1985).

Summary

Improvements in health status are less likely to come from technological breakthroughs than from improvements in environmental and social conditions, changes in lifestyle and behaviour, and participation of people in maintenance of their own health. As the leading causes of morbidity and mortality have shifted from infectious diseases and other acute problems to chronic illnesses such as cancer, the need to focus on environmental conditions and health-promoting behaviours has increased. Identifying ways of modifying unhealthy conditions and behaviours is particularly germane to the improvement of women's health.

As nurses, we can do little to influence the social changes that will affect women's health in the years to come. Increasing numbers of women will be poor, more women will work, and women will continue to live longer than men. However, nurses can play an important role in educating women to be knowledgeable about their own health and to seek care for their symptoms. In the future, the numbers of women diagnosed with cancer will continue to increase, as women live longer and therefore are in the more common age range for cancer. However, with the exception of lung cancer, large increases in rates for the common forms of cancer among women are not apparent (Devesa, 1987). The lung cancer mortality rate among women is now increasing faster than that among men. Clearly, nurses have a critical role to play in prevention and detection practices related to those cancers of utmost importance to women: lung, breast and cervical cancer are the most common. To increase our effectiveness, we should adopt recommended health practices ourselves in order to become role models for our patients, family members, friends and neighbours.

References

Bader, J.E. (1985) Respite care: temporary relief for care-givers, *Women and Health*, Vol. 10, pp. 39–51.

Bullough, B. (1980) Discovery of the first signs and symptoms of breast cancer, *Nurse Practitioner*, Vol. 31, pp. 31–47.

Derogatis, L.R. (1986) The unique impact of breast and gynaecologic cancers on body image and sexual identity in women: a reassessment, in *Body Image, Self-Esteem, and Sexuality in Cancer Patients* (2nd edn), Karger, Basel.

Devesa, S.S. (1987) Cancer mortality, incidence, and patient survival among American women, *Women and Health*, Vol. 11, pp. 7–22.

Edstrom, S. and Miller, M.W. (1981) Preparing the family to care for the cancer patient at home: a home course, *Cancer Nursing*, Vol. 11, pp. 49–52.

Ekberg, J.Y., Griffith, N. and Foxall, M.J. (1986) Spouse burnout syndrome, *Journal of Advanced Nursing*, Vol. 11, pp. 161–5.

Elwood, J.M. and Moorehead, W.P. (1980) Delay in diagnosis and long-term survival in breast cancer, *British Medical Journal*, Vol. 280, pp. 1291–4.

Feldman, J. (1966) *The Dissemination of Health Information*, Aldine, Chicago.

Funch, D.P. (1985) The role of patient delay in the evaluation of breast self-examination, *Journal of Psychosocial Oncology*, Vol. 2, pp. 31–9.

Germino, B. (1984) Family members' concerns after cancer diagnosis. Unpublished doctoral dissertation, University of Washington, Seattle, Washington.

Gould-Martin, K., Paganini-Hill, A., Casagrande,C., Mack, T. and Ross, R.K. (1982) Behavioural and biological determinants of the surgical stage of breast cancer, *Preventive Medicine*, Vol. 11, pp. 429–40.

Gove, W.P. (1984) Gender differences in mental and physical illness: the effects of fixed roles and nurturant roles, *Social Science and Medicine*, Vol. 19, pp. 77–91.

Gove, W.P. and Hughes, M. (1979) Possible causes of the apparent sex differences in physical health, *American Sociological Review*, Vol. 44, pp. 59–81.

Green, C.P. (1986) Changes in responsibility in women's families after the diagnosis of cancer, *Health Care for Women International*, Vol. 7, pp. 221–39.

Hackett, T.P., Cassem, N.H. and Raker, J.W. (1973) Patient delay in cancer, *New England Journal of Medicine*, Vol. 289 pp. 14–20.

Hibbard, J.H. and Pope, C.R. (1986) Another look at sex differences in the use of medical care, *Women and Health*, Vol. 11, pp. 21–36.

Horowitz, A. (1985) Sons and daughters as care-givers to older parents: differences in role performance, *The Gerontologist*, Vol. 25, pp. 612–15.

Huguley, C.M., Jr and Brown, R.L. (1981) The value of breast self-examination, *Cancer*, Vol. 47, pp. 989–95.

Lierman, L. (1987) Discovery of breast changes: women's responses and nursing implications forthcoming, *Cancer Nursing* (in press).

McCorkle, R. and Quint-Benoliel, J.Q. (1983) Symptom distress, current concerns and mood disturbance after diagnosis of life-threatening disease, *Social Science and Medicine*, Vol. 17, no. 7, pp. 431–8.

Magarey, C.J., Todd, P.B. and Blizard, P.J. (1977) Psychosocial factors influencing delay and breast self-examination in women with symptoms of breast cancer, *Social Science and Medicine*, Vol. 11, pp. 229–32.

Marshall, J.R. and Funch, D.P. (1986) Gender and illness behaviour among colo-rectal cancer patients, *Women and Health*, Vol. 11, no. 34, pp. 67–82.

Mechanic, D. (1976) Sex, illness, illness behaviour, and the use of health services, *Journal of Human Stress*, Vol. 2, pp. 29–40.

Merritt, D.H. and Kirschstein, R.L. (eds.) (1985) *Women's Health*, Report of the Public Service Task Force on Women's Health Issues, Vol. II, US Department of Health and Human Services, PHS.

Miller, D.B. (1985) Women and long term nursing care, *Women and Health*, Vol. 10, pp. 29-37.

Nathanson, C.A. (1975) Illness and the feminine role: a theoretical review, *Social Science and Medicine*, Vol. 9, pp. 57-62.

Nathanson, C.A. (1977) Sex, illness and medical care: a review of data, theory and method, *Social Science and Medicine*, Vol. 11, pp. 13-75.

Quint, J.C. (1963) The impact of mastectomy, *American Journal of Nursing*, Vol. 63 no. 11, pp. 29-34.

Sandelowski, M. (1981) *Women's Health and Choice*, Prentice-Hall, NJ, USA.

Stetz, K. (1986) The experience of spouse care-giving during advanced cancer. Unpublished doctoral dissertation, University of Washington, Seattle, Washington.

Strafford, F.P. (1980) Women's use of time converging with men's. *Monthly Labour Review*, Vol. 103, no. 12, pp. 57-9.

Strauss, A. (1975) *Chronic Illness and Quality of Life*, C.V. Mosby, St Louis.

Vachon, M., Freedman, K., Formo, A., Rogers, J., Lyall, W. and Freeman, S. (1977) The final illness in cancer: the widow's perspective, *Canadian Medical Association Journal*, Vol. 117, pp. 1151-4.

Verbrugge, L.M. (1979) Female illness rates and illness behaviour: testing hypothesis about sex differences in health, *Women and Health*, Vol. 4, pp. 61-79.

Verbrugge, L.M. (1982) Sex differentials in health, *Public Health Report*, Vol. 97, pp. 417-37.

Watson, M., Greer, S., Blake, S. and Sharpnell, K. (1984) Reaction to a diagnosis of breast cancer: relationship between denial, delay and rates of psychological morbidity, *Cancer*, Vol. 53, pp. 2008-12.

Chapter 16

Transcultural Aspects of Cancer Care

CHRIS EBERHARDIE-SAMPSON TD, RGN, RNT

Nurse Tutor, Continuing Education (General)
St George's Hospital, London

Introduction

The movement of populations around the world has accelerated dramatically over the past fifty years. The increased speed of travel and its decreasing cost have made international movement more popular and places more accessible than ever before. In 1986, 26 million international passengers flew into and out of Heathrow airport alone, so the United Kingdom total must be very much higher. This trend will be mirrored in most other countries. The millions of visitors included in such a total will comprise tourists, visitors to family and friends, businesspeople, students, refugees, immigrants, professionals and others travelling for work experience. Any one of them could at any time become a hospital patient and some may have already undergone investigations or treatment for cancer. Visitors who suddenly become ill present many difficulties that would not be faced by the indigenous population. And, even among expatriates, those who have been migrants to one country or another for several years can have very different cultural problems compared with short-term visitors. This point is developed later in the chapter in some detail.

The Health Care Problems of Immigrants

Health care problems of immigrants are now being studied more closely because of their transcultural impact and because immigrants and visitors from other continents and climates bring with them diseases and disorders previously unknown, or a least rare, among the indigenous population. Because immigrants have tended to collect in certain inner cities and metropolitan conurbations, some readers may not have much experience of the transcultural aspects of caring for them. Table 16.1 shows the numbers and ethnic origin of most immigrants in 1985 to Great Britain. There were 3 million immigrants within a total population of more than 54 million and, of these, 2.3 million are non-white. These figures do not include non-immigrant visitors, some of whom come to Britain especially to seek medical treatment. The penultimate column shows the percentages in each ethnic group were born in the United Kingdom. These percentages are substantial, which is important because they give rise to additional cross-cultural problems, as is explained later.

Immigrant Health Care Professionals

A substantial proportion of doctors, nurses and other health care professionals are also from different ethnic groups. Some hospitals and clinics are heavily dependent on them and their ubiquity adds a new dimension to the transcultural scene. This can either aggravate an already complex problem or even create a new one where potential difficulties could otherwise be contained.

So within hospitals, clinics and wherever patients live, receive treatment, work or relax there is a network of cultural factors which plays an important role in the well-being of patients (Figure 16.1). The ability of individuals to cope with the pressures exerted by this network of cultural groupings can be greatly disrupted by illness. A sensitive awareness on the part of practitioners can anticipate and defuse some of these problems and, even if they cannot entirely prevent them, at least they can support patients and their families with greater understanding and thus alleviate their impact. Practitioners can also become more tolerant and understanding of each other and of their differing reactions to the transcultural needs we are discussing – and which can become a part of the problem.

Transcultural and Cross-Cultural Factors

At the beginning of this chapter, the notion was introduced that long-term immigrants can present with very different cultural

Table 16.1 Population* of Great Britain by ethnic origin and age, 1985

	Percentage in each age-group					Total* all ages (= 100%) (000s)	% born in UK	Number of males per female +
	0–15	16–29	30–44	45–59	60 or over			
Ethnic origin								
White	20	22	20	17	21	51,222	96	0.95
West Indian or Guyanese	26	33	15	19	7	547	53	0.90
Indian	32	26	24	13	5	689	35	1.00
Pakistani	43	25	18	12	2	406	44	1.10
Bangladeshi	51	18	14	16	1	99	28	1.30
Chinese	27	25	30	13	5	122	24	1.10
African	28	28	36	6	2	102	32	1.30
Arab	17	48	21	10	3	61	12	2.70
Mixed	55	25	11	6	2	232	76	1.10
Other	24	26	34	12	4	117	26	0.80
All non-white	34	28	20	13	4	2,376	42	1.05
Not stated	31	23	17	14	15	637	69	0.90
All origins	21	22	20	17	20	54,235	94	0.95

* Population in households.
+ Figures are rounded to the nearest 0.05.

Source: Office of Population Censuses and Surveys (1985) *Labour Force Survey* with kind permission.

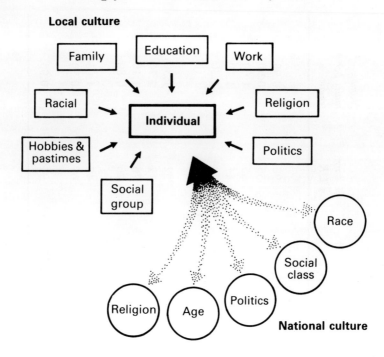

Figure 16.1 Network of cultural factors.

problems to short-term visitors. Considerable thought needs to be given in the application of cultural factors when making professional judgements.

Because this is a facet of care that is relatively new, the components of which are still being analysed, some important terms are being used ambiguously by the few real authorities on the subject. These differences can be crucial both to an understanding of the subject matter and to a diagnostic approach to the problems that arise. The terms 'cultural', 'transcultural' and 'cross-cultural' are sometimes incorrectly used synonymously. At best, this gives rise to much confusion and is positively misleading when important distinctions are concealed beneath their synonymous use. Getting these distinctions clear is fundamental to developing understanding and making judgements that are accurate, sophisticated and practical.

USE OF THE TERMS 'CULTURAL', 'TRANSCULTURAL' AND 'CROSS-CULTURAL'

While claiming no authority that goes beyond the force of the argument that follows, an attempt is made to explain the distinctions between these three terms. The term *cultural* is used in a more general way than the other two terms and it subsumes the following distinctions as to what is also 'transcultural' or 'cross-cultural'. It applies to a culture at its root and in its pure form. *Transcultural* is used to describe the cultural phenomena which result when a cultural factor is transposed into a different ethnic environment, either by visit or by immigration. *Cross-cultural* is used even more specifically to apply to those modifications to root cultural attitudes that ensue when an individual from one culture has been not only transposed into another ethnic environment, but has either been born there, educated there or has lived there for a sufficient length of time to create in that individual a mixture of attitudes that may follow no consistent pattern. One attitude may derive entirely from his or her original ethnic background, another more or less completely from his or her land of adoption and others may fall somewhere between the two in varying proportions or may even create a new synthesis in particular cases. A consensus will no doubt emerge in time as to the definition of these terms. Meanwhile the above definitions hopefully serve a purpose. The examples and case histories that follow are intended to vindicate this approach.

CULTURAL AND CROSS-CULTURAL EXPORTATION

There is a further complication in that many root cultures are themselves being diluted or modified in their own homelands by the importation of ideas, attitudes, language, education and institutions from abroad. One has only to think of the American impact on Japan or of the much longer influence of the British in South-East Asia and in the Caribbean to know that this is the case. Hence cross-cultural effects can be considerable even within the homeland of a root culture and this is especially so within the better-educated upper and middle classes, many of whom still send their children either to British schools in their own homelands or to native schools. These are so British in their administration, curricula, language and customs as to be almost indistinguishable from them. There is nevertheless a considerable difference between the impact of cross-cultural effects within the homeland of a root culture and the impact of, for example, a United Kingdom-based cross-cultural attitude. This is partly due to all the all-pervading influence of the majority culture on all its subcultures, transcultures and cross-cultures and to the legal framework in which they exist and to which they must perforce adapt.

Cross-cultural attitudes can be very misleading, especially those which are overseas grown and which can introduce a whole range of new effects. For example, visitors who have had a British education abroad but who are setting foot in the United Kingdom for the first time, may appear on the surface more British than the British and be at pains to foster this impression once in Britain. But they will be ignorant of many of the daily realities of life in modern Britain (they may well have inherited some rather archaic British attitudes) which long-term immigrants take for granted. This may be the case even if they are from a different social class, less well educated and not speaking English nearly as well. Cross-cultural visitors may not be prepared for the way in which the British law responds to the religious and cultural imperatives that govern their life in their own homeland and where the law not only reflects the local custom but is formed largely by them. The tensions which arise between the different subcultures and cross-cultures and between them and the law, are entirely different. These are not pedantic theoretical abstractions. Brushes between imported cultures and the law do happen and are many and varied. They range from the failure to register births, deaths and marriages to the 'disposal' of unwanted wives and daughters; in the sociomedical field, from invoking the law to implement blood transfusions, to the performance of sterilization and termination of pregnancies; in life-saving situations, to the treatment of undernourished and abused female children, simply because they are regarded as unimportant.

Changing British Attitudes to Imported Cultures

An example of the ways in which attitudes are changing to this considerable movement of individuals throughout the world is considered below. Although the example used is that of the United Kingdom, similar situations exist elsewhere.

The intercultural equation is a dynamic one and British attitudes towards imported cultures do not remain static. An amusing example is provided by a tall and elegant Indian naval captain whose professional education alternated between Indian and British service academies. He had been a student at the Royal Naval Staff College, Joint Services Staff College and Royal College of Defence Studies. When asked how he found things in Britain he replied, after a rather long interval, 'Well, last time I came to England everybody thought I was at least a Maharaja. This time I come to England everyone knows I am a bus conductor.' While this may be a humorous response from a highly educated and distinguished gentleman, it nevertheless touches on a common source of tension which is generated by the host population in its immigrants and visitors – through its failure to recognize social class, education, professional qualifications and other attainments or status. Contrary to popular belief, most Eastern and West Indian people are very sensitive to status, even in their own countries.

Cultural Diagnosis

Cross-cultural effects can considerably complicate an accurate 'cultural diagnosis' based on an accurate assessment of how an individual is likely to react to various aspects of the hospital environment, medical condition, treatment, staff, fellow patients and so on. Ideal management includes the foresight to forestall problems that may arise and create favourable psychosomatic effects that help patients to respond positively to treatment.

DEGREES OF COMPLEXITY AND EXPERTISE

It is difficult enough for practitioners to acquire sufficient knowledge of all the cultural attitudes and potential consequences found in the many different racial, cultural and religious groupings. One can be sympathetic with any impatience that may develop in confirming that these cultural stereotypes are further diluted or distorted in one way or another, probably as often as they exist in anything approaching a pure form. The question is, how seriously do you want to take this subject and how successfully do you want to practice those aspects of medical and nursing care that are covered in this chapter? Happily, it is not a case of 'a little knowledge being a dangerous thing'. While serious mistakes can be made, they can be avoided by a mixture of observation, common sense, goodwill, a little knowledge, some humility and, above all, an alertness to cultural needs. Expertise will grow after practice and experience have been applied to basic knowledge. At an elementary level, one can avoid putting a Pakistani Muslim in a bed next to an Indian Hindu. This requires no more than common sense, practical sensitivity and a minimum knowledge of current affairs. It requires more knowledge to understand the present antipathy that exists between Sikhs and Haryana Hindus and a good deal of knowledge to realize that ancient feuds between Sikhs and Muslim

Pakistanis are now being modified as they find themselves becoming increasingly natural allies in the face of Indian hegemony.

AN EXAMPLE OF TRANSCULTURAL AND CROSS-CULTURAL COMPLEXITY

To illustrate the complexity, distortions and difficulties that can be created by a cross-cultural background, a specific example is considered.

The patient is a 16-year-old Omani Arab girl, born and educated in Britain. Her parents are strict Muslims, whereas she has absorbed some completely different attitudes from her British environment at school. This applies to her ideas about relationships between the sexes although, in some other respects, she remains true to her ethnic and religious origin, including the traditional deep respect for her parents, especially her father.

After becoming pregnant by a white English boy, a clandestine visit to an antenatal clinic reveals an early cervical carcinoma. On her admission to hospital, the admission interview reveals that she has been afraid to tell her parents of the situation. It may also be presumed that they do not even know where she is. It is explained that the hospital is bound to inform her parents of her whereabouts and that the proposed treatment for her cancer will usually require their consent. She is obviously much more distressed about her parents being informed than by her condition itself or its medical outcome.

As expected, the father disowns her and refuses to visit. The mother remains sympathetic but will not oppose her husband, although she does send messages via the girl's elder sister, who was also born and educated in Britain and who shares much of the same cross-cultural attitudes as the patient. However, she also visits clandestinely. The older brother, who is heir and future head of the family, though cross-cultural and fond of his sister, spent his one visit berating her for her iniquity. However, he became the go-between with the father in the matter of consent for treatment. When the father refuses to allow a termination of the pregnancy, the girl is made a ward of court so that effective treatment can proceed. The strength of the father's feelings can be judged less by him hazarding his daughter's life than by his preference for enduring the family shame of an illegitimate pregnancy to disobeying the Koran's prohibition of abortion. He is incensed at his parental and Muslim rights in the matter being overruled by the court. The English boy, although not keen on emphasizing his responsibility in the matter, is fond of the girl and visits regularly, but care must be taken that his visits do not coincide with those of the family, as verbal or physical aggression could result.

In the above example, the equation might have been further complicated by the introduction of a doctor from a society with a more fatalistic approach to life, and/or a nurse from a society with strong views on the sanctity of life.

During her traumatic stay in hospital, the patient's strongest attachment is to her sympathetic and understanding nurse from whom she derives her greatest comfort and support. The experienced ward sister, foreseeing the inevitable social problems that will follow, calls in the medical social worker at an early stage and arrangements are made for the girl to be taken into care on leaving hospital. The nurse, recognizing a candidate for suicide, does not regard the case as finishing at the hospital gates but instead befriends the girl, retains contact with the family and becomes instrumental in the girl's eventual rehabilitation when she becomes a student nurse.

It may be considered that the role of the nurse here has been extended too much into one of social work. That is not meant to be the message. What is advocated is a more holistic approach to medical and nursing care and a greater concern among staff with the eventual sociomedical outcome of a case. The nurse is in a unique position here because of the patient's dependence on her, because of her frequent and intimate contacts with the patient and because of her sociomedical overview of all aspects of the case. All the other staff, including the medical social worker where appropriate, are involved with their specific part of the whole case but all of them are at a disadvantage in comparison with the nurse. The close attachment that can be forged at the bedside between nurse and patient can become a potent psychosomatic element in treatment and rehabilitation.

Using a Problem-Solving Approach to Plan Care

The specifics of cultural and religious difficulties and the knowledge, understanding and form of care required are best presented, and taught, by reference to individual patients using a problem-solving approach. This helps to identify transcultural issues that may arise in the care of patients suffering from various forms of cancer. Reference to individual patients cannot provide a comprehensive coverage because of the permutations of race, culture, illness and circumstances. However, it is the most illustrative and useful approach for initiating readers into the kind of knowledge required to handle these matters and into the kinds of judgement that may flow from this knowledge. To set out all the racial, cultural and religious factors that may impinge would require a book of its own. However, a small selection of references is supplied at the end for those who wish to read further. The case history approach which follows, and which deals exclusively with cancer patients, is complementary to these more compendious analyses. The examples are taken from life, although names and some of the patients' details have been altered or transposed to preserve their anonymity.

ANALYTICAL FRAMEWORK

To identify the problems that may arise in any particular case, it is useful to check systematically through the twelve activities of daily living in the Roper, Logan and Tierney (1980) model of nursing — and then link these with the main cultural headings that may apply to the nursing management of the patient. These two lists are given in Table 16.2.

Table 16.2   *Checklist for analytical framework*

Roper's activities of daily living	Main cultural headings
Maintaining a safe environment	Country of origin
Breathing	Country of education
Communicating	Language
Eating and drinking	Race
Eliminating	Socioeconomic factors
Cleansing and dressing	Religion
Controlling body temperature	Familiarity with the nation's
Mobilizing	health system (in the
Working and playing	United Kingdom, the
Expressing sexuality	NHS)
Sleeping	Attitudes to treatment and
Dying	care
	Attitudes to men and women
	Attitudes to cancer
	Politics
	Relevant life experience

CASE HISTORY 1

Mr J.W., age 69 years, came to London in 1946 following release from Auschwitz. He is a Lithuanian Jewish refugee. His first wife, son, daughter, two brothers and a sister-in-law all died in concentration camps. He has remarried. His second wife is also a Lithuanian Jew. They have one son by the marriage. He runs a small business in a London suburb. He has recently been admitted to hospital suffering from carcinoma of the lung with liver metastases. His condition is deteriorating.

What cultural care will he need? Following the analytical methodology outlined above, the nurse responsible for the assessment and planning of Mr J.W.'s care should check through the above-listed factors.

Maintaining a Safe Environment

No cultural factors involved.

Breathing

No cultural factors involved.

Communicating

Problem: J.W.'s previous life experience may induce painful reactions when he is questioned directly about his country of origin and religion. He and his family have suffered the worst possible racial and religious hatred.

Nursing intervention: J.W. has obvious Jewish features which give the nurse her first clue and she should look out for signs of tattooed numbers on the forearm or the faint scars of their removal.

Problem: English is not his native language but he has lived in London for more than 40 years. His vocabulary is limited and, when his blood oxygen level drops, he becomes confused and lapses into Yiddish or Lithuanian.

Nursing intervention: locate staff who speak Yiddish or Lithuanian. Ease alternative phrases and expressions into the conversation so that J.W.'s comprehension is improved without embarrassment.

Eating and Drinking

Problem: J.W. is a liberal Jew and does not adhere strictly to the dietary laws, but he will not eat anything from a pig, including patés, sausages or bacon. He does not eat shellfish either, but does not insist that his food be prepared by the Kosher method.

Nursing intervention: ensure that J.W. is not served shellfish or any pig derivative. The nursing staff should facilitate access to dishes or delicacies from his homeland in amounts that his liver can cope with.

Eliminating

No cultural problems.

Cleansing and Dressing

These present no cultural problem except that J.W. likes to pray with his head covered. He is sensitive about the number tattooed on his arm and prefers to keep it covered.

Controlling Body Temperature

No cultural problems, although heat may cause distress.

Mobilizing

Problem: J.W. has some residual neuropathy due to malnutrition while interned. This makes him clumsy when walking and handling objects because of impaired sensation in his hands and feet.

Nursing intervention: ensure that J.W.'s feet and hands are protected from harmful objects and substances. The bath water should be tested before he steps in.

Working and Playing

Problem: as a self-employed businessman, J.W. will need access to those who are caretaking his business. He also wishes to sort out his affairs with his solicitor.

Nursing intervention: strike a balance between assisting J.W.'s attention to his business affairs and achieving peace of mind. Try not to let him overtire himself.

Expressing Sexuality

No cultural problems.

Sleeping

Problem: respiratory difficulties prevent J.W. from sleeping well. He often has nightmares.

Nursing intervention: allow J.W. to sleep when he can do so. Discuss his nightmares with him.

Dying

Problem: the prognosis is very poor. J.W. is not afraid of death but is afraid of dying. He has witnessed so much horrifying death that he finds it hard to believe that one can die peacefully.

Nursing intervention: create opportunities for J.W. to discuss his feelings about death in general, and his own death in particular, with anyone he chooses – nurse, rabbi, family or friends.

Problem: J.W. has a profound faith which is simply expressed. He wishes to receive the rites of his faith in the terminal stages of illness.

Nursing intervention:

a Ensure that J.W. has the religious artifacts he requires – the Torah, the Talmud, prayer book, prayer shawl and skull cap (yarmulke). His wife will bring these in from home.

b Do not disturb his time of prayer. Ensure the rabbi's access to him and his family and their privacy together.

c Ask the rabbi in advance what the procedure will be if J.W. dies on the Jewish Sabbath or other holy day. The family may ask for him to be kept alive for the Sabbath as some Jews are alarmed at the prospect of dying on any holy day.

d After death, gloves should be worn when straightening the body, lying it flat and removing all tubes and intravenous infusions.

e Call the rabbi if he was not present at the moment of death. Jews prefer burial to cremation and this should take place as quickly as possible.

CASE HISTORY 2

A.A. Singh, aged 30 years, is a married man with one son (age five years). He is admitted to a ward specializing in oncological surgery. He was born in the Punjab and, when twelve years old, came to live with his parents in a small town in southern England. He is a devout Sikh and, like all male Sikhs, has the family name suffix 'Singh', which means 'lion'. He speaks English fluently but with a marked Asian accent. He also speaks fluent Punjabi. He is now the head of his branch of the family both here and in the Punjab. After a series of investigations he is found to have a malignant laryngeal tumour. He needs to undergo a laryngectomy and radiotherapy.

Maintaining a Safe Environment

Problem: racial, religious and political passions run high in the Indian subcontinent and can erupt quickly into violence. In the hospital environment the patient needs to feel secure from threat from other patients and staff.

Nursing intervention: do not put a Pakistani or another Indian next to him if they identify strongly with opposing politico-religious factions. While nurses cannot be expected to know all the potential causes of tension in the different ethnic groups, they can know enough about it to play safe and avoid putting him next to another patient from the Indian subcontinent. This principle applies even more strongly to the allocation of nursing staff to his care.

Breathing

No cultural problems.

Communicating

Problem: difficulty in understanding A.A. Singh's accent.
Nursing intervention:
a Allocate the same nurses to care for the patient before and after surgery.
b Make an allowance for his intonation which may cause many statements to sound like challenging questions. In many Asian accents, the voice rises interrogatively at the end of a sentence.
c Postoperatively, nurses must allow for difficulty in lip reading A.A. Singh and vice versa. Alternative forms of communication must be explored.
Problem: there may be potential communication difficulties with his family and friends some of whom, especially the women, may speak much less English than he does.
Nursing intervention: ask A.A. Singh which members of his family speak English well and whether any have particular difficulties to be considered, for example a bad experience of communications in hospital, harassment or racial aggression.

Eating and Drinking

Problem: some Sikhs are vegetarians, others refrain from eating beef or beef products. A.A. Singh eats some meat but not beef and adheres to this strictly. He is anxious about the contents of nasogastric tube feeds.

Nursing intervention: ensure that the patient has a diet free from beef products. Avoid sausages, meat loaf, steak and kidney pies, minced meat, beef-based drinks and soups. Check especially the constituents of commercially made nasogastric feeds.

Eliminating

Problem: no cultural problems except if the patient continues to wear his Kacha, a pair of white shorts which are one of five Sikh religious symbols. He may have difficulty removing them when using the toilet or a bedpan.

Nursing intervention: the Kacha, along with the four other religious symbols, must be treated with great respect. Remember when giving intimate assistance that Sikhs are exceptionally modest.

Cleansing and Dressing

Problem: A.A. Singh has very long hair and a full beard, which are well groomed and of great religious importance. To keep his hair in place he wears the Kanga or comb (another of the religious symbols) under a traditional turban. This need not be a problem until he requires surgery.

Nursing intervention: explain to the patient that he must have some or all of his beard shaved off before surgery. This should be broached early, probably in the outpatient department, so that he can prepare himself for what will arouse strong emotions about his manhood and religion. Clear explanation of the reasons for the request must be given. Ensure that he is wearing a clean, fresh turban before he goes to the operating theatre.

Problem: like many Asian men, A.A. Singh is very modest so, whenever possible, he should be encouraged to wash his genitalia himself.

Nursing intervention: nurses should keep a discreet distance while he is washing or using a urinal or bedpan and he should be well screened.

Problem: A.A. Singh insists that all five of his religious symbols accompany him to the operating theatre.

Nursing intervention: identify the five 'K' religious symbols; Kes, uncut hair; Kanga, the comb; Kara, a steel bangle; Kirpan, a dagger, often symbolic or replaced by throwing rings; Kacha, white shorts. Three of these symbols have already been discussed, the remainder could be wrapped in a sealed packet and attached to the patient's notes during surgery. They should not remain on his person because of the danger associated with metal and diathermy.

Controlling Body Temperature

No cultural factors, although A.A. Singh may feel the cold more than some other patients. Conversely, he may cope with hot weather better than other patients and staff.

Mobilizing

No cultural problems.

Working and Playing

Problem: A.A. Singh keeps a shop within the family business. He can return to some kind of family employment appropriate to his condition but he is anxious about being able to fulfil his role as head of the family. He finds it difficult to discuss this problem.

Nursing intervention: encourage the patient to discuss his socioeconomic problems with nursing staff or a medical social worker. In most Sikh communities this kind of problem is taken in hand by the family or wider community. Sikhs are an exceptionally supportive and well-organized group.

Problem: while awaiting surgery and when he has recovered afterwards, and is awaiting supplementary treatment or is learning to cope with feeding himself, A.A. Singh will need distraction and entertainment.

Nursing intervention: discuss with the patient his hobbies, pastimes and interests. He may like Indian music and may wish to use a cassette recorder, but should be encouraged to use headphones. Encourage him to indulge his interests so long as they do not impede his recovery from surgery or disturb fellow patients.

Expressing Sexuality

No cultural problems.

Sleeping

No cultural problems.

Dying

The long-term prognosis for A.A. Singh is poor and he may express fears for his future.

Problems:

a What is A.A. Singh's perception of his illness and prognosis and what part does Sikhism play in his ability to cope?

b When A.A. Singh reaches the terminal stage of his illness what special religious observances will he expect?

Nursing interventions:

a Encourage the patient to express his feelings about his illness and prognosis.

b Ask him or his wife if they have strong links with the local gurdwara and if any of the elders will be visiting. Find out if he needs additional spiritual help.

c Ensure privacy when prayers are read to him.

d Be aware that Sikhs prefer cremation to burial.

Conclusion

In this chapter I have tried to introduce the burgeoning discipline of nursing anthropology as it affects cancer patients. The relationship between health care professionals and the patient suffering from cancer is an intimate and demanding one. It is a relationship in which racial, transcultural and cross-cultural harmony can be fostered, not only for the benefit of the individuals concerned but for that of society as a whole. An enlightened practitioner can be an important catalyst for intercultural understanding, tolerance, harmony and integration.

References and Further Reading

Helman, C. (1984) *Culture, Health and Illness*, Wright, Bristol.

Neuberger, J. (1987) *Caring for Dying People of Different Faiths*, the Lisa Sainsbury Foundation/Austin Cornish, London.

Roper, N., Logan, W.W. and Tierney, A.J. (1980) *The Elements of Nursing*, Churchill Livingstone, Edinburgh.

Sampson, C. (1982) The neglected ethic: religious and cultural factors in *The Care of Patients*, McGraw Hill Book Co. (UK) Ltd, Maidenhead.

Index

Volume One

Pathology, Diagnosis and Treatment

Table of contents of the first volume of this three-volume work

Series editor

Robert Tiffany OBE, RGN, RCNT, FRCN
Director of In-patient Services/Chief Nursing Officer,
The Royal Marsden Hospital,
London and Surrey,
and President, International Society of Nurses in
Cancer Care

Volume editor

Phylip Pritchard BA, RGN, RMN
Assistant to the Director of In-patient Services/Chief
Nursing Officer,
The Royal Marsden Hospital,
London and Surrey

CONTENTS

Chapter 4   The General Pathology of Tumours
Noel Gowing MD, FRCPath
Emeritus Professor,
The Institute of Cancer Research,
University of London
and
Cyril Fisher MA, MD, FRCPath
Consultant Histopathologist
The Royal Marsden Hospital,
London and Surrey.

Chapter 5   Immunity and Cancer
Joe Hall MB, PhD, DSc, FRCPath
Honorary Consultant Pathologist to
The Royal Marsden Hospital,
London and Surrey.
Chairman, Experimental Unit, Section of Medicine,
The Institute of Cancer Research,
The Royal Marsden Hospital,
London and Surrey and
Professor of Immunobiology,
University of London

Chapter 6   Systemic Manifestations of Malignant Disease
Ian Smith MD, FRCPE
Consultant Medical Oncologist,
The Royal Marsden Hospital,
London and Surrey

Chapter 7   Screening for Early Detection of Cancer
Joycelyn Chamberlain, MB, FRCP, FFCM
Director, DHSS Cancer Screening Evaluation Unit,
Epidemiology Section, and
Professor in Community Medicine
The Institute of Cancer Research

Chapter 8   Imaging in Oncology
Colin Parsons, FRCS, FRCR,
Consultant Radiologist,
The Royal Marsden Hospital,
London and Surrey
and
Michael King, FRCR
Consultant Radiologist,
The Royal Marsden Hospital,
London and Surrey

Chapter 9   Surgical Oncology
Gerald Westbury, FRCP, FRCS
Professor of Surgery,
The Institute of Cancer Research,
The Royal Marsden Hospital,
London and Surrey

Volume Three

Cancer Nursing

Table of contents of the third volume of this three-volume work

Series editor   Robert Tiffany OBE, RGN, RCNT, FRCN
Director of In-patient Services/Chief Nursing Officer,
The Royal Marsden Hospital,
London and Surrey,
and President, International Society of Nurses in
Cancer Care

Volume editor   Derryn Borley RGN, RCNT, OncCert
Senior Officer, Royal College of Nursing (North East
Thames Region)

CONTENTS